DEPRESSION

The disorder and its associations

DEPRESSION

The disorder and its associations

by

B. Mahendra

Consultant Psychogeriatrician,

Hope Hospital (University of
Manchester School of
Medicine)
Salford

and

Prestwich Hospital,
Manchester

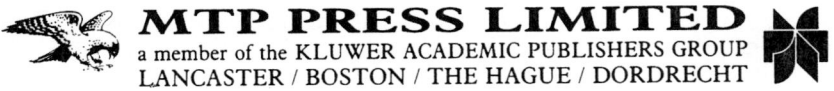
MTP PRESS LIMITED
a member of the KLUWER ACADEMIC PUBLISHERS GROUP
LANCASTER / BOSTON / THE HAGUE / DORDRECHT

Published in the UK and Europe by
MTP Press Limited
Falcon House
Lancaster, England

British Library Cataloguing in Publication Data
Mahendra, B.
   Depression: the disorder and its
   associations.
   1. Depression, Mental
   I. Title
   616.85′27   RC537

Published in the USA by
MTP Press
A division of Kluwer Academic Publishers
101 Philip Drive
Norwell, MA 02061, USA

Library of Congress Cataloging-in-Publication Data

Mahendra, B. (Bala), 1950—
   Depression: the disorder and its associations.

   Bibliography: p.
   Includes index.
   1. Depression, Mental.   I. Title. [DNLM:
1. Depression.   WM 171 M214d]
RC537.M33   1986   616. 85′25   86–27536

ISBN 978-94-010-7947-1   ISBN 978-94-009-3225-8 (eBook)
DOI 10.1007/978-94-009-3225-8

Typeset by Witwell Ltd, Liverpool

Contents

Acknowledgments   vi

Preface   vii

1   Depressed minds, discursive thoughts:
From melancholia to depression: a brief historical sketch   1

2   Depressed minds, distressed folk:
The nature and onset of depression   25

3   Depressed mind, disordered brain -
I: The neurobiology of depression   65

4   Depressed mind, disordered brain -
II: The neuropsychiatry of depression   95

5   Depressed minds, disputed cures:
The management of depression   119

6   Depressed minds, disordered cells:
Malignancy and depression   159

7   Depressed minds, dastardly acts:
Violence and depression   177

8   Depressed minds, diverse souls:
Transcultural aspects of depression   203

9   Depressed mind, distinguished art:
A pathography of depression   227

References   251

Index   271

Acknowledgements

The material for this book has been collected over nearly 10 years, and during that time it has been my good fortune to be able to avail myself of the services of several libraries. I would like to express my thanks to the Librarians and staff of the Institute of Psychiatry Library at the Maudsley Hospital, the St Bartholomew's Hospital Medical Library at West Smithfield, the John Squires Library at the Clinical Research Centre at Northwick Park Hospital, the Royal Cornwall Hospital Library in Truro, the County Library at Morpeth, Northumberland and, most recently, the Prestwich Hospital Library in Manchester. Without the material they obtained for me, this book would not have been feasible.

Dr J.M. Brewis, Acquisitions Editor, of MTP Press Ltd, Lancaster, commissioned this book and also undertook to arrange the thankless task of having the manuscript typed. I must thank him and his staff for their assistance and for the expeditious result they have brought about.

Preface

The purpose of this book is to acknowledge the universality of depression, to throw some light on those aspects of depression which are neglected in the more conventional treatments of the subject and also to attempt to provide a synthesis between the biological and socio–environmental factors which lead to the onset of depression and modify its course.

A book devoted to depression has the advantage that it has the space at its disposal to explain and clarify concepts and promising ideas that a chapter in even a comprehensive textbook does not have. A single author writing about all the relevant aspects of a subject brings with him the merit of uniformity, continuity and lack of repetition. He is also more fallible in some areas than others, which finds an exact parallel in the experience of clinicians in their practice. A multi-author, multi-specialist work portrays an air of omniscience and omnicompetence which many clinicians find dispiriting. It is likely a considerable number of practising clinicians will have a greater knowledge and experience in some areas of the subject of this book than I have and will feel emboldened to approach others.

The entire work is informed by historical considerations. The lesson of history is to be open-minded and not to judge too harshly those that have gone before. The proper reading of history should induce a salutary humility, and impress upon one the need to distance oneself from even the most alluring theories, which sadly are too often to be found in psychiatry. Nature is said to abhor a vacuum, and that which has been created by the decline of magic and conventional religion appears occasionally to be filled by some psychological doctrine or other.

In this book depression has been presented as a medical subject having considerable social and environmental overtones. There is no medical subject which is free of social and environmental considerations. The distinction between general medicine and psychiatry, in this respect, is therefore, falsely made, and the subject of depression is dealt with here as one which most interested medical practitioners can study if they set their minds to it. The practical importance of this is that a very large number of depressed patients in medical and surgical wards, and in the community, can have their conditions recognized, understood and effectively treated by non-psychiatrists. It is an enduring source of mystery that doctors who can fathom, say, the classification of epilepsy and the mysteries of the EEG, are apparently bemused by something considerably more straightforward as depression. Part of the reason may lie in the attempts of some in the psychiatric profession to project depression as something mysterious requiring arcane knowledge to unravel it, which is further evidence that vacuums can be filled by pseudo-priests, too.

Despite what the books might say, our knowledge of depression is far from complete and any dogmatic certainty is unwarranted. For instance, the alarums and excursions surrounding various classification schemes appear to be really a sophisticated version of 'blind man's buff'. Depression may appear to be the final common pathway of events that occur in the mind and, as the evidence reveals to an increasing extent, may also be due to subtle changes in the brain. To create elaborate schema on the basis of what are only superficially observed phenomena is something akin to amateur weather forecasting, amusing and satisfying to a band of enthusiasts but of little use to farmers, controllers of air and shipping traffic and others who rely on the fruits of a more exact knowledge of basic processes. This book encourages the pursuit of knowledge and speculation, but with a critical and sceptical spirit.

Trainee psychiatrists preparing for both parts of their membership examination will find there is sufficient material for that purpose, but one hopes some of them can be induced to wander down the by-lanes of the subject. The more senior psychiatrist who wishes to refresh his memory, the research worker who needs an overview of subjects other than his own, the interested general practitioner who nowadays is likely to treat more and more depressed patients, and the medical student who wonders what it is all about may find this book of some value. As with my earlier work on dementia, the chapters on history and pathography may be of some interest to the general reader.

Having studied depression for over 10 years in a variety of settings – university departments, district general hospitals, a specialized psychiatric hospital, mental hospitals and in community practice both in urban, inner city and rural areas – in Britain and a Third World country, the book also reflects my personal experience of the subject.

Manchester,   B. Mahendra
July 1986

1
Depressed minds, discursive thoughts: From melancholia to depression: A brief historical sketch

The history of the term 'melancholia', as with the concept of dementia, has been a chequered one. In general, an over-inclusive term has been narrowed with age. Like 'dementatus', 'melancholia' originally embraced the whole range of madness, and it is possible that this meaning survived at least until Elizabethan times. In his magisterial survey of the concept of melancholia, Aubrey Lewis (1934a) pointed to the difficulty in extricating the ideas relating to melancholia from those general to the whole history of psychiatry.

However, a reading of the history of melancholia is a more than salutary exercise as it becomes clear that, over-inclusion apart, the concepts surrounding melancholia do not seem to have materially changed with the passage of time. Quite apart from inquiring into the nature of the condition, there has been a determined speculation, qualified only by the *zeitgeist*, about the origin, the localization, the progression, the course, the effect of treatment, the natural history and the prognosis of the constituent elements of melancholia. Every age appears to have produced the credulous and the sceptical; the interventionists and the detached observers; those hidebound by the facts and those carried away by speculation; the reductionists and the expansive social theorists. And every age has produced what we, from the vantage of the second half of the twentieth century, would consider the insightful and the prescient.

When a historical survey of ideas pertaining to any subject is undertaken, two broad approaches are available to the inquirer. He may study these ideas and concepts in the context of other ideas in existence at the time, or in terms of the insights and attitudes of the present day. The latter approach has been decried for, among other reasons, its essential 'unfairness' to those who have lived, thought and practised in another age. It is surely unreasonable, say, to expect a practitioner whose ideas are founded on a specific doctrine to be sceptical and open-minded in his inquiries or in his practice. If one believes the devil gets into the soul to

1

produce melancholy, the next logical step surely would be to speculate on the nature of the soul that has attractions for the devil, a beginning which, as one knows, may lead anywhere. Criticism of this form of retrospective analysis is, therefore, valid. However, one imagines practising clinicians will have little patience with history in the abstract. The social attitudes, the cultural norms, the philosophical traditions, the politico–economic environment and theories of bodily structure and function, all of which influence our ways of thinking about disease, will nevertheless hold little attraction for the average clinician who would prefer historical inquiry to throw light on his present day practice rather than illumine the dark corners of the past. Hence, this brief historical sketch has a deliberate egocentricity, the result of a fascination with the more prescient of the ancient thinkers. It need hardly be added that our current ideas and practices will be subjected to a similar future scrutiny.

It may also be mentioned in passing that it is striking to anyone who surveys the past, in however sketchy a fashion, that it is not merely the currency of ideas which we believe might reflect the contemporary view but the diversity of views that are present. While a general account of melancholia may reflect the majority view, the deeper one delves the more likely one is to discover not merely dissent but notable enlightenment. Nowhere is this better illustrated than in the period when one is led to believe that the whole population was zealously combing the land for witches who were to be sought, tried and eliminated. The dissenting views of Scot, Weyer, and not a few others, proclaim not merely humanity but quite advanced and insightful psychiatry.

It must be clear that all aspects of the study of any subject may be enriched by historical considerations. Therefore, reference is made throughout the rest of the book to pertinent historical detail. Special mention may be made of Chapter 5, where a brief historical reference is made to the more specific treatments of depression, which has been essentially a development of the past 50 years; Chapter 6, where emotional aspects of malignancy have attracted long-standing attention; Chapter 8, where the dubious historical antecedents of transcultural psychiatry are noted, and Chapter 9, in which pathographic considerations are taken up.

EARLY DAYS AND THE MIDDLE AGES

The Old Testament (1 *Samuel* XVI, 14–23) refers to an early example of depression and its 'cure' by psychotherapeutic means.

> But the spirit of the Lord departed from Saul, and an evil spirit from the Lord troubled him.

This malaise was subjected to musical therapy, with an earnest search for a competent and acceptable therapist:

> ... to seek out a man, who is a cunning player on an harp, and it shall come to pass, when the evil spirit from God is upon thee, that he shall play with his hand, and thou shalt be well.

In interesting contrast to modern-day assessment of the patient or client, it was Saul's prospective therapist who had to undergo vetting, and indeed Saul's servants undertook this, vouching for the therapist thus:

> ... is cunning in playing, and a mighty valiant man, and a man of war, and prudent in matters, and a comely person, and the Lord is with him.

Having passed muster, he undertook his treatment with remarkable success:

> And it came to pass, when the evil spirit from God was upon Saul, that David took an harp, and played with his hand: so Saul was refreshed, and was well, and the evil spirit departed from him.

Hippocrates (?460 BC–?359 BC) made an early reference to the relationship between mood and the related affect of anxiety: 'If fear (phobos) or distress (dysthymia) last for a long time it is melancholia' (Lewis, 1934a). Employing the concepts of his time, he alluded to the importance of temperament and constitution, noting the alteration of the brain by black bile and phlegm, so darkening the spirit and causing melancholy. This localization was necessarily crude as the substance of the brain was deemed important for mental activity only in the sixteenth century. However, Hippocrates' view of melancholia was certainly over-inclusive in modern terms and his reference to the relationship between epilepsy and melancholia was in terms of the connection between two forms of madness rather than between cerebral disorder and a specific mental disorder.

To Aristotle (384 BC–322 BC) the 'sensorium commune', located in the anterior ventricle, was a functional part of the soul, attracting sensations from everywhere and producing higher mental activity which radiated elsewhere (Meyer, 1960). Aristotle might be said to have produced an early neuropsychiatric synthesis.

Aretaeus of Cappadocia (2nd century AD) is generally credited with having made one of the earliest observations of what we understand as mania and depression. He also commented on the diversity of melancholia: 'Those affected with melancholy are not every one of them affected according to one particular form'. He detailed the various associated symptoms of melancholics – 'suspicions about poisoning', unsociability ('fleeing to the desert'), they become ritualistic, get fed up with life and speak of dying or killing themselves. He refers to the symptoms of apathy, withdrawal, psychomotor slowing, irritability and insomnia. He pointed to what a later age would call 'endogenous' – the manifestation of these symptoms without apparent cause. He spoke of the recurring nature of the condition and, in a major advance for his time, excluded disturbances of consciousness or delirium in making this diagnosis. Aretaeus also described gastro-intestinal symptoms, and while his speculations on aetiology were in terms of the movement of black bile, his emphasis on the stomach and gut led him to believe that both mania and melancholia were to be localized in the region of the hypochondrium.

Galen (AD 130–201) helped revive the brain as the organ of prime importance in melancholia, and believed that excess of black bile in the substance of the brain caused melancholia. If indeed he did say this it would be remarkable, as it is claimed (Meyer, 1960) that it was only after 1543, when Vesalius published his *De Fabrica*, that the substance of the brain was generally considered to have any importance in mental activity. Two to three centuries *after* Galen, at least in general terms, the 'animal spirits' were assumed to reside in the ventricles for which the brain substance simply provided a covering capsule. Be that as it may, Galen was in broad agreement with Hippocrates as to the importance of the brain and also confirmed the relationship between melancholia and epilepsy.

According to Skultans (1979), the Galenic or Aristotleian interpretations of melancholy were still current in Elizabethan England as alternative explanations of phenomena and behaviour in melancholia. The Galenic tradition, based on explanations of an excess of black bile, a viscid and highly tenacious substance, produced the melancholy man who is 'morose, taciturn, waspish, misanthropic, solitary, fond of darkness, (suffering) from grotesque hallucinations ... he is extremely wretched and often longs for death' (quoted by Skultans). The Aristotleian tradition is altogether more romantic, associating melancholy with poetic inspiration and wit. Aristotle asked:

> Why is it that all those who have become eminent in philosophy or politics or poetry or the arts are clearly of an atrabilious temperament and some of them to such an extent as to be affected by diseases caused by black bile? (quoted by Skultans).

This, of course, is a contemporary concern and will be given a more up-to-date airing in Chapter 9.

A curious interlude associating hallucinations with depression led to the founding of St Bartholomew's Hospital in London (Clare, 1985). The monk, Rahere, undertook a journey to Rome to expiate his sins. He fell ill and 'thought his last hour was drawing nigh'. He became depressed, tearful and vowed that if he should be allowed to return alive, he would build a hospital to serve the poor. On his return journey he had a 'vision' of St Batholomew who commanded him to build a church as well in Smithfield. On his return he was charged by Henry I with founding the hospital and the priory of St Bartholomew the Great in 1123.

Hunter and Macalpine (1963) refer to Bartholomaeus Anglicus who published his encyclopaedia *De proprietatibus rerum* in manuscript in the 13th century. The still (in modern eyes) over-inclusive use of the term melancholia is evident as it covered anxiety states, hypochondriasis, depression and delusional states.

We shall presently devote a brief section to the subject of diabolical possession. Suffice it here to note that most witches would appear to have been vulnerable, suggestible and eccentric females. However, a few do appear to have had mental states suggestive of depression, and a colourful example, occurring before the epidemic of unreason swept through Britain, is recounted by Summers (1926) and involves the Franciscan penitent, St Margaret of Cortona, who was 'long and terribly tormented'.

Following her to and fro up and down her humble cell as she wept and prayed, (the devil) sang the most filthy songs, and lewdly incited Christ's dear handmaid, who with tears was commending herself to the Lord, to join him in trolling forth bawdy catches ... but her prayers and tears finally routed the foul spirit and drove him far away. (quoted by Summers).

By the end of the 15th century, anecdotal evidence suggests that some vague delineation of the condition we would recognize as depression was taking place in some places, more by accident than design. Rosen (1964) describes the case of the Flemish painter, Hugo van der Goes. About 1475 he appears to have joined the monastic community of the Roode Clooster near Brussels. Five years later he suffered from an affliction which is unmistakably a depressive illness – 'a disorder of the imagination'. He was incessantly self-reproachful and self-damnatory; he was suicidal and had to be restrained by his companions. The prior of the community suspected this malady was a latter-day version of that experienced by King Saul. He gave orders that music be constantly played in Hugo's presence but, perhaps the condition being beyond psychotherapeutic reach, there was no improvement in the patient's state. He continued to ramble in the most self-denigratory fashion, eventually recovering with the passage of time. A contemporary account exists, speculating on the causes of the painter's illness. The document seems to suggest that melancholia could be the outcome of several causes, and that the manifested form of the illness may be related to the original cause: food which produces black bile; strong wines which may heat the body juices and turn them into ashes; restlessness, sadness, anxiety or excessive exertion; the virulence of noxious juices in the body of a vulnerable man who is susceptible to melancholy.

The distinction between the melancholic temperament and the symptoms of melancholia was the basis of a further attempt at clarification by Andreas Laurentius in 1597. All melancholic men were not infected by the 'miserable passion' called melancholia, he said. He urged the study of the diversities of the melancholic constitution, pointing to the wide range possible in the attributes of the melancholic temperament and its compatibility with the normal. This was one of the earliest attempts to distinguish between physiological variation and pathology.

By the 16th century, some of the ideas that had held sway for two thousand years or more were being seriously questioned at least in some circles. The cornerstones of aetiological speculation until that time were theories of the humours and the temperaments. These ideas were challenged, most notably by Paracelsus (1493–1541) and Francis Bacon (1561–1626) who suggested that melancholia, and other mental disorders, might be natural diseases. Also, by the early 16th century the localization of the source of melancholia had moved downwards again, to wit the hypochondrium. Following Aretaeus, the early emphasis was on the stomach and gastro-intestinal systems but another constituent of the hypochondrium – the spleen – acquired increasing importance in the 18th century. However, Hieronymous Mercurialis (1530–1606) suggested an involvement of the heart, on the basis that some of the fears displayed by melancholic patients could be traced to that organ.

Hunter and Macalpine (1963) refer to Philip Barrough and his *Methode of Phisicke* (1583), an influential work which has also been referred to in the historical section of a book on dementia (Mahendra, 1984a). The over-inclusive nature of the concept of melancholia is clear in the vivid description in the work, but once again one of the verities in the speculation on melancholia (the other is the relationship with mania) is retained, namely the absence of fever. Melancholia is described as 'an alienation of the mind'. The prominence of anxiety is noted as is the presence of delusions, some not quite congruent with a depressive mood. Suicidal feelings and fears and fascinations regarding death are mentioned. 'Moreover they desire death, and do verie often behight and determine to kill themselves and some feare that they should be killed'.

The same authors (Hunter and Macalpine, 1963) also refer to Thomas Bright's (1551–1615) *A treatise of melancholie*, published in 1586, where the author's classifications of melancholia and its appropriate treatment have a modern ring to them. Bright wrote of one form of melancholy where 'the perill is not of body ... (but) proceedeth from the minde's apprehension ... (requiring) cure of the minde', which four centuries later would have been construed as a case of 'psychogenic' depression requiring psychotherapy. The other variety of melancholy, '... being not moved by any adversity present or imminent ... (the humour) ... deluding the organicall actions, abuseth the mind'. Here, 'no counsel of philosophy, nor precept of wise men were comparable to calme these raging passions, unto the purging potions of physitians'. Hunter and Macalpine believe that while this distinction was made partly on clinical grounds, there was also theological doctrine to be taken note of. There could be no disease concept of the mind as that was equated with the immortal soul which was incorruptible and not susceptible to disease; the body, on the other hand, could be affected to produce an affliction of the mind. It is not difficult to trace the threads of some contemporary objections to the medical model of mental disorder to views such as these. It is also salutary to remind oneself that an important component of the ethical furore surrounding the first heart transplant in 1967 was that medical technicians and clinical engineers might be interfering with an organ vital to the emotions and, hence, with individuality.

In the 17th century, while clinical descriptions occasionally displayed an enviable sophistication, neuropathological speculation remained less distinguished. Thomas Willis published his *Cerebri Anatome* in 1664, and claimed melancholia was caused by the degeneration of animal spirits (Meyer, 1960). 'Animal spirits' were secreted from the blood in the regions of the cerebral and cerebellar cortex. It has been suggested that by speculating if 'stupidity' could be caused by anatomical lesions of the cerebrum as well as by the disintegration of the 'animal spirits', Willis had probably anticipated the dubious distinction to be drawn between 'organic' and 'functional' lesions, a subject further taken up in Chapter 3.

This distinction was related to speculations about the mind and body, a subject which has, of course, exercised numerous writers through the ages. But a fresh impetus was given to the argument by the burgeoning subject of psychology. The influence of G.E. Stahl (1660–1734) in particular has been noted by Lewis (1934a) to have been exercised through his animistic doctrine. He held that mental disorders were an aberration of the soul which had its regular activity inhibited by a strange idea which might have arisen from the senses, or from other bodily functions, or from the mood.

The view that an association, if not a relationship, exists between mania and melancholia has persisted in virtually every age in the past 2000 years. In the 18th century, Richard Mead (1673–1754) attested to this phenomenon, and he also demonstrated the rapid switches in the mood state that were possible in the affective disorders.

WITCHES AND DEMONS

No history of any aspect of mental disorder can be complete without reference to one of the more than usually unedifying chapters in history – witchcraft, its alleged practitioners and their tormentors.

Discrimination was sometimes attempted between witches, to be hunted down and despatched as agents of the forces of evil, and melancholics, recipients even then of rudimentary compassion. King James I and VI, a considerable scholar, an indifferent king and a demonologist, attempted to be fair in his *Daemonologie*, published in 1597.

> For as the humor of Melancholie in the selfe is blacke, heavie and terrene, so are the symptoms thereof, in any persones that are subject thereunto ... feeding thereby their humor in that which they think no crime...

Despite these insights, James's book was written as a 'counterblast' to Reginald Scot's (1538–1599) *Discoverie of Witchcraft* (1584) which questioned, heretically, the whole basis on which witches were being persecuted. Passages from Scot's work with their insistence on natural explanations for the behaviour of witches are given by Annear (1979). What witches really needed, Scot maintained, was 'physick, food and necessaries'. He observed,

> ... in truth this melancholike humor (as the best physicians confirm) is the cause of all their strange, impossible and incredible confessions – which are so fond, that I wonder how anie man can be abused thereby.

Scot's cases included a farmer's wife with severe depression, agitation and insomnia. She 'confessed' she had given her soul to the devil, had bewitched her family and that the devil would come to her on a certain night as part of the bargain that had been struck. That night she made a recovery upon being startled by a loud noise which she discovered had been made not by a prowling devil on a nocturnal visit to collect his dues but by a dog attacking a sheep's carcase.

> She now being recovered, remaineth a right honest woman, far from such impietie, and shamed of hir imaginations, which she perceiveth to have growne through hir melancholie ... how best she was

7

brought lowe and pressed downe with the weight of this humor, so as both hir rest and sleepe were taken awaie from hir, and hir fansies troubled and disquieted with despaire, and such cogitations as grew by occasion thereof'.

Scot's was by no means a voice in the wilderness. Other distinguished dissenters included Johann Weyer (1515–1588) whose book *De Praestigiis Daemonum* (1563) suggested the confessions of witches were in reality misinterpretations, oddly held ideas or delusions due to mental disorder. Another who sought to explain the behaviour of witches in terms of depressive phenomenology was John Webster who published *The Displaying of Supposed Witchcraft* in 1677. He explained the 'confessions' of witches as 'passive delusions' which were imposed upon their 'depraved fancies' as *melancholiae figmenta*. He castigated the witch hunters who were taken in by these 'absurd, idle, foolish, false and impossible' ideas, ascribed them to the devil and proceeded to punish, torture and put to death those women whose delusions were 'intrinsically wrought' (endogenous).

Scot and Weyer were virtual contemporaries but Webster came nearly a century after. But despite them witchhunting continued, the last witch to be executed in England was in 1684 and in Scotland in 1722.

MELANCHOLIA INTO DEPRESSION: THE INTERREGNUM

Robert Burton's *The Anatomy of Melancholy* (1621) was an influential work that continued to dominate thought for decades afterwards. It was a child of its age and melancholy was still largely equated with madness. Nevertheless, the insights contained in it were significant. Burton made the distinction, as Laurentius had done, between the melancholic temperament and the state of melancholy, calling them, respectively, *disposition* and *habite*. Some people have transient mood disturbances ('transitory melancholy') in response to the relatively trivial events of life. This disposition could lead to a 'habit' and in this change Burton acknowledged the importance of perception of stresses and life events in those of a vulnerable disposition – 'For that which is but as a flea biting to one, causeth unsufferable torment to another ...'

Burton classified melancholia into three forms. In the first the primary lesion was thought to be in the brain – Head Melancholy, a category which also included Love Melancholy, Lycanthropia and Religious Melancholy. In the second category, called simply Melancholy, a global or generalized affection of the body was suspected. However, this global view of the body excluded not merely the head, but the bowels, liver, spleen and the mesentery. These latter organs were the seat of the third category of Melancholy, Windy or Hypochondria-Melancholy. All these disturbances were, it must be noted, characterized by an exaggeration of function which was not necessarily depressive in origin. He further noted that symptoms such as obsessions, delusions, suicidal behaviour and hypochondriasis could be part of the syndrome of melancholia as much as sadness could.

The speculations of Burton as to constitutional factors in both the temperamental trait and the pathological condition went a step further in

8

ascribing importance to heredity. Burton wrote that both temperament and the malady could be inherited from one's parents, revealing no stigmata on the body or its functions – '... this doth not so much appeare in the composition of the Body' – but affecting the constitution of the mind and its predisposition to afflictions –'... but in manners and conditions of the Minde...'

Not surprisingly Burton was a creature of his age, and the preoccupation with diabolical influence and, indeed, aetiology found this echo in him: 'How farre the power of Divels doth extend, and whether they can cause this or any other Disease, is a serious question and worthy to be considered...'

Another of Burton's insights into the causation of melancholy is the role of upbringing – a man 'may be undone by evill bringing up'. The preoccupation of three centuries later already exercised his mind – what kind of upbringing was most likely to produce a child that would grow into a stable adult? The child may be the father of the man but the man who is father of the child – and, to be fair, Burton did make specific references to 'parents and such' – has the power to shape the child. Burton took the middle of the road, castigating a too strict, or too lax, upbringing: 'Parents and such: ... offend many times in that they are too sterne ... others againe in that other extreame doe as much harme...'

A more sternly organic view than was hitherto current was taken by Nicholas Robinson (1697–1775). Robinson believed melancholia was a real affliction of the mind which arose from a real, tangible, mechanical causation in the brain. The constitution of the brain thus affected caused changes in matter and motion which led to 'melancholy madness'.

Melancholy, most especially in its hypochondriacal variety, was long considered a peculiarly English disease. In his book *The English Malady* (1733), George Cheyne (1671–1743) considered the reasons for this apparent frequency, and also implied that the incidence of melancholia had actually risen in the 18th century. His reasons for both the apparent increase as well as the preferential incidence in the English were the atmospheric humidity, the variability of the weather, the peculiarities of the soil and its fertility, the rich and heavy food, the wealth of the inhabitants, the inactivity and sedentary occupation of the higher social orders (here Cheyne made the percipient point that the malady was commoner in the upper classes) and the tribulations of living in large, populous and insalubrious cities were some of the reasons he adduced. With one or two qualifications this is almost exactly the contemporary explanation for the high incidence of ischaemic heart disease in Britain, a state of affairs which probably reveals more about the unchanging nature of sociological speculation rather than the truth about the causes of disease.

Preoccupation first with witches and then with speculative sociology slowed down the systematic inquiry into the neuropathology of mental disorders. Among the contributors who helped pick up the trail was Haslam who asserted 'that madness has always been connected with disease of the brain and its membranes', and is revealed *post-mortem* in every case of mental illness (quoted by Meyer, 1960). Haslam's views were influenced by the high incidence of organic brain disorder in mental hospital patients of the time – about a third of these are estimated to have been patients with general paresis and Haslam is generally credited with the first clinical description of the condition – and it is suggested that an extrapolation to all mental disorders including melancholia took place. Haslam, in 1798, like others before him, also discussed the relationship between mania and melancholia and with insight disputed the assertion that the two conditions were opposed. He suggested the 'association of ideas' in both were equally incorrect and argued that only the passions (affect) that accompanied the ideas were different in the two conditions, anticipating to a degree by a century and a half the view that depression and mania have common origins and lay at opposing poles only in manifest clinical presentation.

A more sophisticated delineation of melancholia was presented in the late 18th century by several authors including Thomas Arnold (1742–1816) whose *Observations on Insanity* were published in two volumes between 1782 and 1786. Starting with a classification of insanity with hallucinations and delusions, 'ideal' and 'notional' insanities, he placed melancholia under the latter category. He further sub-divided the condition into *hypochondriacal* insanity and *pathetic* insanity. In the former, the major feature was the patient's preoccupation with his state of health, his dysphoric state and his anxious, unrelenting attention to both. A sense of distress is evident. In *pathetic* insanity, a 'master passion' takes over the mind, conquering and enslaving all other features ('exercises a despotic authority over all other affections'). This delusional melancholia is accompanied by distress, dejection, anxiety and restlessness of the mind. The emphasis on clinical features involving prominent positive symptoms such as hypochondriasis and delusions illustrates the changing nature of depressive presentations over time. Though both hypochondriasis and delusions are accepted features of depression in the present day, neither feature would strike a modern worker considering a classification of the disease as cardinal points in categorizing it. Even allowing for the mongrel nature of melancholia as understood at the time, these symptoms convey more the socio–cultural influence on, rather than relating to the biological origin of, depression. Eagles (1983) studied the records of delusional depressive in-patients between 1892 and 1982 and showed that while there had been no great change in the number of delusional depressives being admitted to hospital over 90 years, changes in the content of depressive delusions had occurred. Between 1892 and 1942 delusions of disease and sinfulness increased in frequency. Delusions of persecution, common in 1892, appeared as the most common form of delusion in the 1982 samples. As with melancholia in the 18th century, contamination of the depressives of 1892 was suspected with schizophrenia. The *raison d'etre* for transcultural psychiatry was the study of differences in clinical presentation of mental disorder, and some of the changes in the symptomatology of depression over time in a culture are taken up further in Chapter 8.

The origin of the concept of neurosis is traced to William Cullen (1710–1790) whose influence countered some of the more extreme views of those who proposed an apparent and exclusively organic basis to melancholia. Cullen's contribution to the study of melancholia was in aiding in distinguishing it from hypochondriasis. He also noted the invariable association of melancholia with anxious fears, and the occurrence of the condition in those who were constitutionally predisposed – i.e. in persons of a melancholic temperament. In the wider scheme of things, Cullen noted, it was a partial insanity and the accompanying symptoms merely reflected the causative agent of the melancholia. His groupings of the symptoms of the condition are multiple and reflect the thought of the day. Pride of place in the classification goes to preoccupations and anxieties regarding health (indeed to Cullen, melancholia was partial insanity without dyspepsia). Other symptom clusters included the patient's belief in his impoverishment, superstitions, anxieties, an increase in libido, restlessness and irritability, weariness with life and despondency. It is quite apparent that despite the relegation of hypochondriasis to the place of a symptom rather than a disease entity on a par with melancholia itself, the term was still a hybrid one. It is probably correct to say that while the actual incidence of hypochondriasis might have fallen because of changes in the socio–cultural environment, some of the falling off was due to the change in diagnostic concepts used by such clinicians as Cullen.

Further contributions to the symptomatology and psychogenesis of melancholia were made in the 18th century by John Ferriar (1761–1815) and Benjamin Rush (1745–1813), respectively. Ferriar pointed to the possibility of the patient starving himself to death in melancholia. The reason for this was not severe psychomotor retardation and an attendant inability or unwillingness to take nourishment, but paranoid fears on the part of the patient who suspected that he might be poisoned.

Benjamin Rush speculated about psychogenesis, and tried to account for the fact that an obvious cause was not always evident. He worked from first principles and analogy. Diseases always needed causes; bodily illness may arise from causes that are not always apparent, or are overlooked. In like manner melancholia may be caused. But, he added, the cause of the distress may lie below the surface of memory, an early reference to the possibility of unconscious causation of depression.

MODERN STIRRINGS

Between the end of the 18th century and the beginning of the 19th, several attempts were being made to clarify the concept of melancholia and bring it closer to that which we would now equate with depression. One of these was by Dreyssig (1770–1809) who believed melancholia was caused by a disturbance in the balance between the power of judgement and the power of imagination. Melancholia formed a triumvirate with mania and imbecility. It was thought to be a partial insanity, or a partial failure of judgement and reasoning capacity, limited to one or a few subjects. Melancholia could be true or false, the former being associated with a persistent lowering of the mood; in false melancholia, indifference or, indeed, cheerfulness raised the suspicion of what moderns might call a 'pseudo' state; raging melancholy, when severe, approached mania (Lewis, 1934a).

11

Not for the first time, credit for an attempt at accurate delineation of a condition is due to Esquirol (1772–1840). He gave his views in *Lypemania or Melancholy* published in 1820. He divided melancholia, or partial insanity, into lypemania and monomania, or true partial insanity. Affective disorder came under lypemania; monomania had sub-categories of 'intellectual', 'affective' and 'instinctive' which correspond in modern parlance to paranoid disorder, hypomania and psychopathy. In explaining the distinction he excluded monomania, dementia and idiocy by the presence of ideas and the ability to reason, i.e. on intellectual grounds. The idiot could never have reasoned; the dement was once able to reason but now had a poverty and confusion of ideas because of debility; the monomaniac has ideas but these are delusions and his affect is cheerful and expansive. This narrowed the field to mania and lypemania. In the former there is generalized delirium and sensibility and intellectual functioning may seem elevated; in lypemania the delirium is partial and the affect is invariably a sad one. As others before him had done, Esquirol confirmed there was no fever in lypemania and held the condition to be cerebral in origin.

In parallel with Esquirol's attempt at clarification of the concept of melancholia was the work of Samuel Tuke, who in 1813 brought the concept to the state that is recognizable to the modern clinician. '... under the class melancholia, all cases are included in which the disorder is chiefly marked by depression of mind, whether it is, or is not, attended by general false notions'. Burrows, the director of the Clapham Retreat, further emphasized that mania and melancholia have a common origin and, essentially, are one and the same disease.

An idiosyncratic work by George Nesse Hill, *An Essay on the Prevention and Cure of Insanity* (1814), further emphasized the 'organic' nature of melancholia. He wrote that all forms of insanity had a bodily, if not necessarily cerebral, origin, and in a tellingly visionary maxim wrote, insanity being as curable as anything found in the rest of medicine, '...the first and indeed principal object of the medical artist is to explore organic mischief'. On the eve of the 21st century, it will serve well as a dictum for psychiatrists.

These 19th century views were emphatically summarized by Conolly in his Croonian Lectures, *On some of the Forms of Insanity* (1849):

(Melancholia) is governed by the same laws as mania and often alternates with it. The precise character assumed by the mental disorder is often evidently determined by what is commonly called the temperament of the patient — sanguine or melancholic.

There then follows a carefully detailed description of depression in all its forms, which is quite acceptable even today.

Conolly was speaking at a time when the growing use of the microscope was opening new vistas in neurohistological research. New anatomical structures were being seen, and functions were being speculatively attributed to these entities; what was not yet seen was envisaged. Conolly had little doubt as to the future:

The future scope of the psychological physician may be more ambitious and rest on new and broader foundations, formed out of the result of researches now made by many physiologists, aided by the use of the microscope, by chemistry, and other auxiliaries, still accompanied by the close observation of phenomena during life. The yet unsettled state of many important questions relative to the nervous system, and the revolution even now taking place in its theories... tend at least to enforce caution, to lessen one's reliance on mere experiments, and direct our attention more closely to structure and function in health and disease.

The advent of neurohistology about this time prompted the notion, especially in Germany, that insanity was related to anatomical brain lesions. Microscopic study of brain tissue was still a rudimentary art but speculation, untempered by scepticism, led to unwarranted dogmatism based on the few details proffered by the infant science of microscopy. The chief disputants appear to have been Griesinger, Meynert and Schroeder van der Kolk. Griesinger appears to have been the most cautious of the trio. Having divided the psychotic disorders into those of the emotions and those of false modes of thought and will, Griesinger conceded that it was rare to find organic change in the former group under which melancholia was classified. Meynert believed the cerebral cortex had an exclusively psychic function, and that mania and melancholia were due to cortical irritation. Schroeder van der Kolk was the most certain in his localization, claiming invariable pathological changes in the upper and hind lobes of the brains of melancholics (Meyer, 1960).

Henry Maudsley took Schroeder van der Kolk's claims to task, preferring, like Conolly to put his faith in the unknown and in the future, '... it is beyond doubt that important molecular or chemical changes may take place in those inner recesses to which we have not yet gained access'. Maudsley's more general views on melancholia were expressed in his *The Physiology and Pathology of the Mind* (1868). They were not startlingly original and might indeed have appeared over-inclusive at a time when determined efforts were being made to narrow the field of conditions being subsumed under the rubric of melancholia. In terms of symptoms he grouped the conditions into 'affective insanity', i.e. conditions without delusions, and 'ideational insanity', i.e. conditions with delusions, a classification of limited value even for the period, and remarkably conservative in view of what has been said of Cullen and Esquirol's work. However, Maudsley's view of the cognitive change associated with depressive disorder is remarkably percipient, and his statement regarding this relationship serves even today in the arguments against 'functional' illness and the disputed concept of 'pseudodementia' (see Chapters 3 and 4).

The affective disorder is the fundamental fact; in the great majority of cases it precedes intellectual disorder; it co-exists with the latter during its course; and it frequently persists for a time after this has disappeared.

13

In a recent paper, Berrios (1985) has pointed out that 19th century psychiatrists had emphasized disorders of thinking at the expense of the affect. Psychiatrists of the time held the same view of mental disorder which had come down from the Greeks, as disorders to be seen in terms of irrationality and overt behavioural disturbance. Melancholia itself was seen as a disorder of unreason with reduced behavioural output, and a depressed mood was deemed secondary. The conceptual advance, in Berrios' view, was that in the 19th century, for the first time, depression began to be seen as a primary disorder. He explains the confusion as being due to two distinct meanings of the term melancholia in the 19th century. On the one hand there was the popular usage in which melancholia was associated with sadness, suicide and nostalgia. Then, there was the more technical usage which considered melancholia to be a form of delusional insanity.

The Faculty psychologists maintained that the affect constituted a 'primary, autonomous and irreducible' faculty of the mind and thus, like other faculties, could be susceptible to primary pathology. Thus, in Berrios' view, emotional or affective forms of insanity came into being, and melancholia had to be redefined to fit into this category. Berrios quotes Heinroth on the primacy of the affect even in the presence of delusions.

> The presence of an *idée fixe* does not mean that the disease is an affectation of the intellect; the intellect is the mere servant of the sick disposition ... the *idée fixe* may not be present but melancholia remains what it is; depression of the disposition, withdrawal into oneself, detachment from the external world.

Berrios also claims that Kraepelin's (1913) distinction between dementia praecox and manic-depressive psychoses was based not on the disorders of thinking and affect but on features of psychopathology such as the uniform and good prognosis in the latter, the differential heredity and the presence of primary excitement or inhibition.

CYCLES OF FASHION: INVOLUTIONAL MELANCHOLIA

The concept of involutional melancholia has suffered vicissitudes of fashion over its 100 year history. The involutional period corresponds to the perimenopausal years in women, i.e. between the ages of 40 and 55; it is generally thought to occur at a somewhat later period in men. Controversy as to its nosological position had begun soon after Kraepelin (1896) delineated involutional melancholia as distinct from manic-depressive psychosis. Lewis (1934a) describes how in the fifth edition of his *Lehrbuch*, Kraepelin (1896) divided all insanity into acquired disorders and those arising from constitutional factors or morbid predisposition. Involutional melancholia featured as one of the former disorders. In the latter category, periodic insanity is classified as one of the constitutional mental disorders, and the constitutional mood disorder is described as one of the psychopathic degenerations. Included in the term 'periodic insanity' are the manic, circular and depressive forms of mental disorder.

Thus the distinction between involutional melancholia and manic-depressive psychosis was made not merely in terms of symptomatology but on the basis of the former being acquired and the latter belonging to the endogenous or constitutional psychoses.

It is interesting to note that when this form of specific melancholia in later life was being suggested, active work was going on on a variety of pre-senile and senile psychoses. The two decades between 1890 and 1910 were among the busiest and most productive periods in the history of the study of dementing disorders, and the early cases of the eponymous dementias were of patients in the involutional period of life. Not for the first time one sees the emergence of a particular disease concept not simply in terms of inspired clinical insight on the part of the individual physician but in keeping with the climate of thought of the period.

Patients diagnosed as having involutional melancholia had to satisfy several criteria: the onset of the illness was in the involutional period, there having been no previous episodes of depression or mania; symptoms such as fear, anxiety or apprehension were prominent; there was a conspicuous presence of hypochondriacal ideas or delusions; the condition was of lengthy duration and, at least in the period before modern physical treatments, of poor prognosis. In 1923, Eugen Bleuler claimed the disorders grew slowly, remained at their height for several years and, then, if recovery took place at all, took time to decline.

The concept was attacked within a few years of unveiling, first by Thalbitzer (1902) and, then, more notably by Dreyfus (1907). Dreyfus re-analysed 85 of Kraepelin's cases and found a history of previous manic-depressive illness in 54% of the cases and a recovery rate of 66%. It is generally believed that it was Dreyfus' views that led to Kraepelin changing his mind, and by the time of the 8th edition of his textbook (1909), Kraepelin had restored involutional melancholia to the group of manic-depressive disorders; from a disease in its own right it had descended to being merely a clinical picture. In doing so Kraepelin might have paid heed to Dreyfus' and others' criticisms, but, as has been pointed out, he was also working in a period when organic factors such as senile degeneration and 'arteriosclerotic' change were being shown to be important in the causation or precipitation of the psychoses of this age group. These degenerative processes were hardly acquired, and it is possible that these ideas influenced the change in the view of involutional melancholia as an acquired or exogenous psychosis. Thus, at most, the role of the involutional period was seen as pathoplastic, not causal.

Dreyfus's re-examination of Kraepelin's material was itself subjected to serious criticism by British and American authors, chiefly on the grounds of incompleteness in the analysis and of special pleading in emphasizing very doubtful manic-depressive features (Tait et al., 1957). Following this criticism of Dreyfus' re-analysis, involutional melancholia was partially restored as a distinct entity (e.g. Kirby, 1909; Hoch and MacCurdy, 1922) but the controversy continued, especially among French and German workers to whom Lewis (1934a) has referred.

The doubts and uncertainties sensed by research workers as to the condition's nosological position were not conveyed in the textbooks which, in the nature of things, require clearcut statements of fact and opinion. The

15

result was that for several decades involutional melancholia was accorded the dignity of a separate syndrome. It was taught that the clinical features to be noted in involutional melancholia, namely marked anxiety and apprehension, bizarre hypochondriasis and nihilistic delusions, helped distinguish it, at least in terms of symptomatology, from cases of depression in younger patients who displayed psychomotor retardation with ideas of guilt and self-reproach. But conventional teaching had to concede that an embarrassingly large overlap existed between the age groups.

A case was also being made by Titley (1936) as to the importance of the premorbid personality in involutional melancholia. Where manic-depressive patients in younger age-groups had personalities closer to normal subjects, a distinct personality profile was being suggested for involutional depressives. They were, it was claimed, premorbidly rather rigid, methodical, meticulous, obsessional, with a narrow range of interests and emotional response and with a limited capacity to adapt to change, i.e. vulnerable to stresses and life events. Genetic factors were mooted for both this allegedly characteristic pre-morbid personality and the ensuing form of depression in the involutional period. The nature of psychological stress in the involutional period in terms of the losses of role, the end of the period of production, the approach of retirement (this was, mercifully, before the age of mass involuntary redundancy in the involutional period, circumstances which, on the basis of the argument, should have precipitated an outbreak of involutional melancholia in this age group but have apparently not) and the imminence of senility were all suggested as stresses peculiar to those in this age group but from which younger depressives were largely spared. The obvious endocrine changes of the involution, well established in women but popularly suspected in males too, were also considered in the listing of aetiological factors which might separate those in the involutional period from those who had depression at a younger age.

The textbook accounts were challenged by sceptics. One group among the latter, Tait et al., (1957), re-analysed Lewis's (1934b, 1936) data and tabulated patients according to whether they were under or over 40 years. They found that self-reproach, far from being a symptom predominating in the younger age group, was actually equally distributed between the two groups. As for hypochondriasis – and including the most bizarre form of this symptom – it seemed, if anything, to be commoner in the younger depressives. While agitation appeared to be commoner in older patients and retardation in the younger age group, the differences between them were not statistically significant. The authors' scepticism was well-founded. Even clinically, age did not seem to provide a point of distinction between one form of depression and another. They quoted other authors as having come to a similar conclusion.

However, some attempt had to be made to account for the persistence of the concept in textbooks and the prevailing orthodoxy. One possibility, as always, was that series of cases under study had been contaminated. Were unremitting or recurring cases of involutional melancholia really one or the other of the schizophrenias? It is generally thought that schizophrenias emerge less commonly in later life, the conditions then having a lower genetic loading, and remitting more frequently, even if not permanently. However, the symptoms of this condition are very different to the classically portrayed involutional melancholia. A more valid explanation appears to be contamination by cases of cerebral degeneration. These cases would have an obvious impact on the prognosis of any group of patients, although deterioration and increased mortality were not features noted in the classical descriptions of involutional melancholia. One recalls that Kraepelin was encouraged to change his mind as to the existence of involutional melancholia as a separate entity by the realization that organic change in the insanities of the involution made the concept of an acquired psychosis untenable. A more telling point appears to have been the emergence of physical treatment. However much they might be an artifice in considerations of the natural history of a disorder, the availability of electroconvulsive treatment (ECT) from the 1930s had dramatically altered the condition in terms of both curability and prognosis. As for the question of distinctive premorbid personality, it is possible to detail the unsatisfactory nature of the retrospective analysis of personality. After all, premorbid personality is always evaluated when the patient is ill, and what biases may creep into such a method performed at such a time cannot be estimated. No-one is reported as proffering the results of a prospective follow-up of rigid, meticulous and obsessional persons, many of whom would have been seen to ascend to the higher reaches of the civil service or other areas of bureaucracy and live largely blameless and uneventful lives. In any case the type of personality alleged to predispose to involutional melancholia is a largely culturally-determined profile, when what was required to support the case that the condition was a distinct entity would have been a feature that was universally applicable.

A genetic element was introduced early into the debate, but it had to wait till the late 1950s when the findings could be appraised in the arguments between the proponents and opponents of the idea of involutional melancholia as a distinct disease entity. Kallman (1959) claimed to have found a high incidence of schizophrenia, but not manic-depressive psychosis, in the families of patients with involutional melancholia. This might have made a significant contribution to the controversy had it been confirmed, but Kallman's findings were disputed by Stenstedt (1959) who found merely a history of depression in relatives of those who suffered from involutional melancholia. Winokur (1979) noted a genetic difference between early-onset and late-onset depressive illness. This claim is important, firstly, because it brings with it the consequence that depressive illness may be seen within the framework of the interactionist model which is now in vogue. Put simply it means the greater the genetic loading, the lower the need for an environmental input to make the brain cross the necessary threshold to manifest the clinical features of depression. Conversely, a reduced genetic loading would require a commensurate increase in such factors as environment-provoked stress to bring the brain to the disease threshold. Secondly, there are interactionist parallels with other disorders, not only in psychiatry, but in neurology and beyond. Schizophrenia is one group of conditions in which a heavy genetic loading is

17

alleged to produce the onset of the disorder at a younger age. Parkinson's disease and Alzheimer's disease are two examples of neurological conditions in which younger patients with the disease may well have a greater genetic contribution than patients whose disease has a later onset. In general medicine, the examples of hypertension and diabetes mellitus come to mind. Invariably, or so it seems, patients who contract these disorders when they are younger are not merely exceptional in being less common as a class but have more severe forms of the illness. These distinctions do not seem to apply to forms of depression allegedly distinct in the two age groups. Moreover, at least with schizophrenia and Alzheimer's disease, the neurobiological features are more prominent in younger patients with earlier onset of illness and a more malignant course. This distinction, too, does not appear to hold for the two supposedly separate forms of depression. A curious Kraepelinian footnote may be essayed here. If the interactionist argument is upheld for depressive illness, the stronger environmental features necessary for involutional melancholia – or its equivalent of a late-onset depression – make it relatively more 'acquired' than other depressive illnesses. Even though his concept was misconceived Kraepelin, it would seem, might well have been right in this respect the first time round.

Eschewing comparison, Post (1962) made a direct study of a consecutive series of patients over 60 years of age. When he took those whose depression developed after the age of 50, he found that ideas of poverty and guilt, and pre-morbid personality were not over-represented. He could also find no relationship between a particular pre-morbid personality and the developing clinical features. He concluded that, 'A few conformed in terms of aetiology, symptomatology and outcome to textbook manic depressive involutional or senile melancholia, but our study suggests strongly that these stereotypes are nowadays of little help to psychiatrists'.

The cycle of fashion has not turned full circle to the belief once more in involutional melancholia, but Brown *et al.* (1984) have attempted to re-establish the validity of the concept. They found that patients who first experienced depressive episodes in the involutional period had more somatic symptoms and hypochondriasis, less guilt, fewer complaints of decreased libido and less suicidal intent than patients with an earlier onset. The involutional-onset group had a lower incidence of family history of affective disorder. To the authors it appeared that the clinical picture seen in depressives with early and late onset of the first episode might have been different, and that genetic loading might have determined the age of first onset. The findings and arguments remain unconvincing. Somatic symptoms, hypochondriasis and decreased libido are explicable in terms of features of age alone; the lack of guilt and the assessment of suicide intent are culture-, and sub culture-bound to such an extent that the findings of a single series are insufficient to make a case for their general presence or absence. The view must be that at the present time involutional melancholia is not accepted as a separate disease entity.

These authors, like numerous others, have made the point that early treatment, drug as well as ECT, might have resulted in a decline in the

18

incidence of involutional melancholia. The same claim could not be made for schizophrenia, as the fall in incidence and the improvement in prognosis appears to have preceded the introduction of neuroleptic therapy, but a symptom, catatonia, indeed a species of schizophrenia dignified as catatonic schizophrenia, has had its reduced incidence and virtual elimination explained in terms of social therapy. Plausible alternative explanations have been suggested in purely environmental terms for this decline (Hare, 1974; Mahendra, 1981). Similar alternative suggestions might equally reasonably be put forward for the decline in involutional melancholia. Not only have society and culture changed, but the personalities of those who are potentially depressive might have changed. If, as it was claimed, premorbid personality is an important factor in the manifestation of symptoms, it would appear only reasonable to expect the personality change one expects in the majority of a population who have lived through cultural change to respond *differently* to stresses from outside. It is possible that the resulting neurobiological substrate which gives rise to depressive illness and the emerging constellation of depressive symptoms have undergone corresponding change. The acknowledged translation of florid hysterical symptoms into more subtle and covert forms is a case in point.

The influence of cultural factors is indeed demonstrably powerful. Writing in 1956, the anthropologist-psychiatrist, Field, surveyed witchcraft in the Gold Coast (West Africa) and reached the conclusion that the elderly West African witch had the stigmata of the involutional melancholic. He compared her features with the agitated depressive in British practice and was struck by the resemblance. And this at the time when the African was being portrayed as a carefree savage who did not become depressed or, if by some chance he did, the depression was masked by gross somatic symptomatology. Not for the first time, the cynic may say, one is led to the conclusion that many of the manifestations of mental illness are largely in the eye, and the mind, of the beholder.

This interlude in the history of depression is a salutary reminder that concepts of illness are the product of the age in which they are conceived. Society, culture and personality change. Ideas about illness change, sometimes bringing the cycle full circle. Therapies appear, more or less specific, for the condition under consideration. Laws of the land change, turning what once was criminal into something to be tolerated, if not accepted. And diseases may be mutable, too. The primary qualification for the responsible clinician is the possession of an open-mind. Nothing illustrates this requirement better than the saga of involutional melancholia.

PSYCHOANALYTIC VIEWS ON DEPRESSION

The psychoanalytic views on depression form an extensive and complex literature. For the limited purposes of this historical sketch, the ideas of Freud and Karl Abraham must suffice. Freud's view stems from his analysis in *Mourning and Melancholia* (1917). In this work Freud traced the resemblance between grief and depression. The psychic mechanisms in both could be

19

linked to the real or imagined loss, real in grief and symbolic in depression, of the 'love object'. The ego is in fact mourning for somebody or something that has been lost and with whom the ego now identifies itself. This mechanism of identification alone is insufficient as the lost object needs to become a 'bad object' – in case the loss became unbearable. In mourning, the libido originally invested in the lost object is slowly re-invested in other objects and a form of restitution takes place. In melancholia, on the other hand, the patient regresses to an earlier stage of emotional development when the love object has been incorporated into the ego. This introjection of the lost object accompanies the withdrawal of libido into ego which is then subjected by the superego to unrelenting attacks, threats, criticism, condemnation or punishment. This is the basis not merely of the depressed mood but of the feelings of despair, hopelessness, self-reproach and guilt. The ego's helplessness is accompanied by aggression directed against those considered responsible for the state in which the ego finds itself. These symptoms would be prominent while a hold on reality persisted, but if this hold weakened, psychotic features such as hallucinations and delusions would appear. Delusions of punishment are commonplace in depression for this reason. A further result of the break with reality is the impulse to destroy the self. Suicide results when the superego orders the ego to kill the self.

Karl Abraham (1924) summarized his earlier views on depression, speculating on a number of aetiological factors. There was, firstly, a constitutional element in that an overemphasis on oral erotism might be inherited, a tendency which leads to the libido being fixated at the oral level. Both melancholia and mania involved a regression to the oral level of fixation. There is a further predisposition in that pre-oedipally there has been a loss of a love object and ensuing disappointment; and if there is a repetition in later life of this primary disappointment by a more immediate cause of loss, the sadistic impulses which have been set in play by the original loss might be re-awakened. These sadistic impulses are then directed inwards on the ego and depression results. Although the cause might be something immediate, the depressive's anger is directed against the original 'love object'. Given time the sadistic impulses are appeased, the introjected 'love object' ceases to be part of the self and regains its place in the world outside.

Later analytical thinkers emphasized the loss of self-esteem in producing depression, and recently, Storr (1983) has criticized the emphasis on love, pointing out that Freud himself emphasized the importance of, and the satisfaction in, work as a protective factor against depression. While orthodox analytic views are obviously highly speculative and have severely limited heuristic value, the emphasis on work – or, for the loss of it, in depression – has considerable importance in the changing nature of employment and is discussed in Chapter 9.

THE NATURE OF DEPRESSION: AN ONGOING CONTROVERSY

From the time in 1896, when he differentiated involutional melancholia from manic depressive psychosis, to 1909 when he replaced his supposed entity in the wider category, to 1913, when he expanded his ideas in the widest possible terms to include all melancholic and manic illnesses, Baillarger's *folie a double forme*, Falret's *folie circulaire* and the morbid fluctuations of mood which exceeded what might reasonably be considered to be variations of the normal mood state, Kraepelin did not lose faith in the ultimate constitutional basis of manic-depressive illness. His views were also the basis of the debate between the nature of 'endogenous' and 'exogenous' illness. He believed that even if an exogenous event could be deemed to be an apparent precipitant, a manic depressive illness ran its own course, uninfluenced by the turn of events outside the patient and not affecting him, even favourably. In the exogenous or psychogenic depressions, on the other hand, events and circumstances had a material, even if transient, effect on the patient's mood state.

Kendell (1968) has reviewed the influence of Kraepelin's views on British psychiatric thought in the decade following. Two schools of thought sprang up to champion the causes of, as they came to be known, 'endogenous' and 'reactive' depression. To Mapother (1926), however, there was no real distinction, these categories merely being stratagems to circumvent administrative and legal inconvenience. Mapother claimed that certification and asylum treatment, in order to justify such drastic actions, labelled those liable to receive them 'psychotic' depressives; if outpatient care or no treatment at all were deemed necessary, the type and degree of depression were held to merit the term 'neurotic' depression. Mapother trenchantly claimed he could find no other feature of distinction, whether it be the degree of insight, the co-operation of the patient in treatment or suitability for psychotherapy.

Not surprisingly, this emphatic opinion was challenged by several who claimed there was a valid distinction to be made between the two forms of depression, even though some had to resort to that old standby of the authoritarian and dogmatic physician to make their point: experienced clinicians were able to discern the difference.

Gillespie (1929) emphasized the feature which Kraepelin had noted as the point of distinction between 'endogenous' and 'psychogenic' depressions. The endogenous depressions ran an autonomous course, but the psychogenic depressions tended to fluctuate in one or the other direction, in response to changes in the environment and the reaction to these on the part of the patient. This feature was called 'reactivity' and it is necessary to stress the nature of the term as coined by Gillespie, and anticipated by Kraepelin, that reactivity meant not, as some later disputants claimed, the initial precipitating event or stress, but the subsequent variability of the mood in reaction to changes in the world outside or to the patient's inner life. Indeed Gillespie stressed the lack of a necessary relationship to precipitation and agreed with Mapother in as much as the presence of insight or the accessibility to psychotherapy were not always points of distinction.

Lewis (1934b, 1936) based his conclusions on detailed clinical study and follow-up of patients. His view was that the more closely a patient was studied, in detail and with follow-up, the more easily one came to the conclusion as to the universal nature of the symptoms of depression. On follow-up, there were no distinctive features regarding prognosis and little relationship between the symptoms of a depressive illness and its outcome. He had little doubt that the distinction between endogenous and exogenous depressions was a false one. An early interactionist, he accepted that constitutional and environmental factors combined, in more or less degree, to produce a depressive illness. He decried the 'either/or' claim implicit in those who were more actively involved in the dispute. To attempt to set up a sharp distinction, when such was not found in nature, Lewis admonished, '... is no help to thought or action'. Lewis' authority attracted considerable support but did not entirely stifle the dispute which continued to smoulder in the background. Some 20 years later, Garmany (1958), exploring the literal distinction between 'endogenous' and 'reactive' depression, found the incidence of 'stresses' of various kinds was not significantly different in the two forms of depression, and concluded the alleged differences were unreal. When those of this school examined the presence of other features which had been put forward as points of distinction, a similar overlap was to be found in the two forms of depression. Kendell (1968), admittedly a not entirely disinterested reviewer, notes that those who found no difference in forms of depressive illness examined series of consecutive cases, while those who were convinced the division was valid argued either from the authority of their clinical experience or illustrated their case with selected material, and, by claiming the necessity for making the distinction, may almost have fulfilled it by showing that differences existed. Kendell also notes a factor which, as history has shown us, is not an inconsiderable one in any passionately disputed idea, not least in medicine or psychiatry. In this one, personality and the influence of institutions might have played a crucial role in keeping the controversy alive. The disputants on the separatist side such as Ross, Gillespie and Rogerson were directors of the Cassel Hospital, while the other side fielded Mapother, Lewis and Curran, all products of the Maudsley Hospital.

Early genetic evidence seemed to favour the idea of distinctive forms of depressive illness. It was natural that the protagonists sought evidence from more than purely clinical findings. The general belief in the 1940s was that neuroticism – the trait that allegedly predisposed to reactive or neurotic depression – was multifactorial, the result of an accumulation of a number of genes. Not only did neurotic illness appear to have a constitutional basis which could be inherited, but the heredity seemed to be graded. Psychotic depression, on the other hand, seemed to be transmitted by an autosomal dominant gene with incomplete penetrance. This explained the fact that while the incidence in the general population of manic-depressive illness was about 1%, about 15% of parents, siblings and children of depressive psychotics could expect to have the illness. These findings strengthened the hand of the separatists, but why the presence, apart from type, of constitutional disorders did not support the view that all depressive illness appeared to have a constitutional basis, a general point of greater significance it would have seemed, is not clear. It might have been imagined that the fact of constitutional predisposition would have been thought of as a common denominator rather than a locus of difference.

Lewis' (1938) view was that the distinction between the two alleged forms was essentially the distinction between acute and chronic, and mild and severe depressions; manic depressive psychosis displayed the characteristics of acute, severe depression and neurotic depression was a mild, chronic depression.

Kendell (1968) also notes that the controversy between the two schools was a largely British pre-occupation. He sees the explanations for the passion devoted to it by British psychiatric workers, and the indifference of others in continental Europe, North America and elsewhere, as lying in the relative strengths of the Kraepelinian and Meyerian traditions in this country. The separatists and their opponents subscribed to the two traditions respectively. In a more tolerant climate, the two schools flourished, though not with equal vigour. The Kraepelinians followed the master's pre-occupation with delineating discrete disease entities, the Meyerians being interested not so much in disease entities as in less definite 'reaction types'. On the European continent, the supremacy of the Kraepelinian tradition was in general established and gave rise merely to several complex classifications of disease. In North America, the influence of Adolf Meyer and, later, the immigrant psychoanalytical disciples of Freud led to work and practice based on the crucial importance of the psychosocial environment and psychodynamic mechanisms.

For 30 years, from the 1920s to the 1950s, both schools continued the dispute on the validity of the entities in depression in terms of the symptomatology of depression and were not reconciled. Then, for a period, the dispute continued with the assistance of statistical techniques imported from the world of psychology, but no great edification resulted – the methodologies of statistics, themselves the subject of controversy and criticism among pure mathematicians, seemed simply to afford more points of dispute. Kendell himself employed some of these techniques, and his conclusion was that depressive illnesses are best regarded as a single continuum extending between the traditional neurotic and psychotic stereotypes.

Then in the 1970s, new hope arrived in the form of possible biological markers. Here, at last, were objective measures, emerging from laboratory tests carried out on the blood and other tissues, read off from mechanical gadgets and free from the influence of philosophical traditions, the biases of clinical practice and the distortions of personality. What could be more sensible than correcting aberrant chemistry with replacement chemicals, or disturbance in the psychosocial milieu with psychology applied to the patient or manipulation of the environment to make the patient feel better? However, the putative markers, by and large, soon proved to be a mirage in which swam several red herring. These issues are discussed further in Chapter 3.

A more valid, and less controversial, classification was proposed by Leonhard (1959) to deal with categories associated with the more severe forms of manic depressive illness. The distinction was made between depressive illness associated with, or free from, preceding or subsequent

23

mania. The case for the validity of these entities was buttressed not only by demonstrable differences in the symptomatology of the two groups but in terms of the genetics and pre-morbid personalities of the patients. Further studies from a variety of angles helped produce an even more convincing case for the separation of bipolar and unipolar manic depressive illness. These included, apart from genetic and pre-morbid personality factors, such elements as precipitating factors, childhood experiences, marital status, response to treatment, the length of treatment, rates of relapse, mortality rate and such physiological indices as flicker and sedation thresholds. Unlike the virtual century-long controversy as to 'psychotic' and 'neurotic' depression, the distinction between unipolar and bipolar depressive illness was soon accepted, and passed without much controversy into the literature.

Non-medical hypotheses on the causation, nature and progression of depressive illness tend to be cyclical in their appearance. The period after Freud and the early psychoanalysts was followed by much speculation as to the nature of early influences that might predispose or, indeed, lead to depression. As in all fashions, the socio-cultural climate plays an important part in these revivals, and it is of interest to anyone working in the area to look deeper into the philosophico–political debates of the period. A later revival was associated with the rapid social changes, liberating or amoralizing, as taste would have it, of the 1960s and 1970s. It was a period in which intense introspection was paradoxically allied to interest in the workings of the wider world.

This was reflected in a more detailed interest in patients' early lives and their formative influences. Although of intrinsic interest, and relatively accessible to lay persons, these ideas remain, needless to say, speculative. They include, among a host of others, the view that the loss of a father between the ages of 10 and 14 leading to depression and suicide in females in later life; the loss of a mother before the age of 15 leading to depression in later life; loss of a mother before the age of 20 leading to severe as opposed to moderate depression; loss of a mother before the age of 11 predisposing to depression in women. Some of these ideas are further referred to in Chapter 2.

Other sociological theories on the causation of depression have included alienation in the inner cities, especially of the new 'underclass' consigned to live in unsatisfactory housing, in social isolation brought about by geography as well as by material deprivation, the lack of emotional support especially in the parents of one-parent families, the expected mobility in search of education, employment and fortune and the consequent rootlessness, the rise of drug and alcohol abuse, crime and violence. Then in the 1980s, mass unemployment returned, the consequences of which are not yet fully apparent in terms of the incidence and nature of depression. Two generations after the last bout of mass idleness in an industrial society the social and mental consequences on the growing and the grown must await future analysis.

2
Depressed minds, distressed folk –
the nature and onset of depression

Feelings of sadness and disappointment are part of the human condition, experienced by everyone at some point in their lives. The boundary between normal state and abnormal symptoms, if it exists at all, is a far from well-defined one. For practical purposes, features which are intense, pervasive, persistent and which interfere with day to day functioning are considered pathological. The clinician usually attempts to discern a break or discontinuity in the habitual patterns of affect or behaviour before he draws a distinction between, say, a depressive temperament, which might be subject to a transitory dysthymia and a clinically defined depressive illness. This disjunction might be apparent if the individual in whom it is sought has previously made a good adjustment. But a previously unhappy person can also become depressed, when the change becomes an apparently quantitative one. The depth of the depressed mood is a matter of degree as are the symptoms which are discussed in later sections of this chapter. The cognitive change of common unhappiness does not differ from that in depression; poor attention and concentration may lead to impaired memory in both instances; intellectual functioning and judgment are also impaired in both states. Suicidal behaviour is possible in both. Biological dysfunction does not yield the expected clue – sleep, appetite, sexual desire, menstrual and bowel functioning may all be affected in both states of unhappiness and depression. Even response to antidepressant therapy (see chapter 5) does not help one make a distinction. The only form of depression which may be said to differ in more than a quantitative direction from unhappiness is that which has true psychotic features, i.e. delusions and hallucinations. (Even here the distinction is not absolute – visual hallucinations may be seen in grief reactions).

Thus, the evidence for the argument that depression is a disease state and unhappiness merely a variant of a physiological reaction is sparse. Moreover, although it is usual to consider unhappiness to be the reaction to adverse events in the world outside, the considerable incidence of

Table 1 The distinction between unhappiness and depression

	Unhappiness	Depression
Lowered mood and its associations	present +	present + + +
Biological dysfunction	+	+ + +
Cognitive dysfunction	+	+ + +
Psychotic features	very unusual	occasional (< 10% of cases)

unhappiness in those who are materially and socially provided for makes such aetiological theorizing suspect. As with depression itself, the more closely one looks for a distinction between unhappiness and depression, the less likely one is to find it.

A broad diagnosis of depression would take in both the clear-cut disease entity as well as the more prevalent dysthymias of ordinary life. If one attempts to bring in a concept of depression which excludes the relatively mild and brief disorders and defines the condition more narrowly, one will find a 'disorder' which is homogeneous with a more or less characteristic symptomatology, course, prognosis and, perhaps, even aetiology. This may be satisfactory for research purposes but is of little help to the average clinician in general or hospital practice who must observe, diagnose and manage large numbers of unselected cases who appear before him. Highly selected and exclusive forms of depression may say little about the overall universe of depression – possibly bearing the same relationship as a carefully described, Kennel Club authenticated breed of dog to dogs of the world.

DISTRESS AND DEPRESSION

Copeland (1985) makes the distinction between 'simple distress' and 'morbid distress' and between these two forms of distress, which he sees as belonging to the same sphere as normal behaviour, and which he would like to distinguish from depressive illness. When individuals develop psychiatric symptoms as a normal response to a life's problems, this is 'simple distress'. If these features increase, due to the severity of life events as well as in any failure to cope, even if they did not satisfy the diagnostic criteria for depressive illness or anxiety states, they become instances of 'morbid distress'. 'Depressive neurosis', in its generally understood meaning, would include these cases of morbid distress as well as those of the 'psychotic' variety (e.g. depression with symptoms such as early morning wakening, a morning exacerbation of mood), but the clinical picture in these cases would be dominated by 'neurotic' symptoms. 'Depressive illness' would refer to cases of 'psychotic' and 'neurotic' depression.

Copeland further describes the properties of cases of distress. The onset of morbid distress is usually gradual, although rapid onset is possible. Depression and anxiety may be present with impaired social functioning. Features that are absent are hallucinations, delusions, loss of insight, slow or muddled thinking, feeling like crying but unable to, feeling worse in the morning, early morning wakening and severe weight or appetite loss. Common symptoms are – frequent weeping, depression worse in the evening, feeling numb, irritable, angry with others, loss of concentration and early insomnia. In the slow onset type a mild onset, precipitating major life event within 3 weeks of onset, insidious development, marked exacerbations, frequent life events after onset, major long term difficulties, personality disorder and symptoms between episodes may be prominent. These symptoms of morbid distress are though to be akin to the dysthymic disorder of DSM-III (American Psychiatric Associaton, 1980).

There are criticisms of this approach in at least two respects. Firstly, there appears to be a denial of a 'biological role' for cases of distress. It must be evident that there is sufficient overlap between cases of 'distress' and depression to make a distinction between them on the grounds of alleged biological involvement in one group and not another suspect. The consequence of narrowing the intake of the depressive group is to produce a more homogeneous group which may well also show a more uniform neurobiology. However, a biological basis to distress cannot be wholly excluded. Secondly, although the basis of the distinction between forms of distress and forms of depression appear to be on the basis of symptomatology and the clinical course, the formation of the symptoms appears to be due to the interaction of personality with the environment. This is an entirely subjective assessment as an inadequacy of personality may be determined by adverse environmental factors. For instance, a person of borderline subnormality may function perfectly satisfactorily in a rural community which makes little demand on his abilities or capacities. When he is translated into an urban, inner-city environment, his capacities are eroded and then overwhelmed. He becomes inadequate, finds it difficult to cope and then becomes distressed. We are faced with the old bugbear of psychiatry – personality disorder. In practice it will be impossible to consider the symptoms of distress without taking into account coping ability, a wholly subjective appraisal bringing in train a whole host of subjective evaluations, not least the philosophical, ideological and doctrinal background of the psychiatrist. Moreover, the distinction between 'simple distress' and 'morbid distress' appears to be made in terms of the need for professional intervention. A person who seeks 'treatment' selects himself; if he is in the community intervention may not be available. The distinction between simple and morbid distress may, therefore, not only be subjective but be determined by purely social factors as the availability of professional help and its accessibility in the community.

It might be imagined that there is a gradation from the kind of case seen in general practice to those referred to, and treated in, hospital. The hypothesis might be that cases of unhappiness and distress are more likely to be seen in general practice, and the full range of depressive illness be seen in hospital wards, day units and out-patient departments. This has more than academic interest as it is possible that general practitioners might be using antidepressant drugs inappropriately, whereas, if they indeed were seeing mainly unhappy and distressed citizens, they should resort more to social and psychological interventions rather than chemotherapy. The properties of drugs and their efficacy are, after all, attested to, in the vast majority of cases, from hospital practice.

However, Sireling *et al.* (1985) found that most cases of depression treated by general practitioners satisfied criteria for psychiatric disorder, even though these tended to be relatively mild and borderline in quality. However, these patients received standard antidepressant drugs and the outcome on the whole appeared good. These patients were less severely ill, had shorter illnesses, a lower incidence of primary, endogenous or retarded major depression, and milder symptoms of depressed mood, biological and psychomotor changes. Where 86% of an out-patient sample reached a total score of 17 on the Hamilton Scale, which is used as a cut-off for inclusion in antidepressant trials, only 36% of the GP patients treated with antidepressants did so. It appeared that GPs used the criterion of severity as the basis for the decision to treat with antidepressants, with reactivity of mood and sleep disturbance as ancillary symptoms. The more severe and less reactive the depressed mood, the more likely the GP was to prescribe antidepressant drugs. The more mildly depressed and those with depression secondary to some other diagnosis were more likely to receive other treatment. It was also shown that groupings of symptoms, the degree of stress and the patient's social circumstances did not appear to influence the GP in his decision to prescribe antidepressants.

Less than 20% of depressives seen in general practice are ultimately referred to psychiatrists (Fahy, 1974; see also Figure 1). This no doubt forms the basis for the common observation that psychiatrists see the more severe cases of depression. There appears to be, then, a gradation in

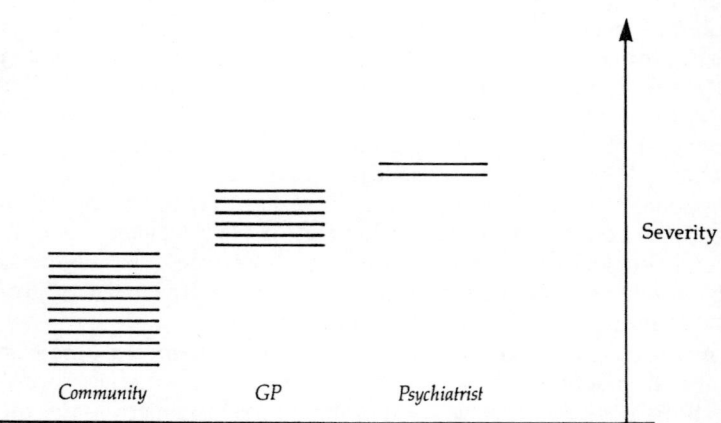

Figure 1 The 'filter' for cases with depression

severity seen when one goes from the community through the GP to the psychiatric hospital. As we have seen, GPs appear to use severity as a criterion for treatment decisions. The least severe forms of depression in a GP sample are not likely to receive antidepressant treatment. The evidence may not be wholly satisfactory but there seems little doubt that in the clearing house for depression, the GP surgery, the pragmatic distinction between what is depression and what is not is based on the severity of symptoms.

BEREAVEMENT

In moving from what might be termed distress and into depression, a distinction arguable in its conception, bereavement may be a convenient half-way station. In the first place, the vast majority of individuals suffer bereavement of one kind or another at some point in their lives. There is statistical normality, therefore, in the experience, and the manifestations of grief are worth studying for their distressing but physiological importance. However, even uncomplicated grief has its pathological sequelae, as has been suspected for a quite considerable time. Bereaved individuals have been shown to be more likely than non-bereaved controls to develop both physical and psychological complaints during the first year of bereavement (Maddison and Viola, 1968). Rees and Lutkins (1967) showed that, in the first year of bereavement, 12% of the recently widowed died compared to less than 1% in a control group. The difference was significantly greater for men, especially in the first 6 months of the bereavement. Shepherd and Barraclough (1974) noted that over 5 years the survivors of suicide had a greater risk of dying than those who had survived death by natural causes. Clayton (1982) believes the increased mortality of bereavement occurs only in men over 55 and that there is no increase in mortality in other groups. Although the figures for increased mortality in the bereaved may be equivocal, there seems little doubt that there is an increase in secondary mental disorder including an increase in alcohol abuse, cigarette consumption and use of psychotropic medication. Furthermore, a significant minority of the bereaved show 'abnormal' grief, which is a recognizable pathological state. For these reasons, a discussion of bereavement may serve as a useful bridge between an introductory section on distress and depression and the sections that follow on the more pathological aspects of depression.

The stages of normal bereavement reactions have been delineated by several authors, including Clayton (1982) and Parkes (1985). There appear to be two major components – an acute episodic disorder on a chronic background disturbance. The first stage, which may last from a few hours to a few weeks, consists of a stage of numbness which follows upon the impact of loss. The bereaved person is dazed and his life goes on automatic pilot, as it were. He needs to get on with his own life, look after his family, go to work, perhaps run his household and, of course, prepare for the disposal of the dead person. In addition to the funeral arrangements, there may be more distressing actions required such as identifying the body,

29

agreeing to the switching off of a life support system, authorizing the removal of organs for transplant, giving assent to an autopsy, helping the police, attending the coroner's inquest and speaking to (or hiding from) the press. Not surprisingly, perhaps there is little retrospective recollection of what was said or done, often with financial repercussions.

The second stage of this acute phase may be characterized by yearning for the dead person. There may be the pangs of grief, characterized by restlessness, anger, pining for the dead person, anxiety, all produced by any reminder of the dead person, and accompanied by the autonomic features of anxiety. This stage resembles the 'separation anxiety' seen in young children when they are separated from their mothers and are also seen in animals when they are separated from other members of their group. There are also parallels to be seen with patients recovering from amputation or loss of organs, especially those which may have an important emotional or symbolic role (see Chapter 6). This stage may normally last up to a year. Apart from the symptoms of irritability, restlessness and anxiety, most of the symptoms of depression may also be seen. It is also the stage at which defence mechanisms may come into excessive play, helping to store trouble for the future. Grief may be unnaturally repressed, avoided or postponed. Recovery is to be expected from normal grief after 6–12 months, and the intensity, frequency and duration of the 'pangs of grief' tend to diminish with the passage of time. Parkes equates this with the reduced behaviour by 'extinction of non-reinforcement'. Thus the final stage involves the acceptance of the death of the person and a reversal to the activity and behaviour before bereavement. Even after the resumption of the premorbid levels of behaviour, some involvement of an irrational kind with the dead person may be seen – e.g. the dead person's room being kept in the state in which the person left it – and these may be continued for several months or years and are considered essentially normal variants of behaviour.

The chronic background disturbance of grief is characterized by feelings of loss of any sense of purpose or meaning in life, social withdrawal, difficulties in concentration, impairment of memory, and disturbance in appetite, weight and sleep.

As Clayton and Darvish (1979) have shown, the symptoms of depression may be present at one month following bereavement. In over a third of cases there is crying, sleep disturbance, depressed mood, loss of appetite, fatiguability, poor memory, loss of interest, weight loss, restlessness, nocturnal exacerbation of diminished mood, irritability, anger and a tendency to blame others. By the end of one year some of these symptoms might have subsided. This is particularly true of the somatic or physiological symptoms, but the psychological symptoms such as suicidal ideas, hopelessness, feelings of anger and worthlessness may not diminish and may actually increase. This is related to the bereaved individual looking outwards and attempting to restructure his life. In the early stages the level of arousal and autonomic disturbance may be high, giving way to an emotional reaction later on.

Clayton (1982) points to those symptoms of depression which are rarely seen in bereavement. Suicidal thoughts, though observed, are uncommon. Guilt is often noted, but it is related to things that were not done or done during the last illness or just before death e.g. a bereaved man blamed himself for not feeding his dead wife enough, though she died of advanced carcinoma of the oesophagus and could not feed normally for several months before death. Psychomotor retardation is also rare and of pathological import.

There seems little doubt that a sizeable minority of bereaved patients seek psychiatric help and satisfy the criteria for formal mental illness (Stein and Susser, 1969; Weissman and Myers, 1978a). However, natural remission is the rule. At one year most bereaved persons have adjusted to loss. Appetite is said to return early, though sleep disturbance may persist longer. Libido follows increasing appetite for food. A low mood may also persist but is not sustained, and the mood is especially adversely affected at times such as anniversaries and dates of note.

As for physical morbidity, recent prospective studies have shown there to be less illness than had been suspected from earlier studies. Older men appear to be particularly at risk of dying in the first 6 months of bereavement. There are explanations of a more sophisticated kind rather than non-specific stress, and these are outlined briefly in Chapter 6. Parkes (1985) has also noted the increase in mortality from heart disease during the first year after the death of a wife. This implies that it may be unproductive to consider increased mortality generally, but that a consideration of specific physical pathology may yield important results. There are also still to be clarified links between bereavement and other physical and psychosomatic disorders such as malignancy and arthritis. The relationship between depression and malignant disease is considered in Chapter 6, and the discussion may well apply to the morbid sequelae of bereavement.

The best predictor of poor outcome following bereavement appears to be prior morbidity, of a physical or psychiatric kind. If the bereaved person has been physically ill before the bereavement he will be more likely to fall ill again, require care in hospital and, perhaps, even die. Those who have been previously mentally ill and have abused drugs and alcohol before will be most vulnerable to psychiatric illness after bereavement. This finding also accords with studies which have involved other trauma such as being rendered homeless or a refugee, undergoing a hysterectomy or being a victim of rape. It appears that those who exhibit prior vulnerability before stresses of any kind respond adversely after the event.

Other factors which may be of some importance include a poor social network to which the bereaved person is linked, socio-economic deprivation, youth, lack of previous experience with death and other concurrent life events.

Pathological grief has often mistakenly been dealt with as if it were a homogeneous entity. Parkes (1985) has criticized this somewhat simplistic notion and points to at least two common types – delayed (or avoided) grief and chronic grief. He has further elaborated this distinction and now favours a subdivision into three.

(1) *The unexplained grief syndrome:* This follows unexpected and untimely bereavement. These give rise to a defensive posture which delays the full emotional reaction but still allows relatively high levels of anxiety to surface. This grief reaction is characterized by the persisting sense of the presence of the dead person, feelings of self-reproach and feelings of continued obligation to the dead person which impedes the bereaved person putting the past behind him and resuming his life.

(2) *The ambivalent grief syndrome:* follows the loss of a relationship which has been ambivalent and uneasy. The bereaved person experiences an initial reaction of relief. There is little anxiety at the beginning but with the passage of time, higher levels of anxiety get through, and despair and intense pining may come to the surface. The reaction may be prolonged and self-criticism may be prominent. Though impelled to make restitution, the bereaved person may not be able to go about it.

These two form most of the delayed grief reactions seen in practice.

(3) *Chronic grief:* is expressed in full from the start but goes on for an abnormal length of time. It is associated with bereavement that ends a relationship which has been characterized by a high level of dependency, and feelings of helplessness in the bereaved person may be a major feature. It does not seem to matter whether the surviving partner was the dominant or stronger individual in the relationship.

Combinations of the three forms of abnormal grief reactions occasionally occur.

In the management of bereavement and its complications, several authors have commented on the cultural determinants of the act of mourning, which usually involves rituals. These rituals, although superficially different across cultures, have several themes in common. These help the bereaved to express their grief, and then to make the transition into the new roles they are expected to play. Many of these rituals have been abandoned in Western culture with the result that several of the bereaved have had to take on another role in its place – the sick role. The features of grief are then seen as symptoms of illness needing medical attention. If the doctor responds medically, i.e. by prescribing drugs, the 'patient' may have his views confirmed and continue to play the sick role. This may well prolong the sense of distress which might have otherwise undergone a natural remission.

Bereavement, when uncomplicated, therefore requires no treatment. The only medication that might be required is a hypnotic used in the short term. There is no evidence that active therapy in the form of specific drug treatment or one or other form of psychotherapy benefits simple, uncomplicated grief. It is, however, probably true that the bereaved benefit by being allowed to talk about the terminal illness of the dead person soon after death. This may allow them to see things in proper perspective, absolving themselves of unnecessary blame, helping ventilate their anxieties and, in concluding their account of the version of events, confirm the death of the loved person.

The management of bereavement may usefully start before the death of the person to be grieved. It is important to be able to identify those who might be at risk (see Table 2). Prior physical or mental illness in the bereaved, or about to be bereaved, has already been mentioned. It may well be possible to identify the person and so begin a process of pre-bereavement counselling.

Sudden death or an unexpected one, especially one which has been painful, traumatic or questionable (where medical mismanagement or hospital mishap is a factor) and where the survivor may be reasonably expected to shoulder the blame make it more likely that an abnormal grief reaction will take place.

Where a difficult or ambivalent relationship comes to an end or where a spouse or young child or mother (of a young child) dies, there is greater likelihood of a pathological grief reaction taking place.

Table 2 Features in those 'at risk' after bereavement

Previous physical or mental ill-health.
Sudden or unexpected death.
Painful, traumatic or questionable
    circumstances surrounding death.
End of previous difficult or ambivalent
    relationship.
Abnormal personality.
Culture that inhibits expression of grief.
    - or alienation from 'normal' culture.
Unemployment.
Presence of dependent children.

Those who have an abnormal personality (anxious, insecure, depressive, angry) or a personality which for socio-cultural reasons is unable to express emotions at times of grief may be at risk. This has been given as one reason why men are more likely to suffer abnormal grief reactions than women.

Lack of intimacy within a family setting, alienation from traditional social, cultural and religious supports (as with immigrants), unemployment, and dependent children at home are also factors that may be important in prolonging grief. It is of some interest to note that several of these factors are also considered as making some individuals prone to depression following other life events.

With 'at risk' individuals, wherever possible, as with terminal stages of an illness, staff in hospital wards and other institutions should endeavour to give as much information as possible about the clinical condition of the dying patient. It must be indicated what is and what is not possible for the relatives to do at this stage of the patient's illness. It may be helpful to let the relatives participate in the care of the dying patient and repair whatever omission they might believe they are responsible for. Access to staff at this time to ventilate any feelings is important.

During the phase of actual bereavement, the expression of grief is one aim of those caring for the bereaved. The other is to provide reassurance about the physical and psychological symptoms the bereaved person might experience. This is relatively easy when explaining a symptom such as insomnia or loss of weight. But quite a few lay persons – and not a few general practitioners – are alarmed when the bereaved claim that they can 'sense' or actually 'see' the dead person. Over-strict interpretation of the significance of the symptom of hallucination – a criterion of psychosis – is largely responsible for this. A sound working knowledge of the natural history of bereavement is therefore required. The personality of the counsellor is also important. A detached, non-judgmental person is superior to the one who reinforces cultural biases against grief – 'pull yourself together' – or one who takes an egotistical view of matters – 'Now, if it was me ...'.

In the later stages of bereavement the emphasis shifts to the more practical aspects of the bereaved person's life and his attempts to resume or restructure it. Here a working knowledge of financial and social security matters is useful for the counsellor as a high proportion of the bereaved, even the seemingly well-off, need advice and guidance. The counsellor, therapist or adviser must not hesitate to recruit the specialized knowledge possessed by the social worker and the bank manager. Groups of bereaved persons may usefully assist one another collectively.

For pathological grief, specialist techniques of psychotherapy may be indicated. For ordinary practitioners, drugs, when appropriately used, are a valuable standby. Even in uncomplicated grief they have a role in symptomatic management, e.g. of insomnia or intolerable anxiety. When the features of depression emerge, especially with such atypical features, in bereavement, as retardation and suicidal ideation, antidepressant medication and electroconvulsive therapy may be considered. It becomes a matter of judgment if a medical intervention in that respect is a necessary one as there are dangers of 'pathologizing' the grief. Hospital admission is best avoided for such patients and the management carried out in the community, where the patient, as he now has become, will be more easily and more rapidly rehabilitated and allowed to get on with the business of resuming his life.

STRESS, LIFE EVENTS AND REACTION

A very simple model of depression, or indeed any mental disorder, holds it to be the outcome of stress acting upon personality. 'Stress' may be susceptible to different interpretations. At one level there is the objectively assessed event or situation, e.g. bereavement or loss. At another there is the response, both cognitively and unconsciously, of the person who faces the stress, and here clearly the interpretation of the meaning of significance of stress is less objective and more personal. Thirdly, we have the outcome of the stress which may be, in broad terms, mental disorder, but also have as responses physiological correlates which may be the result of the effect of stress on bodily mechanisms, e.g. the limbic–hypothalamo–pituitary–

34

adrenal system, or the result of the individual's response to the stress, e.g. the catecholamine response. As it has been shown in the previous section on bereavement, and will be referred to again in Chapter 6, stress and its effects may also produce consequences of a physical kind including disease, and influence the progress of pathological processes.

It has been said the significance of any stress can be only partly objectively measured. This is especially true in relation to depression. Stress antecedent to depression is assessed in the course of the disorder when there is likely to be distortion in the retrospective recall of significant stressful events. The mood state, characterized by guilt, pessimism and self-denigration, may magnify the subjective importance of any stressful event. Moreover, the fact of depression and the associated mood state may lead the patient into situations which may be construed as stressful. These stresses are, then, the consequences rather than the causes of the depression. Furthermore, in those depressive conditions in which delusions are a feature a stress may well be part of the delusional system. In an effort to minimize the incidence and effect of such stresses, various methodological rules have come to be adopted. One obvious step is to ensure that the experience of stress was actually in limited time periods before the onset of depression. Another is to ensure that the stresses that are studied have occurred independently of the patient and his mental state (Brown and Harris, 1978).

There is little to relate stress to the symptomatology of depression. This argues for non-specific effects of stress, and it helps us to consider a synthesis between social causation and the biological manifestations of depression. As Freeman (1984) has remarked, results of animal study data show that a wide range of pathological conditions may emerge following change in the social milieu. The susceptibility to disease in general rather than an aetiological influence of a specific disorder may be enhanced. The manifestation of disease in an individual will depend on the characteristics of the individual – e.g. genetic predisposition – and the response to the stress – e.g. endocrine or metabolic state – and the symptoms will vary accordingly.

Dolan et al. (1985) studied the relationship between antecedent life events, the clinical profile of patients and hypothalamo–pituitary–adrenal function in depressed patients. They found that antecedent life events were associated with first episodes of depression and with greater severity of illness, and urinary free cortisol levels were higher in those patients suffering life events and difficulties. They felt the increase in the 24-hour urinary free cortisol levels in patients with life events was a reflection of the role of stress in hypothalamo–pituitary–adrenal function. It would also appear that these changes are an adaptive response to environmental stress rather than an effect secondary to other biological processes. This and other studies, to which reference will be made in Chapter 6, suggest that a point of interaction between biological and social phenomena may well be the neuroendocrine system.

The role of stress in depression has been studied in comparison with non-depressed patients as well as general population controls. Paykel et al. (1969)

35

found that in depressives, in the 6 months before the onset of symptoms, there were three times as many life events as in controls.

Brown and Harris (1978) have defined as their 'provoking agents' events with markedly threatening long-term implications or those that are associated with long standing social difficulties. The severe, long-term life events are distinguished by the experience of actual or threatened major loss. A second group of aetiological factors are 'major difficulties' which are defined as being severe, lasting at least 2 years, and not involving health, e.g. poor housing (e.g. overcrowding, extreme physical deprivation, problems with noise, and lack of security of tenure). Although both severe events and major difficulties have been found in working class women, this in itself was not sufficient to explain the excess of psychiatric disorder in them. For this, another set of factors called 'vulnerability' factors had to be invoked.

As was mentioned before, there is little evidence that stresses of any kind are specific for depression. Both schizophrenia and the neuroses may be preceded by stress. The strongest association between stressful life events and depression involves events rated as 'markedly threatening' or 'undesirable'. Brown et al. (1973) found depressives had an increased occurrence of markedly threatening events in the year before the onset of symptoms when compared to controls in the general population. Moderately threatening events were in excess only in the 3 weeks before the onset of the depression.

Both Brown and Harris (1978) and Paykel (1978) attempted to quantify the causative effect of stress. The former concluded that the effect of stress on depression was formative, in that it had advanced the onset of a bout of depression by 2 years (for schizophrenia, the figure was only 10 weeks, more reasonably considered to be precipitating). The latter found a considerably increased risk for depression as compared to schizophrenia in the 6 months after the most severe stress.

The relationship between stress and the clinical picture is not a consistent one. Certainly the distinction between the common diagnostic categories of 'reactive' and 'endogenous' cannot be made on the basis of stressful life events experienced. Thomson and Hendrie (1972) found endogenous depressives had experienced as much stress as reactive depressives. Dolan et al. (1985) found that antecedent life events did not distinguish patients as diagnosed as 'endogenous' or 'neurotic'. In their study patients with 'endogenous' depression were as likely to have a preceding life event as those with 'neurotic' depression, and they emphasized that their study was in line with previous reports in the literature of the difficulty in distinguishing between 'endogenous' and 'neurotic' depression on the basis of the presence or absence of a precipitant.

As further evidence of the non-specific nature of stresses is the knowledge that not all stress can be classified objectively as adverse or threatening. Promotion at work, a move to a more desirable house, a financial coup and more personal triumphs may all produce depression. It has been argued that some of these events hold concealed threats - promotion at work may mean shouldering more responsibilities, the larger house involving greater financial commitment and so on. But this kind of argument in search of the anti-conscious as opposed to the unconscious does not lead very far. It would seem more reasonable to accept the impact of the stress, rather than its content, as being important in bringing about the neurobiological changes necessary to produce depression. A related example of an event that is generally considered to be desirable is childbirth, yet the incidence of depression is elevated in the three months following it (Kendell *et al.*, 1976).

A stress may have an effect on a person and then fade away or it may persist. Common examples of chronic stress include material deprivation, physical disability and an unhappy marriage. It is as important to assess the effect of this form of stress as to evaluate those that have allegedly formative or triggering effects. Brown and Harris (1978) rated the presence of existing stresses as well as those that had been experienced recently. Apart from health, difficulties which were seen as threatening and had lasted 2 years were associated with depression. As might be expected, when life events and continuing difficulties were both present, there was an increase in the depression greater than for each alone.

Although the effects of the results in one culture, as regards largely sociological findings, may not be capable of being translated to another, this has not proved so with life event research in depression. These studies have been replicated in East Africa (see Chapter 8), and Fava *et al.* (1981) attempted a replication in Northern Italy. They obtained similar results, finding that uncontrolled events, unwanted events and 'exits' played a substantial role as precipitants of depression in some patients. Also, Campbell *et al.* (1983) tested Brown and Harris' model on working class women with children in Oxford and found results which provided general support for the model.

There may also be a relationship between stress and 'organic' disease which may be mediated by psychiatric illness including depression. Malignancy is a case in point and is the subject matter of Chapter 6. Murphy and Brown (1980) studied the relationship between life events and the onset of 'organic' physical illness in a group of women in the general population. They found that the association between severe life events and the onset of 'organic' illness, limited to women younger than 50 years, was not a direct causal one but required the mediation of an intervening affective psychiatric disorder, all occurring within a 6-month period. The average length of time between the psychiatric disorder and the organic illness was 7 weeks; the time period between the life event and organic illness was about 6 months. These results suggested that severe events required the development of psychiatric disturbance before the onset of organic illness and they wondered if psychiatric disorder without the life event could be sufficient to lead to the physical illness.

They had to explain why the results held only for women below 50 years of age. They speculated the reason for this might be that beyond the age of 50 years such biological factors as ageing and the consequences of the habits of a lifetime such as diet and smoking may play a more important role in the causation of physical illness, obscuring the effects of more immediate emotional factors. Their failure to find a link between chronic psychiatric disorder and organic illness may therefore be due to the association of the former with chronic rather than abrupt onset. They felt that disorders such as hypertension may develop gradually as a result of chronic and sustained levels of high physiological arousal. It may well be that a certain threshold has to be breached whether by a severe stress of relatively sudden onset or a more eroding, sustained stress. Murphy and Brown also seek to explain the finding that some 60–80% of medical in-patients and outpatients may suffer from psychiatric disorder of sufficient severity as to require specialized psychiatric intervention (Lipowsky, 1967). It is possible that this is due to those non-specific factors needing physical intervention leading to a psychiatric consultation as well, but it is feasible that a substantial component is due to a causal relationship between psychological and physical illness.

Criticism has been directed as to whether cases studied by Brown and Harris' model satisfy the diagnostic criteria for *clinical* depression, and whether their subjects might have reported distress rather than depression, a distinction of limited validity as might have been gathered from the discussion in a previous section. The other criticisms have been based on methodological grounds. However, a possibly unfair criticism is in respect of the fact that all forms of depression are not explained by this model. In particular, the concept of reactive depressive psychosis lies unexplained. This is a largely transcultural concept, and has its theoretical roots in the work of Jaspers (1913). Jaspers proposed that for a reactive disorder there should be a *meaningful* connection between the content of the experience and that of the reaction; that the precipitating stress should be sufficient to account for the reaction and be found in close temporal relationship; and when the cause of the reaction was removed, the reaction should subside. These criteria are claimed to be necessary for *ab initio* emergence of psychiatric illness; Brown and Harris' model is an additive and interactionist one, requiring stresses and vulnerable personality factors (see below).

But the concept of reactive or psychogenic psychosis was in practice an interactionist one requiring the presence of defined stress and vulnerable personalities (Mahendra, 1977a). The concept and the clinical features are discussed in a later section, but it suffices here to discuss the stress that is alleged to produce reactive psychoses.

In Scandinavian countries the concept of reactive psychoses has a long tradition, with origins from Wimmer. Odegaard (1946) defined the group of reactive psychoses as those which occur in predisposed individuals following more or less severe psychic traumata. Stromgren (1961) pointed out the existence of a great many psychoses which had no features in common with the classical psychoses of manic-depressive illness and schizophrenia, even if there were symptomatological similarities. Stromgren listed the following stresses: death, sexual traumata, loss of money, social traumata such as legal prosecution and imprisonment, external events such as catastrophes or war, and 'contagion' from a psychotic person. Faergeman (1963), however, claimed that it was possible in only a few of his cases to demonstrate that the traumatizing situation was reflected in the content of the psychosis and that Jaspers' criterion as to outcome was not always met.

By 1962, Yap was in a position to note that most European classifications had a place for conditions of acute psychogenic disturbances of unusual degree following psychic trauma. He listed Germany, Holland, Denmark, the USSR and Norway among those countries, and later added Japan. He went on to define the term 'reactive' as one in which an abnormal reaction has been produced by an external traumatic shock of great severity in a mechanical manner, or has been brought into open expression in a predisposed subject by an external, experiential stress.

But considerable opposition persisted, especially in American and British circles, the latter in the immoveable shape of the Maudsley Hospital. The difficulties of introducing the category of reactive psychoses into the International Classification of Diseases by the World Health Organization, the reasons for the opposition and the sequelae to the eventual introduction have been dealt with by Stromgren (1969). Roth (1963) represented the sceptical point of view. He stated the difficulty of the problem lay in evaluating even in a roughly quantitative manner the size of the contribution made by precipitating stress to the causation of the illness. The sequence of the stress closely followed by illness was clearly misleading, some of the most malignant schizophrenic illnesses and undeniably 'endogenous' depressions following traumatic situations.

Mahendra (1977a) found that a characteristic clinical picture was presented in such cases. Following a traumatic event, the definitions of which will be discussed shortly, there was a period of withdrawal, followed by violent excitement, which was transient, and replaced by a severe depression. After a variable period of time – as a rule, relatively short – this depression lifted, and the patient was back to his or her premorbid state. But we had not satisfactorily resolved the question as to whether the stresses that preceded the illness were merely associations – sparks according to Kraepelin – or whether they were causal. An operational definition of stress was made as follows: 'Any event or occurrence that is construed or experienced by a person to constitute a threat to life, status, self-esteem or is likely to lead to the loss, actual or threatened, of a person of emotional significance'. By these criteria, the following categories were established:

(1) Threat to status,
(2) Actual or threatened loss of emotionally significant person,
(3) Pathophysiological i.e. the puerperium, febrile illness, surgery or its aftermath,
(4) Threat to life,
(5) Mixed, and
(6) Others not specified above.

Faergeman (1963) had noted male patients suffered stresses of a different kind. Men appeared to be more vulnerable to pathophysiological stresses (despite the inclusion of the puerperium as a period of stress), while women were more prone to breakdown following the actual or threatened loss of self-esteem or status following domestic arguments. The data also suggested that those informants who knew the patients intimately were prepared to acknowledge the severity of the stress as experienced by the patient.

A substantial proportion of the patients suffered multiple stresses. Anecdotally it could be shown that persons breaking down in a manner suggestive of reactive psychosis rarely did so following a single distressing episode. There was usually a multiplicity of stressful events, understandable in the context of the poor socio-cultural and economic milieu of the Sri Lankan patient (even in the days before the civil war) and a terminal event of relative objective insignificance was merely the last straw for precipitating psychosis. Pathophysiological stress accounted for over 20% of the stresses, largely reflecting the prevalence of physical, especially infective, illness. 'Loss' of a significant person was also very highly significant.

The data cannot merely be dismissed as culture-bound, as comparable results have been noted in a variety of countries, but certainly the picture is rarely seen in Britain, except perhaps in communities with a high proportion of immigrants. The concept of reactive psychosis is now a less controversial one, partly as a result of the general acceptance of Brown and Harris' work and also no doubt influenced by the apparent improvement in the prognosis in the psychoses, especially that of schizophrenia. The immediate clinical picture is not unlike a rapidly switching manic depressive illness, and the widespread use of lithium salts in treatment may have led to the loss of florid psychoses of this kind in clinical practice. But one suspects that those who are attuned as a result of a wide variety of influences – cultural, educational and professional and are part of a certain tradition – are more likely to detect atypical psychoses of this kind. There is a more than passing resemblance of this psychosis to cycloid psychosis and that will be taken up in a later section.

VULNERABILITY

It is not possible to explain the onset of depression solely in terms of stressful life events. Within the framework of an interactionist model a vulnerable personality is required on which stresses can impinge. Clearly, not everyone who is subjected to life events becomes depressed. Brown and Harris, furthermore, found that both severe threatening life events and major difficulties did not suffice to explain the preponderance of working class women in their depressed group. A concept of 'vulnerability' had to be postulated, the result of a number of factors. These factors are deemed to limit a woman's ability, or her perceived ability, to make sense of the world and control it, and they relate to the current environment of the patient and, in the presence of a severe life event or major difficulty, increase the possibility of depression.

Brown et al. (1975, 1977) described four 'vulnerability factors' which they believed increased the predisposition of a woman to depression in the presence of severe life events or major difficulties in life. They were parental loss before the age of 17, especially the loss of the mother before the age of 11; presence at home of three or more children aged less than 14; a poor, non-confiding marital relationship and the lack of full or part-time employment.

Vulnerability is clearly a complex phenomenon which has been considered in a limited social context by Brown and Harris. Genetic endowment makes people vulnerable in another sense, and this subject is important enough to require a section to itself. Vulnerability may be enhanced by prior disorder, physical or psychiatric, and, if the latter, may be through formal illness or through disorders such as alcoholism, drug-related problems or personality disorder. The vulnerability to disorder is paralleled by the susceptibility to the stresses in particular – some individuals may react to events in general, others to events in particular, such as loss. Underlying the interaction between stress and personality is the still uncertain phenomenon of neurobiological status of the individual, which in turn may be influenced by both genetic and constitutional factors and environmental affliction.

The importance of the effects of social relationships and support is reflected in the fact that the single most striking vulnerability factor is female sex. This must be set against the finding of increased vulnerability on most biological indices for the male sex. Depression has a higher incidence in females; depression is higher in mothers with young children; young married women show higher levels of the less severe forms of depression. Women do not necessarily encounter more stressful events. Hence the explanation must take into account both constitutional factors such as genetic endowment and hormonal influences as well as social factors. These include important cultural considerations which may not only affect the onset of depression, but its symptomatology and its expression, an appropriate subject for further discussion in Chapter 8.

It has been traditional to consider the higher social classes as having a greater incidence of depression (Bagley, 1973). This may apply to depression that is clearly an 'illness' i.e. manic-depressive disorder. It is less clear for milder forms of depression or for distress in general which, as the work with stressful life events and vulnerable personalities reveals, may show a higher incidence in working class subjects. In any event, cultural bias is an important factor in the diagnosis and the identification of depression. Numerous studies have attested to the propensity of doctors to make more sympathetic diagnoses in like people, i.e. the middle class and beyond. This applies especially to a condition as eminently treatable as depression. This form of bias is further examined in Chapter 8. Also, a certain kind of successful person may have a tendency to depression, a subject discussed in Chapter 9. There has also been support from a psychoanalytic study (Cohen *et al.*, 1954) for the idea of a vulnerability to depression of individuals from aspirant families. Analysing 12 case histories, these authors showed that the patients appeared to come from ambitious families in which they as children had been chosen to carry the hopes and aspirations of the family. Competition was intense at the expense of such 'softer' values as co-operation and inter-personal relationships within the family. The subject who was later to become a patient strove at the cost of strife. Guilt,

41

insecurity and a reduced capacity for intimacy was the result as well as a tendency to depression. To stretch analytic explanation further, it is possible that those who strive to be successful have to postpone gratification. The ensuing frustration leads to aggression which when suppressed may predispose to depression.

The mere presence of a vulnerability factor does not in itself increase the risk of psychiatric disorder. A provoking agent of some kind is necessary. Thus, early loss in childhood may lead to a later re-awakening by real or symbolic loss in adult life to produce depression. Death in particular may predispose in later life to more severe forms of depression (Birtchnell, 1975).

In men, Roy (1981) found parental loss before 17 years, a poor marriage and unemployment to be vulnerability factors associated with depression. Curiously, it has been thought that, in general, marriage may protect against depression in men (Gove, 1972).

Caution must be enjoined when factors in the family are considered in assessing the vulnerability of persons to depression. Clearly, heredity is shared between parent and child. A parent's depression, disordered behaviour, disruptive influence on family life and tendency to violence (including suicide) may have effects on a child through influences other than the purely environmental. It is impossible in any given case to precisely separate out the influences of biological and social factors and indeed it may not be helpful to do so. The interaction that occurs within the patient must find a reflection in the mind of the practitioner as he assesses the patient's disorder and situation.

The world outside a patient may provide an index to his vulnerability. Henderson et al. (1978) found an association between deficiencies in social networks and less severe psychiatric illness in patients. This was confirmed by Brugha et al. (1982). Patients named fewer good friends, close relatives and attachment figures; they had fewer contacts with these and with other people outside the household. Contrary to expectation, it was not the lack of relationships, but the perception of these as being inadequate under adversity which had by far the stronger predictive power (Henderson, 1981). This may mean that actual conditions in the immediate social environment are not so much important as intrapsychic and personality factors. The relationship is a complex one. Patients may report deficiencies in relationships because of their affective state, because their symptoms may have an adverse effect on their personal networks, or their personality attributes which have rendered them vulnerable to neurosis may also have rendered them less able to establish and maintain mutually satisfying personal relationships. The conclusion is that subjectively adequate social relationships are probably protective in the face of adversity. The crucial property of social relationships is not their availability, but how adequate they are perceived to be when the individual is under stress.

Some vulnerability factors, e.g. low intimacy and a non-confiding relationship may be the same as the provoking agent, e.g. persistent marital difficulties. Brown and Harris treat them as independent variables, and this has been subjected to criticism. The precise delineation of the components is, however, less important probably than the sum of the effects perceived by the subject. If one takes up an interactionist stance, what is presumably significant is the level of stimuli reaching the neurobiological substrate to advance it to the threshold beyond which the symptoms of depression are displayed.

There is a temptation to associate vulnerability factors with life in urban inner-city areas, in which such factors as ineffective social networks, poor intimacy and a non-confiding marital relationship and effects of un- or under-employment may be understood. However, as has been mentioned, studies in other cultures have confirmed the existence of vulnerability factors and provoking agents. It is probable that the details of these factors and agents may differ, but vulnerable subjects may be found in whom depression may be produced by severe life events which might be construed differently in town and country, and across cultures.

Corresponding to the factor of stress in reactive depressive psychosis is the 'vulnerable' personality as opposed to vulnerability factors in patients who are thought to be predisposed to the condition. The high proportion of abnormal personalities in those who suffer reactive psychosis has been commented on by most workers. Noreik (1970) described the categories of schizoid, sensitive–hysteric–neurotic, self-assertive, cycloid, asocial and so on. He described four-fifths of his patients as being abnormal. Similar figures were given by Faergeman (1963), and Welner and Stromgren (1958) mentioned nearly half their cases as being premorbidly abnormal in personality. Mahendra (1977a) was again only able to gather a global impression as to whether a patient was premorbidly vulnerable or stable, but a significant proportion of reactive psychotics were seen to be 'vulnerable' females. It is possible that such vulnerability factors as considered by Brown and Harris were subsumed in a global assessment of the vulnerability of the personality. The interactionist model is thus applicable to reactive depressive psychosis as it is to the less severe, non-psychotic depression observed in the community.

GENETICS

Only a much simplified and general account of this complex subject is possible in a work such as this. The purpose of this section is not only to describe such mechanisms as seem important at present in understanding the genetic basis to depressive illness but also to illuminate the process of interaction that seems to underlie the precipitation of depression.

Over 30 years ago, Kallman (1953) demonstrated the contribution of genetic factors in terms of the 'morbidity risk' in the relatives of patients with manic-depressive illness. The morbidity risk refers to the chances one has of contracting a disease if one lives through the period of risk. For the general population the risk of having manic-depressive illness varies from about 0.5% to about 3%. For parents and sibs of manic-depressive patients, however, it is over 22%. Thus the morbidity risk in relatives of patients is considerably higher than for a member of the general public. Slater *et al.* (1971) showed that the expectancy of manic-depressive illness in first-

43

degree relatives of manic-depressive patients was 11.7% in parents, 12.3% in sibs and 16% in children.

Apart from clinical observation which leads one to suspect a genetic basis, twin studies yield a further clue (Gershon et al., 1976). In monozygotic twins (MZ), assumed to have a similar genetic make-up, there is a concordance of 65% for depression, whereas the concordance for dizygotic (DZ) twins (assumed to have a genetic make-up no more similar than if they had been sibs) the concordance falls to about 14%. The range given in the literature varies from under a third to nearly 100% for MZ twins; and from zero to nearly 40% for DZ twins. Thus, although the precise contribution of genetic factors is in some dispute, there is no doubt that a substantial genetic contribution to vulnerability is present.

It is possible, in theory, to explain the incidence of depressive illness in families in terms of stresses and environmental influences that impinge on the family. Severe material deprivation can obviously affect parents and children; so can emotional stresses related to marital strife and breakdown. Thus it is important to set up experimental models in which the differences in genetic endowment can be compared, e.g. twin studies, as can environmental influences, e.g. adoption studies.

The other piece of evidence for a genetic factor is that the females preponderate over men by a factor of some 1.44.

One form of inheritance may be ruled out with some confidence. Autosomal recessive conditions (e.g. as in some of the rare metabolic disorders) do not occur in successive generations of families; depression does occur; hence it cannot, except perhaps in some rare subtypes, occur by recessive inheritance. There is also no evidence of consanguineous mating (Marriage in close relatives) in depression, a usual occurrence in recessive conditions, as is an increased incidence of the condition in sibs of affected patients.

Sex-linked recessive inheritance (as seen in haemophilia) also does not occur, as males do not preponderate. X-linked inheritance, however, is another matter, to be discussed later.

As successive generations have the disorder and the incidence in first degree relatives of probands is comparable, a case could be made for dominant inheritance. But this will not explain the increased female incidence which is consistently seen. Bucher et al. (1980a, b) concluded that neither a single mendelian autosomal gene nor an X-linked gene is adequate to explain the data.

The simple interactionist model, which was used in the previous section to explain the onset of depression, postulates that stress and vulnerability combine to exceed a pre-set threshold allowing depression to take place. There are two variables, and if the magnitude of one is great the contribution of the other need only be small. Thus excessive stress can overwhelm only a mildly vulnerable personality or one that is not vulnerable at all, a common enough observation in life. A component of vulnerablity that may be assessed with some degree of accuracy is heredity and a hypothesis that can be set up is that those who are faced with severe stress will have less genetic vulnerability. Pollitt (1972) did precisely this by

44

studying a series of depressives. He showed that those who had become depressed as a result of severe viral or bacterial infections, other physical stresses and severe psychological stresses had a lower 'morbidity risk' than those who had little psychological stress or puerperal illness. The interactionist model can also be illustrated by reference to the capacity of reserpine to produce depression in those who are genetically susceptible (Goodwin and Bunney, 1971).

As has been mentioned, an X-linked dominant model of transmission has been proposed. This followed from the common observation that there was little father to son transmission in depression. There was also some support from linkage studies in which some other trait due to a gene in close proximity to the one studied (i.e. gene for depression) is also investigated. The marker affected in this association with depression is a form of colour blindness, protanopia. Both depression and the marker are inherited when the chromosomes divide, so that the relatives suffer from depression and are colour-blind, or are not subject to depression and have normal vision. It now appears that X-linked dominant transmission may account for the disorder in some families, perhaps as a sub-type of depressive illness, and this illustrates the heterogeneity of depressive disorder. The most telling argument against X-linked dominant inheritance is that father–son transmission of manic-depressive illness can occur. This makes it impossible to transmit the gene, as the genes on the father's X-chromosome can only go to the daughter, never a son. However, Mendlewicz et al. (1980) reported evidence of a linkage between manic-depressive illness and glucose-6-phosphate dehydrogenase (G6PD) deficiency. They believed their finding of a close linkage between manic-depressive illness and G6PD deficiency along with the previous reports of a linkage relationship between affective illness and colour blindness, demonstrated the presence of a dominant X-linked inheritance in manic-depressive psychoses. At most, however, it can only be said that the findings and conclusions refer to a sub-group of cases and illustrate the genetic heterogeneity of manic-depressive illness.

The model in current vogue is the multifactorial one which postulates that there are several factors (genes) which contribute additively to an individual's genetic liability. Obviously, different individuals will have a different liability which can be inherited by first degree relatives. There is no requirement for an 'all or nothing' inheritance of a single gene, but a greater or lesser proportion of the predisposing genes may be inherited, perhaps by a variety of mechanisms or by different mechanisms in different families. The great advantage of this model is that it allows play of environmental influences and so is compatible with the interactionist model of depression.

Further discussion of genetic mechanisms must take into account the diagnostic sophistication which now informs the practice of clinical psychiatry. Depression is often seen with manic illness (bipolar illness; unipolar illness, in the absence of this connection), schizophrenic features (schizoaffective disorder) and may be a primary process (primary depression) or secondary to some other psychiatric illness (secondary depression). These are matters considered in the next section, but some reference may be made to them at this stage.

It has been known for some time that 'morbidity risk' for affective illness is greater in relatives of bipolar illness as compared with relatives of unipolar illness. Bipolar and unipolar illness may be found in the relatives of bipolar patients, but only unipolar illness is found in the relatives of unipolar patients.This considerably increases the morbidity risk which may be up to 40%. The relatives of bipolar patients show a greater tendency to bipolar illness, but the incidence of unipolar illness is also high. The morbidity risk in unipolar illness is only about 15%, and this is made up almost entirely of unipolar illness, the risk for bipolar illness not being higher than that for the general population.

The bipolar–unipolar distinction in manic-depressive illness distinguishes between bipolar patients who have had both manic and depressive episodes, and unipolar patients who have had only depression (see discussion in next chapter).

The twin data also illustrates that even when there is concordance in identical twins, some 20% may show discordance for the kind of affective psychoses. Some may have a unipolar illness whilst others have a bipolar disorder, which indicates that while genetic predisposition may be similar, the illness phenotype may differ. Also, a considerable proportion who do not show concordance for illness suggests that there is a variable penetrance. Penetrance indicates the proportion of those who are genetically susceptible and who may show the illness.

There appears to be a single underlying disorder which may manifest as unipolar or bipolar illness, caused by a yet undetermined mechanism. Gershon et al. (1976) showed that bipolar illness may be a genetically more severe form since more illness was transmitted in families of bipolar than in families with unipolar patients. In the families of bipolar probands unipolar psychoses may be more numerous than bipolar illness. Thus the unipolar and bipolar psychoses do not appear to breed true.

The refinement of the multifactorial model of transmission is the postulate of two-threshold transmission models as propounded by Gershon et al. (1976). This model advocates a continuum in the level of liability to affective illness. This liability is based on an interaction between genetic and environmental factors, and there may be two or more thresholds. When the first threshold is passed, an illness results, in the case of affective illness, unipolar depression. When the second threshold is exceeded, a bipolar illness results.

Winokur et al. (1971) divided depression into 'pure depression' and 'depressive spectrum disorders' (see later discussion). This results in an extension of the concept of depression and, in a sense, seeks to study the genetic and biological roots of conditions such as alcoholism and psychopathy, which are then considered to be depressive equivalents. This seeks to inquire into phenotypes, which may be genotypically similar. Whether a widening of the concept, which makes little clinical sense, may yield biological insights remains to be seen.

Gershon et al. (1982) have produced data that schizo-affective disorder, bipolar illness, unipolar illness and normality are all points on a continuum.

46

Thus, from normality one proceeds to unipolar illness, the least severe, through bipolar illness and schizo-affective states, the most severe, and characterized also by psychotic phenomena. However, it appears an analysis does not support their hypothesis (Winokur, 1984).

Where delusional depression is in this scheme of things is not clear. In terms of the presence of a psychotic feature, i.e. delusion, it has affinities with schizo-affective illness. There is also evidence for considering depression with delusions to be a separate entity (see later section and also Chapter 5 on the management of delusional depression).

Winokur (1984) has suggested that the propensity to psychoses is transmitted independently, and is independent of psychiatric diagnosis. If the patient becomes ill in terms of bipolar or unipolar illness, the psychotic features will emerge, but as long as the affective disorder is in remission the psychotic features will be absent. The evidence for this seems to be that each time the patient has a relapse of illness, the psychotic features will appear in some, if not all, of the episodes.

The relationship between schizophrenia and depression is considered in detail in Chapter 4. From the genetic point of view, it has been noted that in successive generations manic-depressive illness has a slight tendency to undergo change into schizophrenia. This is reflected in the work by Rosenthal (1970) who found that in a number of studies there was a higher incidence of schizophrenia in the children of manic-depressive patients. Crow (1984) has considered this finding in terms of a viral hypothesis for schizophrenia. He speculated there might be an alteration in the gene or its location brought about by retroviruses which themselves have similarities to some genetic elements. According to this concept, schizophrenia may arise in three ways:

(1) By inheritance in the usual way of the genes which predispose to schizophrenia,
(2) By inheritance of the gene (modified in the course of transmission) from a parent who has the susceptibility to manic-depressive illness, and
(3) By injection with a retrovirus *in utero*.

The genetics of affective disorder also have some bearing on the question of whether or not depression has any biological advantage, a subject considered in Chapter 9. The fact that parents, sibs and offspring have similar morbidity risks for affective illness suggests that genetic selection is not operative at its maximum.

It also appears that the severity of illness and the presenting symptomatology have little bearing on the morbidity risk in close relatives. On the other hand, age of onset, response to treatment and the severity of environmental stress have some bearing on morbidity risks.

THE NATURE OF DEPRESSION

Depression is a heterogeneous condition due to a variety of interactions and may present with any degree of severity. Traditionally, when a medical or systemic causation has been excluded, depression as a psychiatric condition has been considered to be of 'functional' origin. This concept is critically considered in Chapter 3, and it will be seen that it is now, by and large, an untenable one. However, the term 'functional' still serves a purpose in reminding us that depression can be a symptom of physical disease which is always worth excluding. A practical classification of depression given in Figure 2 in diagrammatic form also takes in some concepts which have been touched on in the previous section and will be dealt with in detail later.

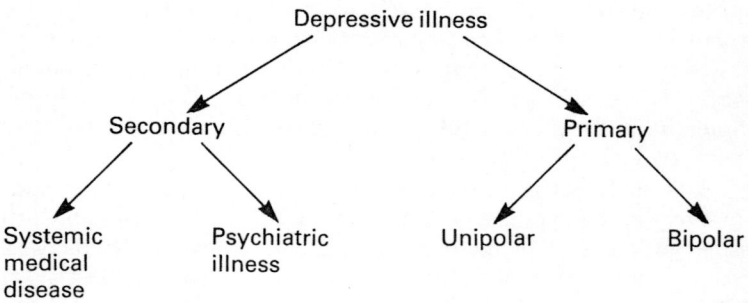

Figure 2 A practical classification of depression

In view of the heterogeneity and complexity of the condition, the epidemiology of depression can only be discussed in relation to other disorders associated with it, e.g. mania (bipolar/unipolar illness), other psychiatric illness (secondary/primary depression), alcoholism and sociopathy (pure depression/depressive spectrum disorder).

It must be clear that when depression occurs as part of the symptomatology of another disease its nature will be different to a depression which arises by itself. Conversely, depression may influence the course of the primary illness, a subject for discussion in Chapter 4. Robins and his group in St Louis distinguished between primary and secondary depression, basing their distinction on priority of time. The primary illness could be physical or psychiatric. Depression here is a symptomatological diagnosis and there are no aetiological considerations such as a role for life events. The ratio of primary to secondary depression appears to be about 2:1 although, of course, the proportions may vary according to the setting in which the diagnosis is made, e.g. a medical ward would obviously yield a higher percentage of cases of secondary depression.

One of the advantages of a symptomatological consideration of depression and its division on the basis of prior illness into primary and secondary categories is that it obviates the need to take up such disputed categories as 'endogenous' and 'reactive'. The controversy regarding this matter was noted in its historical context in Chapter 1. This distinction attracts another line of criticism, quite apart from those raised in Chapter 1.

When considering the interactionist model of depression, we need, in the face of growing knowledge, to take into account the neurobiological basis of depression. The brain is influenced by stimuli emanating from the environment, and it in turn has effects on the rest of the body. Thus stresses and life events must have some 'endogenous' matrix to act upon. Even a purely 'endogenous' depression, if such an entity did exist, once it set in train the various features of the condition, would have those very features acting upon it in the form of further stresses. And, as has been shown, even stress-related mental events can have an autonomy – an 'endogenicity' – of their own.

Objections to the terms 'endogenous' and 'reactive' led to their being seen as clinical descriptive states rather than having any aetiological connotation. Here, 'endogenous' and 'reactive' are used more or less synonymously with 'psychotic' and 'neurotic' or 'biological' and 'psychological' and equated with symptoms traditionally associated with depression, and those seen as the development of the personality interacting with the environment respectively. The distinction has some practical value – response to ECT, lithium and tricyclic and other antidepressant agents on the one hand and MAO inhibitors on the other can be correlated to some extent with the diagnosis. Biogenic amine and neuroendocrine studies offer some limited support in this direction. But clearly there is a need for a better system of clinical classification in advance of a neurobiological one which remains the ideal.

'Endogenous' depression is allegedly an 'autonomous' depression (Rosenthal and Klerman, 1966). Nelson and Charney (1981) suggest there may be at least two autonomous conditions that may be subsumed under 'endogenous' depression – a retarded anhedonic type and an agitated delusional type. There is some support for this distinction from treatment response. Retarded depression responds to tricyclic and related antidepressants, but may be made worse with neuroleptic drugs; agitated delusional depression may respond poorly to tricyclic antidepressants and neuroleptic medication. Nelson and Charney (1981) have suggested that endogenous depression is a depressive state which once developed is autonomous, is associated with neurobiological changes and requires specific biological interventions. They have reviewed the literature and suggest that the symptoms distinctive for so-called 'endogenous' depression are altered psychomotor activity, lack of reactivity to environmental changes, severe depressed mood, depressive delusions, self-reproach and loss of interest. However, as has been referred to in the section on stressful events in relation to neuroendocrine changes and depression, there is little to indicate that stress or its absence is a useful distinguishing variable in any neurobiological classification of depression (e.g. Dolan et al., 1985). Also, as Paykel (1978) has noted, the relationship between life events and symptom pattern is weak. Recent work also suggests that patients with the 'endogenous' syndrome are just as likely to have experienced a major threatening life event in the months before the onset of illness as patients with the 'reactive' condition (Brown and Harris, 1978).

The relationship between mania and depression has been known for some considerable time, as has been discussed in Chapter 1. Kraepelin had noted the symptoms of closely related conditions – periodic and circular psychoses, manias, most depressive illnesses, affective personality disorders and some delirious states – he had studied their good prognosis for the individual episodes of illness and their familial incidence, and had brought them together as the 'manic-depressive psychoses'. Leonhard (1959) and Leonhard *et al.* (1962) suggested a further division into bipolar and unipolar disorders. The concept was further developed by Angst (1966) and Perris (1966).

The unipolar–bipolar distinction in depressive illness therefore depends on a history of mania. Unipolar depression is significantly more common than bipolar depression. In bipolar disorder the incidence is about the same in the two sexes (*cf* the incidence of depression as a whole), the age of onset is earlier than in unipolar cases, the premorbid personality is seen to be more outgoing and the morbidity risk in close relatives, as we have seen, is considerably higher. In unipolar disease there is appreciably greater incidence in females, there is a relatively late age of onset, and there is a quieter, more obsessional premorbid personality. The morbidity risk is considerably less than in bipolar families. The distinction between bipolar and unipolar depression may be made quite easily on clinical grounds but there is now quite substantial support from family histories, and twin and adoption studies, for this separation.

The median age of illness (i.e. the age at which half the susceptible group would have suffered their first attack) is about 30 years for bipolars and about 45 years for unipolars. There are also some differences in symptomatology between bipolar cases and unipolar cases. Bipolar patients have a greater likelihood of some kinds of hallucinations than have unipolar patients (Winokur, 1984). Katz *et al.* (1982) have suggested there is less anxiety in bipolar depression.

Some comment must be made on another traditional differentiation, that into 'psychotic' and 'neurotic' depression. In the strict sense 'psychotic' implies the presence of psychotic features such as delusions and hallucinations. Thus the only valid category nowadays would be the intriguing form of 'delusional depression' which will be taken up in a later section. This form has become considerably less common, accounting for less than 10% of all depressions at any age. As will be discussed later, there are thought to be good grounds for considering this type of depression to be separate from the main body of depression. If this is so, the reduction in incidence cannot wholly be explained in terms of advances in diagnosis and treatment, and may well have implications for ideas for what we now regard as the mutability of disease.

'Psychotic' depression is still equated in some quarters with severe or 'endogenous' depression. Conversely, 'neurotic' depression has been considered to be a milder form of depression. This has also been equated with 'reactive' depression of the neurotic type and the anxiety-laden 'minor' forms of depression have been explained in similar terms. The criticisms applied to the concept of 'endogenous' depression appear to be valid in principle when applied to 'neurotic' depression. Although the response to relatively specific agents was once thought to support the distinction (see Chapter 5), there is in reality considerable overlap. For every treatment failure in a classical 'endogenous' depressive whom one would have sworn was a classic textbook case and who should have illustrated the principle, there is in actual clinical practice one 'neurotic' or 'reactive' depressive who responds to antidepressant drugs and even ECT. This experience argues once again for the heterogeneity of depressive illness, and one cannot do justice to the complexity of the condition by prematurely consigning depression into simplistic diagnostic categories.

Even less clearcut cases of depression abound, as most of us know to our cost. These 'atypical depressions' are occasionally to be considered for psychosurgery, the most drastic of the biological therapeutic procedures we have at our disposal.

Winokur has further divided 'primary' depression into pure depressive disorder with a family history and the usual appurtenances of depression, and 'depressive spectrum disease' in which a family history of alcoholism, psychopathic disorder, hysteria or drug abuse may be found. The characteristics of pure depression are thought to be: late onset, equal incidence in males and females, a moderately increased morbidity risk, and no increase in the risk for alcoholism and psychopathy. In depressive spectrum disease there was a lower age of onset, an increase in incidence in females, a higher morbidity risk for depression in the female members of the family and for alcoholism and psychopathy in the male members (Winokur *et al.*, 1971). It is a moot point, of course, if the cause of clarification of the depressions is served by extending the concept, even if only by implication and indirect genetic considerations. It is a common enough clinical finding that depressives abuse alcohol and occasionally engage in criminal, destructive or antisocial behaviour such as shoplifting, suicide and homicide. There must be considerable sympathy for any attempt which seeks to look beneath the symptoms of depression to seek an understanding of its causes, but it could be argued with some vigour that little justice is done to a complex subject by extending the concept to embrace these secondary behaviours.

EPIDEMIOLOGY

The most striking epidemiological fact is the considerably elevated female incidence. Although there is a variation in figures from study to study, it would appear that in general 1.5–2 times as many women as men become depressed. Virtually every study of depression in industrialized countries has reflected this preponderance. Weissman and Klerman (1977) concluded that this sex difference is a real one and not some methodological artifact, as the predominance of women is found in community studies as well as in 'treatment-based' studies, where, it might have been argued, women sought help more and thus might have been over-represented in studies.

What the explanation might be for this increased incidence is unclear in that socio-cultural factors must be deemed to play an important part until otherwise proved. In the same way the scarcity of women mathematicians and physicists cannot be attributed to differences in the sexes in cerebral hemisphere organization (for which there is evidence). Until we understand the influence of social attitudes, expectations and conditioning, it would be facile to attribute the sex difference in the sexes solely, or mainly, to such biological determinants as hormones. As is discussed in Chapter 8, some transcultural work on depression may help illuminate this point.

Peak incidence and prevalence of depression in women is about 40 years of age, although there may be a minor secondary peak after the age of 55. This contrasts with the pattern for men where incidence and prevalence rise with age. Weissman and Myers (1978b) showed that rates of moderate depression were higher in younger women, and tended to decrease with age, whereas in men the prevalence of depressive symptoms was lower in young men and increased with age.

There does not appear to be an increase of depression in women in the menopausal years (Hallstrom 1973; see also discussion of involutional melancholia in Chapter 1).

The point prevalence of depressive symptoms in the community is about 20%. The risk factors associated with depression are: being a young woman, being an older man, belonging to a lower social class and being divorced or separated. The social class distinction in depression, if it exists, is a problematical one. For unipolar depression there would appear not to be a class difference (Weissman and Myers, 1978a). However, we need to take note of the findings of Brown and Harris (1978) which were discussed in a previous section. It would seem the important variable is children. Women with children and belonging to the working class are at higher risk for depression than middle class women with children. If there are no children, there is no difference in the risk among the classes. When it comes to bipolar disorder, there are suggestions that there is an increased incidence in the higher socio-economic classes. The explanation furnished by Bagley (1973) for this phenomenon was referred to in an earlier section.

Some 'vulnerability factors', as discussed by Brown and Harris (1982) for working class women are outlined in the section on vulnerability to depression. The early environment is a complex issue but there is evidence that when a child's environment is hostile, disruptive and lacking in stability and harmony, there is an increased predisposition to depression when the child grows into an adult (Orvaschel et al., 1980).

Quite clearly personality factors are important in the predisposition to depression. This common sense clinical impression is supported by the work of Hirschfeld and Klerman (1979) who found the following premorbid personalities in patients who had become depressed: previous vulnerability to breakdown under stress, lacking in energy, insecure, being sensitive, worrying, lack of social skills, being unassertive, dependent and obsessional.

The risk factors for unipolar and bipolar depression appear to be different. For unipolar depression, being a woman between 35 and 45 years of age, having a family history of depression or alcoholism, having a negative home environment in childhood, the presence of recent threatening life events, being 6 months into the post-partum period and lacking an intimate, confiding relationship, being working class, having several small children and being under or unemployed all seem to increase the risk.

For bipolar disorder, being a woman (though less of a risk, apparently, than for unipolar illness), having a family history of bipolar illness, being under 50 years of age and being of a higher social class may be significant risks.

CLINICAL FEATURES

It is useful to consider the clinical features of unipolar and bipolar conditions separately before discussing the symptomatology of depression in general.

Unipolar patients are in general older than bipolar patients. The episodes in unipolar disorder tend to be of somewhat longer duration. For bipolar disease, the onset is before 30 years of age, and 88% of patients have had an onset before 49 years (Angst et al., 1973). Although both mania and depression can feature as the initial disorder in bipolar cases there is a majority with a manic presentation. The first attack lasts 2.7 months (Angst et al., 1973), though older patients may have more prolonged attacks. Bipolar illness also appears to give rise to more frequent episodes. As has been noted, there is little to distinguish a depression of unipolar disease from depression of bipolar disease, although a slightly greater tendency to hallucination and a diminished incidence of anxiety has been suggested in bipolar cases. Both bipolar and unipolar depression predispose to suicide, the risk of which is put at 15% (Guze and Robins, 1970). This subject is taken up in Chapter 7. But there is a suggestion that increased mortality in bipolar conditions may involve deaths other than suicide (Petterson, 1977). Thus, suicides and accidents may account for all excess deaths in cases of unipolar illness, but deaths due to malignant disease and cardiovascular disease may be associated with, or related to, bipolar illness (see Chapter 6).

The period of illness is called the 'phase' and the interval between phases is referred to as the 'cycle'. The phase lasts from 6–12 months, and may show an increase with age of onset and there is a positive correlation between length of a phase and the severity of illness. The concept of the phase has some implications for treatment and its maintenance as one might argue that the efficacy of antidepressant treatment is due to reducing the phase of illness, a feature most markedly seen in lithium prophylaxis. The cycle of depression is shortened with age i.e. more frequent episodes occur. It is longer with unipolar depression than with bipolar depression, and there is a tendency for shorter cycles with a later age of onset.

There is a prodromal period before the depressive illness proper which is referred to by many patients. Obviously, features such as insomnia, anxiety or fatiguability could be early, rather than prodromal, symptoms but their existence noted at first presentation may alert the doctor to the impending signs of relapse on subsequent occasions.

To put the effects of treatment into proper perspective it must be stated that the natural history of the majority of depressions is towards remission. However, there is little doubt that the intractable cases, a minority admittedly, continued disabled and depressed in the wards of mental

53

hospitals in the days before specific treatments were available. (ECT, though available from the early 1930s only began to be widely used after 1945; the phenothiazines were introduced in the mid 1950s, the tricyclic antidepressants after 1960, and the lithium salts in the late 1960s). Up to 50% of cases of depression probably remit naturally. This is partly due to such inherent factors as genetic endowment and the self-limiting neurobiological change it gives rise to, and such non-specific influences as placebo factors and the psychosocial impact brought about by contact with a wide variety of services in the hospital and the community. The effect of treatment has been to reduce the length of the illness, diminish the intensity of symptoms and prevent recurrences or prolong the period, i.e. the cycle between episodes. It is appropriate to refer to the state of normality produced by effective drug treatment as a remission as the cyclical nature of both unipolar and bipolar illness is obvious.

When modern physical treatments are used actively, appropriately and effectively, with the mobilization of all relevant non-physical modes of management, there is an expectation that some 85% of depressed patients will have remission of their symptoms and will resume their pre-morbid level of social functioning. This figure compares favourably with any major physical illness.

About 15% of patients do not recover. Whilst there are undoubtedly intractable forms of depressive illness, by far the commonest reason for chronicity is poor prior personality leading to a tenuous adjustment to the world at large or continuing stresses in the family or environment. Chronicity is related to the phase of illness, and there is greater likelihood of a non-resolving depression as the patient grows older.

In the vast majority of cases the essential symptomatology in recurrent attacks of depression remains unchanged, though the frequency, duration and intensity of symptoms may vary. However, a small proportion of patients – less than 10% – show a change in symptomatology over time which leads to a diagnosis of schizophrenia. No methodological or diagnostic artifact can explain this irreducible proportion of cases. It is further evidence of mutability of disease and is discussed in detail in Chapter 4.

The term depression covers a range of phenomena from a mood state within the normal range of behaviour, which is a universal experience, through a symptom that is common in a variety of psychiatric and physical disorders, to a diagnosed illness. The teaching traditionally has been that the central and characteristic feature of depression is diminished mood, and that most or all of the symptoms of the condition must be derived from this central lowering of the mood. The growing realization that several, if not all, ancillary features of depression could exist without diminished mood being present has meant that a different view is now taken of depression. The depressed mood may be absent, concealed by the patient, 'masked' by other features, or find expression through 'depressive equivalents'. It is easy to make sense of this confusion by reminding oneself that depression in all its manifestations is merely the outward and visible sign of neurobiological events. Depression, as will be discussed in Chapter 3, is a common –

probably the most common – mental feature of neurobiological phenomena involving the limbic system and its connections. The almost invariable clinical rule is to find depressed mood within the cluster of features which go to make up the disorder we call depression. If that is the rule, there will be exceptions and these may lead to doubt and error in clinical practice. However, there are no rules which are inviolable in the diagnosis of depression. In ordinary clinical practice, the only practical method of making a diagnosis of depression is by a global assessment of the patient, *with* a semi-quantitative evaluation of the features noted in the ensuing discussion in the next section. For research and more systematic study it is only right to insist upon the definite presence of depressed mood to ensure that only definite cases of depression are included before, say, drugs are tested. This rigour has the effect that a minority of atypical cases are lost, which is not a grievous loss in a research trial, but no help to the clinician who will be confronted by these patients. In these cases the clinician may have to infer depression from changes in behaviour rather than from depressed mood, as may happen with children, the elderly or patients from other cultures, matters which will be explored in Chapter 8.

The clinical features of depression may be conveniently studied in relation to three areas of behaviour:

(1) psychological,
(2) physical and physiological, and
(3) social.

As has been mentioned, it is traditional to derive all psychological disturbance in depression from the central disorder of mood. These would include suicidal ideas and behaviour and disorders in thinking and perception. The physical and physiological effects include impairment in bodily functioning such as disturbance in sleep, appetite, sexual desire, menstrual function, bowel activity, disorders of higher cerebral function, autonomic nervous system functioning and other somatic complaints. In terms of socially disordered behaviour there is a reduced capacity for functioning appropriately in the context of marriage, the family, occupation and in keeping up with social norms.

DISTURBANCES IN PSYCHOLOGICAL FUNCTIONING

The predominant and central feature is depressed *mood*, which may be complained of by the patient, his friends and relatives or elicited by the clinician. It may vary in *severity* and it may show *diurnal variation*, worse at one time of the day rather than another. The distinction to be made between forms of depression on the basis of this variation is less clearcut than was formerly thought. Associated with depressed mood is *a tendency to weep*, another symptom which needs to be assessed in relation to cultural norms. Also related to the depressed mood is *anhedonia*, an inability to derive pleasure from pursuits the patient would have enjoyed in the premorbid state. It used to be taught that *reactivity*, or response to the environment, also characterized one form of depression and set it apart from others which were qualitatively different. This distinction is, again, less definite and one may say only that some depressed patients respond more to events in their environment than others.

Almost universally present is the complaint of loss of energy or *fatiguability* which may be sufficiently marked to produce physical symptoms. There also are feelings of personal inadequacy and a tendency to engage in *self-depreciation*, where the patient has a low opinion of himself and believes – occasionally is convinced – that others take a depreciatory view of him also. This tendency is associated with feelings of *guilt* and worthlessness. These feelings have a cultural bias, as will be discussed in Chapter 8, where it will be shown that feelings of guilt and worthlessness are more common in Western than in African or Asian societies, where shame and complaints of bodily dysfunction are more common.

Occasionally, these feelings of guilt and worthlessness may reach *delusional* levels. Whether a depression with delusions is only quantitatively (i.e. in terms of severity) separated from delusion-free depression will be discussed in a later section in this chapter. These delusions are 'negative', i.e. of worthlessness, monumental guilt and blameworthiness or bizarre interpretations of bodily function and disease and one may imaginatively relate these to the underlying mood state. So can *hallucinations*, characteristically auditory and made up of voices making derogatory remarks and hurling abuse which the depressed patient feels he richly deserves. The relationship of depressed mood to *obsessive–compulsive* features is less readily explained, but these are not uncommon symptoms in depression and even when they appear to run an independent course are almost invariably exacerbated by depression.

The low opinion of self is allied to a mood of *hopelessness and despair* which characterize several forms of depression. The logical outcome of features such as these would appear to be *suicide*. As will be discussed in Chapter 7, the risk of suicide in any form of depression is a serious one. The personality and the circumstances of the patient rather than the severity and characteristics of the depression seem to determine if suicide is successfully accomplished. Suicidal behaviour may take the form of fleeting suicidal ideas, morbid rumination, suicidal plans, attempts and the completed act. The danger of suicide is not necessarily greatest in the depths of depression, but in the period of recovery from psychological and motor retardation. If the patient becomes more active physically whilst he is still depressed in mood, he has the physical means to carry out the act, a case of the flesh being willing while the spirit is weak.

Almost as common as the depressed mood in depression are feelings of *anxiety*. These may be psychological or physical.

DISTURBANCES IN PHYSICAL AND PHYSIOLOGICAL FUNCTIONING

The physical features of depression include problems with motility. Both *agitation* and *retardation* may be found and they may be found in the same patient. Agitation is generally seen in older patients and may take the form of 'static' motility, as in a relatively immobile patient wringing his hands as opposed to the excessive mobility which may be seen in the psychoses such as the schizophrenias and mania. Retardation may extend from a barely perceptible immobility in facial and automatic movements to stupor, through semi-stupor. Stupor is a disturbance in consciousness and whether depression can be diagnosed in a stuporose patient is a moot point. Moreover, there is every indication that stupor is a true 'organic' state, depression merely being an arguable cause (see Chapter 3). The fact that a stuporose patient recovers with treatment for depression is no licence for talk about 'functional' stuporose conditions, as an aetiological factor may affect one part of the brain in less subtle ways than another.

Physical symptoms attributable to organ systems are common in depression, involving virtually every organ in the body. Often extensive investigation may take place and the conclusion 'no organic basis was found' may be reached. There is reason to suspect that these conclusions may not entirely be valid. When 'no organic basis was found' refers to the limits of current medical knowledge, in the same sense the limits of neurological inquiry and practice constrain the concept of hysteria. Recent neurobiological studies have shown that, in individual patients at least, neuroendocrine and psychophysiological change can be demonstrated. A case in point is headache which is a common symptom in depression. Garvey *et al.* (1983) found that patients with depressive headaches were younger, had more somatic complaints and experienced more hypersomnia than other depressives. They tried to explain the association between headaches and depression in terms of 5-hydroxytryptamine (5-HT) abnormality (see Chapter 3). The association between depressive headaches and hypersomnia and somatic complaints may also involve 5-HT abnormality. Tryptophan, a 5-HT precursor, increases sleep time in humans; in animals decreased pain thresholds are associated with changes in levels of brain 5-HT. The relationship therefore is a complex one – hypersomnia appears to involve excess 5-HT, while decreased pain thresholds and some forms of depression may be the result of 5-HT deficiency – but there is evidence on which to formulate hypotheses to test an 'organic' basis to this depressive symptom.

A common *physiological* symptom in depression is sleep disturbance, the vast majority of patients complaining of *insomnia*, the rest of hypersomnia. Insomnia may be divided into initial, middle and late forms, the last sometimes being called early morning awakening. Once again it used to be taught that different types of insomnia could help distinguish between different diagnostic categories of depression. This is no longer held to be the case. The different types of insomnia do no more than reflect the heterogeneity of depression. Insomnia is usually associated with broken sleep, dreams and nightmares, presumably due to the underlying anxiety which is probably also partly responsible for the feeling that a night's sleep has not been refreshing.

Associated with insomnia is loss of weight with *loss of appetite* although, as with hypersomnia, a minority of patients show increased weight and weight gain. There is weight gain during the process of recovery from depression, partly due to the remission of the disorder and partly attributable to the pharmacological effects of antidepressant drugs (see Chapter 5).

Loss of sexual interest is a common symptom, although once again a minority of patients may show an increase in sexual activity, which may be related to feelings of anxiety and tension. Anxiety may also explain impotence, ejaculatory difficulties and anorgasmia which are commonly seen in depression, and may be exacerbated by the undesirable side effects of antidepressant drugs. Irregularity in the *periodicity* and *volume* of the menstrual flow may also be noted.

Bowel function may be disturbed in depression, constipation being the usual feature but where diarrhoea occurs, high levels of anxiety may be suspected.

As a counterpoint to the psychological component of anxiety there is the *physiological* manifestation of anxiety with palpitations or feelings of abdominal discomfort. Some of these features may suggest partial epilepsy.

Disorders of higher cerebral function are common manifestions of depression. These may range from loss of concentration and attention to a cognitive impairment that amounts to dementia, a subject dealt with in Chapters 3 and 4. Interestingly, cognitive disorder involves memory and intellectual functioning but spares cortical functioning such as language function, gnosis and praxis.

DISTURBANCE IN SOCIAL FUNCTIONING

It is to be expected that the impairment in mood and its consequences and the disturbance in physical and physiological functioning will lead to disordered functioning in the social sphere. The lethargic patient with little interest in himself – apart from morbid rumination – or his family, his friends and colleagues performs poorly. There are obvious implications for his marriage, family and occupation. Criminal behaviour is not unknown, a phenomenon not fully explained though some aspects of the violence associated with depression are discussed in Chapter 7. Irritability, anger and hostility are common features. The patient may withdraw from habitual social contacts. Quite apart from the importance of these factors in the initial diagnostic formulation of the patient's condition, the social consequences of depression will influence the management and rehabilitation of the patient. The correlation between symptomatic improvement and social functioning is a tenuous one in all of psychiatry, and the implications of the clinical state of the patient in terms of its impact on his social milieu must be appreciated from the outset if successful rehabilitation is to be achieved.

ATYPICAL DEPRESSIONS

The term 'atypical depression' has a variety of meanings, but for the purpose of this discussion it is taken to mean those depressions that do not show the typical features discussed above. The more usual meaning of the term is in relation to those depressions associated with marked anxiety and, perhaps, for that reason are not merely atypical in presentation but in treatment response. As will be discussed in Chapter 5, the monoamine oxidase inhibitors (MAOI) have been advocated for this form of depression. These depressions are characterized by high levels of psychological and physiological anxiety, initial insomnia, a reversed diurnal variation in mood (i.e. worse in the evenings) and an element of reactivity. Although the syndrome may vary from mild to severe, the depressive component is itself usually mild or moderate. Whether this form of depression ought to be dignified by being allocated a category is doubtful. Some of the reasons for this have been discussed in Chapter 1, and also in a previous section in this chapter. Even the differential treatment response has less than unequivocal backing. While West and Dally (1959) noted that patients with this kind of atypical depression, i.e. chronic depressives with generalized and phobic anxiety, a reversed diurnal worsening of mood, fatiguability, hysterical features and an absence of the more typical features of depression responded to iproniazid, Rowan et al. (1982) found that the basic effects of amitriptyline and phenelzine were similar with, perhaps, phenelzine having some small effect on anxiety symptoms of depression. Thus, although the presentation of this form of depression might be atypical, this may well be due to some features of depression being highlighted. We now know depression to be a biologically heterogeneous condition and there would seem little reason to find separate categories for those depressive conditions showing a prominence of some symptoms.

The idea that depression may be 'masked' by other features has been alluded to before. Masked depression may take the form of a presentation of the condition in abnormal physical or social guise (Paykel and Norton, 1982). Hypochondriasis is one of the forms of a prominent physical presentation. Here the patient highlights or is preoccupied with a physical symptom at the expense of other features of depression. A symptom such as hypochondriasis may precede or be coincidental with the depression, but it is also able to become an autonomous feature which is unrelated to the progression of or improvement in the depression. The head, abdomen and chest provide many of the symptoms in this complaint (headache is seen in between 49% to 84%, of cases of depression, Garvey et al., 1983). Atypical facial pain is another symptom seen in depression, and often responds well to antidepressants. The pain may be associated with anxiety, insomnia and fatiguability instead of the more typical features of depression.

Occasionally, social functioning is affected adversely in the absence of overt depression, and increased irritability, reduced tolerance of frustration and hyperacusis may encourage one to investigate further into an underlying depressive process. The uncommon but well-known phenomenon of the middle aged female shoplifter with depression is another case in point. It is, of course, possible that the condition underlying these symptoms or behaviours is anxiety and the fact that good response to tricyclic and other antidepressants is readily obtained may not be anything more than due to the anxiolytic effects of most of these drugs, or further evidence of the inseparability of the components of affective disorder in practice (see Chapter 4). The dangers of arguing backwards from allegedly specific therapeutic response must be borne in mind.

With the elderly, there may be the possibility that cognitive dysfunction may help mask the other features of depression. This subject is further taken up in Chapter 4.

A phenomenon usually discussed in the same breath as 'masked depression' is 'depressive equivalents'. This is clearly a more dubious phenomenon as inference rather than a detailed clinical appraisal is required to find it. Paykel and Norton (1982) illustrate this by quoting the work that has been done in regard to alcoholism, drug dependence and 'acting-out' behaviour; psychosomatic disorders such as peptic ulcer and skin diseases; the features such as withdrawal, sleep disturbance, school refusal, physical symptoms and conduct disorder in children (see also Chapter 8); and the fact that a high incidence of psychosomatic disorders may be found in relatives of patients with affective disorders. We have also noted that in the concept of depressive spectrum disorder put forward by Winokur, the fact that female depressives are sometimes known to have family histories of alcoholism and psychopathy in male relatives is produced as an argument for widening the concept of depression. All that can be said is that in clinical terms, at least, a concept as wide as that of 'depressive equivalents' cannot be anticipated to have much use. The strictures that were applied in a previous section to the concept of depressive spectrum disorder are relevant here as well.

DELUSIONAL DEPRESSION

Delusional depression is now rare, accounting for less than 10% of all depressions. It is a true psychotic depression. There is now suspicion that delusional depression is not merely a quantitative variation (i.e. a more severe form) but is qualitatively distinctive. Nelson et al. (1984) compared delusional with non-delusional depression, and found there was more family history of depression, less of alcoholism, a greater frequency of cortisol hypersecretion and a poorer response to tricyclic antidepressant drugs among deluded depressives.

Recent clinical studies have shown that delusional depression might be considered to be a distinct subtype of unipolar depression which responds poorly to antidepressant drugs alone but significantly better to a combination of tricyclic drugs and neuroleptic medication. This form of depression may also be characterized by the stability of the clinical picture in each discrete episode of illness. Thus delusion in depression does not merely indicate severity of depression but is probably a biological marker that appears in each subsequent episode.

Winokur (1984) has noted that bipolar psychotic patients were more likely to have symptoms such as hallucination and motor abnormalities than were unipolar patients. They are also less likely to have had a history of multiple episodes on admission and more likely to have more prolonged phases of illness. It was suggested, as has already been discussed in the section on genetics, that a trait or propensity to psychosis is transmitted independently of that for the affective disorder. Charney and Nelson (1981) have confirmed the tendency of delusional depression to breed true in individuals.

Table 3 Features of delusional depression

Incidence	Less than 10% of all depressions
Family history of depression	More than in non-delusional cases Less of alcoholism
Clinical	Clinical features stable in each discrete episode – 'breeds true' Depression severe Fewer multiple episodes Longer phase of illness
Prognosis	Greater chronicity in short-term No significant difference in long-term follow-up
Treatment	Poor reponse to antidepressants alone Better response to antidepressants + neuroleptics, and ECT

Winokur (1984) also suggested that both bipolar and unipolar psychotic patients have fewer episodes of illness, have a post-hospital course with more chronicity and have less complete remission on discharge. However, on 30–40 year follow-up they tended as much as non-psychotic patients to become well. Therefore, he concludes that the immediate course and short-term follow-up is less good for psychotic than non-psychotic patients, but that rates of improvement are similar over the entire lifetime, at least for unipolar depression. Psychotic depression also bears a relationship to schizo-affective disorder, both conditions being characterized by a mixture of affective symptoms and psychotic phenomena, a remitting course and a relatively good prognosis.

Several of these points may be illustrated by the case of an 84-year-old woman who 50 years before had become severely depressed with ideas of pregnancy held with delusional conviction. She recovered over a period of months and went back to working as a legal secretary. Over the next half century she had at least six episodes of severe depression with the same delusion. In the early days the episodes remitted over several months of hospital admission; with the advent of ECT, the phases of illness were ended in a significantly shorter time. At the age of 83 she became depressed again with the same delusion, refusing ECT on this last occasion. She died following a gastro-intestinal haemorrhage. There did not appear to be any material difference between the mental state as recorded on the last occasion and previous occasions. An exclusively psychodynamic formulation might have been feasible for a woman in her thirties who had become depressed and deluded with ideas of pregnancy following a broken love affair. It is carrying imagination too far to attempt such an explanation for a women in her eighties. While the content of the delusion might have been influenced by her life experiences, it seems at least plausible to suggest that biological factors dictated the form, and the onset, of the delusion.

Aspects of delusional depression are considered further in Chapter 3 in the discussion on the biological basis of depression and Chapter 5 on the drug treatment of such conditions.

REACTIVE DEPRESSIVE PSYCHOSIS AND CYCLOID PSYCHOSIS

As has been discussed in the sections on stress, there would appear to be psychoses which follow one or more stressful events and run a benign, short-lived course, recovery being unaccompanied by any residual features. Depression is a major component of these psychoses. The prognosis is that of a self-limiting illness, which may or may not recur and, if it does, does so in relation to a similar, subsequent stress. The conceptual issues have been dealt with above and Mahendra (1977a) presented data on 60 patients with these reactive psychoses and showed that in terms of the clinical picture, its relation to stressful life events and its occurrence in those with vulnerable personalities, it corresponded to the concept of reactive psychosis in Scandinavia and continental Europe.

What relation the condition bears to manic-depressive illness of the usual kind is difficult to say. Stromgren (1961) pointed out that they were distinct though many of the symptoms were shared by both reactive psychosis and manic-depressive illness. Long-term follow-up is not usually available in published series, but it is clear that the illness does not relapse in the absence of maintenance antidepressant therapy. The patient who makes a full recovery from reactive depressive psychosis stays well till the next breakdown and the incidence of suicide is probably less, difficult though it is to judge these matters. (Suicide is often related to the stress rather than the reactive depression.)

Perris (1974) put forward a concept of 'cycloid psychosis', a disorder with benign prognosis and relapsing course that appeared to be distinct from both schizophrenia and manic-depressive illness. The requirements for this diagnosis are a remittent course of illness, swings of mood and the presence of features such as confusion, marked anxiety and delusions and hallucinations which are not in keeping with the mood. First degree relatives appeared to be at high risk for cycloid psychosis, and only one of 65 patients in Perris' series appeared to run a chronic course of illness. Cutting *et al.* (1978) found that females and patients with a puerperal onset were common among patients with cycloid psychosis, which appears to give rise to frequent, abrupt and short-lived episodes of illness with florid psychotic symptoms.

Reactive depressive psychosis may be usefully compared to cycloid psychosis. In both there is an abrupt onset, with confusion, a changeable mood state, a relatively short phase of illness marked by delusions and/or hallucinations which are not in keeping with either the precipitating stress or the current mood state, response to non-specific symptomatic medication or ECT and a full clinical recovery. They differ in that a genetic basis cannot be found in most cases of reactive psychosis and there is no predictable recurrence in reactive psychosis while, as the term suggests, cycloid psychosis is punctuated by frequent episodes. Both the sex difference and the association with the puerperium are common to both conditions. Table 4 summarizes the features of reactive depressive psychosis and cycloid psychosis.

Table 4 Comparisons of reactive depressive psychosis and cycloid psychosis

	Reactive depressive psychosis	*Cycloid psychosis*
Genetics	None determined	High morbidity risk in first degree relatives
Stress	Always present	Stress-related, especially the puerperium
Clinical features	High female incidence	High female incidence
	Abrupt onset	Abrupt onset
	Confusion	Confusion
	Swings of mood	Swings of mood
	Short-lived phase of illness	Short-lived phase of illness
	Florid psychosis – incongruent with mood	Florid psychosis – incongruent with mood
	Marked anxiety	Marked anxiety
Course	Full recovery	Full recovery
Treatment	Non-specific – good response to ECT	Non-specific
	Neuroleptics	Neuroleptics
Prognosis	No definite pattern of recurrence	Occurs in relatively short cycles
	No chronicity	No chronicity

3
Depressed mind, disordered brain – I: The neurobiology of depression

The early division of mental disorders into the organic and the functional, and the inclusion of the depressions within the latter, appears increasingly untenable as a growing number of investigations have provided evidence that there is a cerebral basis to many forms of depression.

'Organic psychoses' refer to mental disorders with a tangible and discernible brain pathology. In another sense, it also suggests disorders with a collection of symptoms which may be characteristic, e.g. disturbed consciousness, disorientation. The 'functional' disorders, as presently perceived, have not been deemed to have a tangible organic basis, although the preservation of consciousness in these disorders has always been a prerequisite for their diagnosis.

As has been said, the whole basis of this distinction has been challenged by the results of modern investigatory techniques, although before these became available it had been known that a form of depression, called symptomatic depression, existed in relation to systemic disease. Some of the features of this condition will be referred to in Chapter 4. It will be seen that when systemic illness impinges on brain function, there may follow disorders in mental state such as impaired consciousness and disorientation as well as depression. However, we may now show that such features of the 'organic' mental state as disordered consciousness and disorientation are not specific to the classical organic psychoses such as delirium and dementia. Reactive and cycloid psychoses, features of which were detailed and compared in Chapter 2, often have a prodromal phase in which disordered consciousness or confusion may be prominent. Undifferentiated puerperal psychosis, preceding the emergence of a recognizable depression, may also present with disturbed consciousness. This used to be attributed to 'toxic' factors associated with parturition and after, but even with modern asepsis and antisepsis, when this factor might be presumed to have been considerably reduced, confusion may still be seen, though gross delirium and severe toxic confusional states are now very rare. As for disorientation, the not uncommon problem of depression-induced and depression-related dementia has been addressed by a number of authors and will also be discussed in Chapter 4. There now seems little doubt that a syndrome of dementia can exist in causal relation to depression. This syndrome also demonstrates the feature of greater or lesser reversibility with the resolution of the depression.

The 'organicity' of depression may be further stressed in relation to this distinction between the 'organic' dementias and those dementias that were associated with so-called 'functional' disease, i.e. the 'pseudodementias'. The commonest form of the latter group is depressive illness. The fact that the distinction had to be made with some difficulty was in itself indicative of the similarity in the clinical picture between progressive, irreversible and untreatable dementias on the one hand, and non-progressive, irreversible and untreatable dementias on the other. The subject has been dealt with in detail by Mahendra (1985a). Psychological testing on patients with depressive cognitive disorder demonstrated that specific functions such as repetition, reading and comprehension, naming, verbal delayed recall and recognition, mathematics, finger tapping and motor praxis were spared. (Caine, 1981). Most impaired functions were tasks dependent on attention, mental processing, speech, spontaneous elaboration and analysis of detail. Taken together, Caine believes that these findings are consistent with a picture of impairment in which cortically mediated intellectual functions are spared in depressive cognitive disorder amounting to dementia. Recent work by Gibson (1981) and Weingartner et al. (1982) has thrown more light on the differences in memory impairment in depressives. It is suggested that in depression there is probably a suppression of otherwise normal memory processes, failures in learning being a function of the intensity of the depression, especially when random or unrelated events are being recalled. Their memory failures are most apparent in tasks that require sustained motivation, effort and active processing operations. The extent and detail of the work noted in these examples indicates that memory impairment is a significant feature of depression, probably part of the disease process and no longer merely to be relegated to a consequence of diminished mood.

Another approach in comparing the cognitive impairment of depression with an 'organic' disorder is by considering the symptomatology of dementia. Clinical and psychological findings support the idea of cognitive dysfunction in depression amounting to dementia but without cortical involvement, i.e. as a form of subcortical dementia. The conceptualization of subcortical dementias (Albert et al., 1974; Albert, 1978) has made possible the inclusion of disorders which may be considered in terms which might also be applied to depressive dementia.

The following are features of subcortical dementia:

(1) Emotional or personality changes (typically inertia or apathy, occasionally with outbursts of anger),
(2) Memory disorder,
(3) Defective ability to manipulate acquired knowledge,
(4) Striking slowness in the rate of information processing.

The subcortical dementias are distinguished clinically from the cortical dementias by the preserved vocabulary and facility with language in the former. No aphasias, agnosias or apraxias are seen in them, unlike the cortical dementias. Thus, the cognitive changes occasionally to be found in such conditions as Parkinson's disease, Huntington's chorea, progressive supranuclear palsy, Korsakoff's syndrome, and the commoner type of Alzheimer's disease may be brought under the rubric of dementia. The arrival of this concept also enables a depressive cognitive change of sufficient magnitude to be called a dementia, and the underlying disease process to be investigated in ways similar to that for any other of a large number of conditions giving rise to dementia. In parallel runs the entitlement to note the 'organicity' of depressive cognitive change. The advent of this concept makes depressive dementia reversible, treatable and a form of secondary, subcortical dementia, but no less 'organic' for that.

The premise of 'functional' illness is logically invalid insofar as it makes use of knowledge of the present and does not – and, to be fair, cannot – take account of the advances that are yet to come. When morbid anatomy was the sum total of observable, pathological change, the distinction between 'organic' and 'functional' might have held some validity. However, that time has passed. Neurobiological advances have opened several windows into the structure and function of the brain, and the light that has been let in has helped illuminate some of the dark corners of the room in which psychiatry has been held prisoner. The room is still uncomfortably murky, but other windows are being opened all the time.

These matters are raised further in Chapter 4.

THE CEREBRAL BASIS TO DEPRESSION

This is a complex subject, not least because the picture is as yet a confused one. No attempt is being made to provide a comprehensive overview in this section, and reference may also be made to Chapter 4, where depression in relation to certain cerebral disorders is dealt with, Chapter 5, where therapeutic considerations in depression, in particular psychosurgery, have a bearing on this subject, and Chapter 7, where aggression and violence in relation to depression are discussed.

The *limbic system* looms large in any survey of the cerebral basis of the emotions. It is a term used to describe a collection of nuclei and tracts which are sited mostly on the medial surface of the cerebral hemispheres. The nuclei involved include the amygdaloid nuclei, the septal nuclei, the hypothalamic nuclei, the anterior thalamic nuclei, the dorsal tegmental nucleus and the nuclei in the mammillary bodies and the ventral tegmental area. The gyri which form the main elements of the limbic system include the subcallosal gyrus, the cingulate gyrus, the parahippocampal gyrus, the dentate gyrus and the gyri of the hippocampal formation.

The pathways of the limbic system include the fornix, the stria terminalis, the stria medullaris, the cingulum, the anterior commissure and the medial forebrain bundle.

The limbic system has close links with the basal ganglia, involving the amygdala and the nucleus accumbens, and with the ventral tegmental region of the midbrain, in which are situated numerous dopaminergic neurones.

These are part of the older brain and have close relations with the olfactory apparatus, hence the term rhinencephalon which has been applied to them. They have also been referred to as the 'visceral brain' (Maclean, 1949). The significance in emotional life of these structures was highlighted by Papez, who defined the Papez circuit of hippocampus – mammillary body – thalamus – cingulate gyrus – hippocampus.

As has been suggested, the limbic system is composed of the older parts of the cerebrum – the archicortex and palaeocortex in distinction to the newer brain, the neocortex. This older structure is reflected in the simple microscopic structure in contrast to the complex arrangement of the neocortex. The separation of the old and the new is far from distinct, however, as the older cortex has links with the parts of the neocortex to which it is anatomically close, such as the temporal and frontal cortex, and has functional links with the basal ganglia, thalamus, hypothalamus and with the midbrain through the medial forebrain bundle. The fornix is a major efferent system from the hippocampus to the septal region and the anterior thalamic nuclei. The septal region has important links with the nucleus accumbens. Efferent fibres from the septal region pass in the medial forebrain bundle to the tegmental area of the midbrain. This bundle contains large numbers of monoaminergic fibres. The septal nuclei are linked to the amygdaloid nuclei by the stria terminalis, and to the habenular nuclei through the stria medullaris.

The limbic system, therefore, is a complex enough structural entity. The functional role it plays appears to be infinitely more complicated and is far from being understood. It is altogether too simplistic, and almost certainly incorrect, to consider the structure and function separately of each of the anatomical structures that go to form the limbic system. At the simplest level, it is safest to say that the whole is more than the sum of the parts; that the limbic system is not the exclusive intermediary in the experience and expression of the emotions, but is probably more intimately involved in emotional functions than other parts of the brain; that a lesion in one structure has effects on the structure and function of other components of the limbic system, and that it is futile to talk of a lesion in one specific structure in the system; noxious or therapeutic agents probably have effects on all even when gross cerebral effects, and their more obvious behavioural manifestations, are not seen.

For depression, the significant components of the limbic system appear to be the orbital surface of the frontal lobe, the cingulate gyrus, the dorsomedial nucleus of the thalamus and the hypothalamus. The orbital surface of the frontal lobe receives afferent fibres from the dorsomedial nucleus of the thalamus and its efferent fibres travel via the medial forebrain bundle to the hypothalamus and the reticular formation. Efferents also project via the cingulum to the hippocampus. The cingulate gyrus also receives fibres from the anterior nuclei of the thalamus, and its efferent fibres project to the anterior thalamic nuclei, the hippocampus and the hypothalamus.

The modulation of the functions of the limbic system is by higher cortical activity, especially that of the frontal lobe. When these fibres are severed, important emotional responses seem both to be suppressed as well as facilitated, and is thus undertaken in psychosurgery. A small lesion in the widespread connections between the cingulum, the orbital surface of the frontal lobe, the hypothalamus and some other parts of the limbic system is sufficient to bring about symptomatic change and is undertaken in psychosurgery (see Chapter 5).

Although the minute structures which comprise the limbic system underlie emotional expression, including depression, it is not usually practicable to study these. The cerebral hemispheres, in their gross structure and general function, have been subjected to inquiry in order to overcome these obvious difficulties. Some of the findings in relation to cerebral hemisphere function and depression are referred to in Chapter 4. A variety of approaches have been utilized, especially non-dominant cerebral function whose activity has been alleged to be impaired in depression. Visual memory, as opposed to verbal memory, is claimed to be a function of the non-dominant hemisphere and said to be impaired in depression. Electro-convulsive treatment (ECT), by alleviating the depression, may be predicted to produce an improvement in this function. However, it has also been long claimed that ECT may produce short term impairment of memory function following its use. Kronfol et al. (1978) found that a number of cognitive functions which have their basis in the non-dominant hemisphere were affected in relation to the depression and appeared to be more affected than dominant hemisphere function, usually of a verbal type. These dysfunctions preceded the use of ECT in those patients. The patients were given unilateral ECT, half of them receiving unilateral dominant hemisphere ECT and the other half receiving unilateral non-dominant hemisphere ECT. The result was that though dominant hemisphere ECT impaired dominant hemisphere-related memory functions, non-dominant hemisphere ECT actually facilitated non-dominant hemisphere-related memory function. The unilateral group showed a highly significant increase on scores of visual testing, while the bilateral group, though showing improvement, did not progress to the same extent. The explanation appears to be that the visual memory problems are due to a lesion in the non-dominant hemisphere which is related, perhaps causally, to the depression and when the depression is alleviated, there is improvement in such measurable non-dominant hemisphere functions as visual memory. It is thus possible to suggest a localization of both depression and visual memory in the non-dominant cerebral hemisphere. Lishman (1968) found that with penetrating wounds of the head affective symptoms were more likely to arise when the lesions involved the right hemisphere, with the frontal lobe being especially prone to manifesting these symptoms. However Keschner et al. (1936) had observed that among their patients with temporal lobe tumours who became depressed, the majority had left-sided lesions.

As will be seen in Chapter 4, the depression associated with strokes appears to be related to dominant hemisphere lesions. The siting of the lesion following a stroke is important in emotional expression. These findings in stroke victims are also related to the aphasia seen in those patients who have sustained a dominant hemisphere lesion. The incapacity with language and the subsequently severely curtailed ability to communicate has been alleged to produce a reactive depression. Lesions of the non-dominant hemisphere, especially those with parietal lobe involvement, may lead to an agnosia regarding bodily incapacity. This morbid ignorance may lead to unconcern, or an 'indifference' that has been noted in another context. However, the gross anatomical setting of the lesion is, perhaps, less important than the functional disruption in limbic system activity, a point which has already been made.

Another approach to the cerebral basis of depression was illustrated by Terzian *et al.* (1964) who injected amylobarbitone sodium into the carotid arteries. Injection into the left carotid artery, in addition to producing obvious neurological symptoms such as transient hemiplegia and aphasia, also produced a depressive reaction – including feelings of guilt, of nothingness, worries about the self, the future and relatives. This reaction was less transient than the neurological features which pass off with the effects of the drug. Thus, it might be claimed that the neurological and psychological features were independently produced by the lesion induced by the drug. When the injection was made into the right carotid artery, the reaction was one of elation, the subjects showing a transient manic picture, which was associated with quite marked, though transient, neurological features of non-dominant cerebral dysfunction.

These lesions – one produced by gross pathology, the other an induced, transient dysfunction – localize depression to the dominant hemisphere. In contrast, and in keeping with the findings of some other studies quoted in the foregoing paragraphs, some work on epilepsy and related EEG studies point to non-dominant or right-sided cerebral hemisphere involvement. D'Elia and Perris (1973) showed that in 'psychotic' depression there was right hemisphere dominance of EEG patterns, which implies the left hemisphere is affected to a greater extent. But in epileptics with involvement of the temporal lobes, Flor-Henry (1969) claimed that psychoses with left temporal lobe involvement are largely of a schizophreniform kind, while manic-depressive psychosis featured in those with the right temporal lobe involvement. A problem in assessing claims such as this is that patients with epilepsy and mental disorder are a selected group and, moreover, dysfunction in epilepsy may indicate increased function at the site of lesion, as in most forms of idiopathic epilepsy, or reduced activity of the lobe which may result from such conditions as trauma.

It is too simplistic to think of either the dominant or non-dominant cerebral hemisphere as having exclusive rights in the matter of producing depression. In reality, a complex balance probably obtains. When a lesion of the dominant hemisphere occurs, there is a tendency for the functions of the non-dominant hemisphere, presumably predominantly depressant, to take the upper hand. When irritative epileptic lesions occur in the non-dominant hemisphere, this naturally depressant tendency is allowed play. But, as has already been suggested, the gross or accessible cerebral phenomena do not take into account the deeper neurobiological reality as projected by the limbic system. It would seem reasonable to suggest that the depression is due to limbic system involvement which may be brought about by dominant or non-dominant hemisphere involvement. This would explain the presence of non-dominant hemisphere associated clinical features, e.g. visual memory impairment even when the pathology is localized to the dominant cerebral hemisphere.

INVESTIGATIONS IN DEPRESSION

The instruments of neuropsychiatric investigation lead to further evidence of the involvement of the brain in depression. The methods of evaluation are necessarily crude and do little justice to the complexities of the neurobiological substrate underlying the condition, but at the very least they provide further support for questioning the justification for considering depression to be part of the 'functional' illnesses. They are also important factors in providing the biological counterpoint to the thesis on which this book rests, that depression results from the interaction of biological and constitutional factors on the one hand, and social and environmental ones on the other. The latter have been discussed in detail in the previous chapter, and this chapter is devoted to the consideration of the case for the former. Although a separation of each element in the equation has been made for purposes of clarity and convenience, the reader must, for the present, provide the synthesis in his own mind as precise details of how such an interaction may come about are, as yet, unknown.

Psychological testing

Investigations of this type extend, refine and quantify clinical assessment in depression. Some psychological test findings have been referred to in the preliminary critique of the 'functional' nature of depression. At one level, the lowered mood and the diminished volition on the part of the patient leads to impaired functioning on psychological testing. Furthermore, the intactness of language function in depression has been commented on; also, reference has been made to differences in hemisphere function, with the relative preservation of dominant hemisphere activity.

Commonsense approaches to interpreting lowered efficiency in completing psychological tests have been challenged by several workers. Coughlan and Hollows (1984) showed that the degree of depression, as measured by a mood scale, did not significantly correlate with performance on memory testing, except for forced-choice face recognition.

However, Rush et al. (1983), when evaluating the neuropsychological performance of patients with mild to moderately severe depression, confirmed previous studies which had reported deficits on cognitive, memory and information processing tasks in depressed patients. They also claimed that 'endogenous' depressives were especially affected in trail-making tasks, when compared to the 'non-endogenous' depressives, which they explained in part by the severity of the condition in the former as trail-making is a timed, visuo-motor task which may be affected by motor function, which is affected by psychomotor retardation.

71

Taylor *et al.* (1981) noted that while neuropsychological testing in schizophrenic patients revealed bilateral hemispheric dysfunction, patients with affective disorder showed mainly impairment on tasks of non-dominant hemisphere function. An extension of the neuropsychological testing of hemisphere function is by dichotic listening techniques in which different information is presented simultaneously to each ear. This technique is also useful in studying cerebral lateralization in normal subjects. On the basis that there is greater evidence of right than left hemisphere dysfunction on neuropsychological testing in depressed patients, Yozawitz *et al.* (1979) used ear asymmetries on dichotic measure as a test for lateralized hemispheric dysfunctions which they hypothesized were different in affective and schizophrenic disorders. Ear asymmetries of affective patients were similar to those of controls with right temporal lobe lesions and differed from those of schizophrenic patients and normal controls. This report presented evidence of ear asymmetries for the dichotic perceptual performance of affective psychotic patients for both verbal and non-verbal stimuli, thus furnishing further support for the hypothesis of right hemisphere dysfunction in these patients.

The benign, remittent nature of manic-depression may also be confirmed by psychological testing. This is especially important in treated patients who may have been subjected to a variety of physical treatments including long-term antidepressant drugs, e.g. lithium, repeated ECT and psychosurgery. To the possibility of unresolved symptomatology is added the hazards of the long-term sequelae of treatment. However, Kerry *et al.* (1983) studied manic-depressive patients and showed that it is a disorder from which the patient can hope to make a complete recovery without any cognitive deterioration in spite of drug and other physical treatment. The manic-depressive patients in their study showed no cognitive deterioration despite long and severe illness. Their patients had had frequent ECT, psychotropic drugs and even pre-frontal leucotomy, all of which might have, in theory, affected their cognitive functioning. In spite of many attacks they had no measurable deterioration. This study confirms that depressed patients can recover without any cognitive impairment due either to their illness or treatments.

Cerebral blood flow

The basis for cerebral blood flow measurement has been discussed by Mahendra (1984a). It is necessary, as that review showed, to be aware of the large number of variables and the normal physiological variation possible when assessing the results of tests. But the results of Uytdenhoef *et al.* (1983) seemed to offer support for the findings of gross dysfunction in the cerebral hemispheres, although the abnormality was limited to certain regions rather than the whole of the hemispheres. These workers used the [133]Xenon inhalation technique to study regional cerebral blood flow in depressed patients, and found a left frontal hypervascularization and a right posterior hypovascularization in depressed patients. This, they found, was state-dependent. The bilateral dysfunction they noted was in keeping with the findings of clinical assessment, neuropsychological evaluation and EEG results. They claimed the results suggested the existence of sub-types of depression, 'major depressive episodes' being related to a bilateral though asymmetrical cerebral dysfunction.

Neuroradiology

Air encephalography produced the early results of any significance in the neuroradiological assessment of depressed patients. Nott and Fleminger (1975) found that a significant proportion of depressed patients with cognitive dysfunction shared minor degrees of sulcal widening or ventricular enlargement on the air encephalogram.

Standish-Barry et al. (1982) demonstrated abnormalities in brain structure in terms of ventricular enlargement in those patients with severe affective illness by both pneumencephalography and computerized axial tomography (CAT). Standish-Barry's group of refractory depressed patients was being evaluated for psychosurgery, but the recurrent ECT which this group of patients is invariably subjected to does not appear to produce ventricular enlargement, a point made by Johnstone et al. (1976).

The advent of the CAT head scan led to its widespread use in psychiatry. Indices such as cortical atrophy and ventricular enlargement were not initially successful in correlating with any diagnostic group (see Mahendra, 1984a for discussion). Jacoby and Levy (1980) using this technique, however, could show that a group of affective patients found themselves intermediate between senile demented patients and control subjects. They also found that a greater number of depressed patients had enlarged ventricles, and attributed this finding to the possibility that a subgroup of elderly patients may exist who have a cerebral 'organic' factor underlying their depression. These patients were also seen to be older, less anxious and more 'endogenous' on the Newcastle scale. In addition these patients, over a period of 2 years from the time of the scan, had a significantly higher mortality rate compared to depressive patients with normal scans. Thus it has been suggested (Jacoby, 1981) that the CAT scan may play a part in prognosticating the course of depression in old age.

A more refined measure on CAT scanning is the attenuation of radiodensity (see Mahendra, 1984a for discussion). Jacoby et al. (1983) studied brain tissue radiodensity by CAT scans in depressed patients, senile dements and controls, and found that the depressives resembled the dements more than they did the controls. Also, when there was ventricular dilatation in depressed patients, this index was found to be associated with lower values of brain tissue radiodensity. Naeser et al. (1980) showed that when the attenuation density (CAT numbers) of patients with depressive dementia had been compared with those with pre-senile dementia of the Alzheimer type, it was possible to distinguish the latter on account of their lower radiodensity numbers.

Jacoby et al. (1983) showed that in depressed patients ventricular dilatation, which they had already shown to predict increased mortality, was associated with lower levels of brain tissue density. This association

73

between ventricular enlargement and low brain tissue density was confined to depressed patients, which suggests that ventricular enlargement does not necessarily correlate with low brain density. It is also not a feature which can be explained by age.

Roberts and Lishman (1984), reviewing the results of CAT head scans of 323 patients referred by psychiatrists, found that more than half the patients appeared to have abnormal scans, and it could also be seen that the group of patients with affective psychosis had the highest percentage diagnosis of 'definite' and 'equivocal' abnormal scans, exceeded only by the group with organic psychosis.

Johnstone *et al.* (1986) suggested that an abnormal ventricular brain ratio found in 19% of their manic-depressive patients might be related to hypothyroidism which might have a direct effect on the central nervous system leading to lateral ventricular enlargement.

Thus it would appear that although CAT scan results in depression do not give rise to unequivocal findings, there seems to be a minority of patients, inhabiting, perhaps, a subgroup of the condition whose radiological appearances put them between normal control subjects and those with definite 'organic' pathology. Apart from providing further evidence for the heterogeneity of depressive illness it calls into question the 'functional' nature of some forms of depression by focusing our attention on the less tangible forms of brain disorder which may be brought to light by technical innovation.

The electroencephalograph (EEG)

Some basic points as regards the EEG have been discussed in the chapter pertaining to that subject in Mahendra (1984a).

There is reasonably good evidence that overall there is greater abnormality in the EEG of depressed patients as compared with normal control subjects, and in particular in depressed female patients. Alpha activity is reduced, in general, with a lower mean frequency in depression. Correspondingly, there is increased beta and delta activity.

However, as with cerebral blood flow and other neurophysiological measures, the limits of normal variation are extensive. Treatment is one possible source of artifact. Thus, the overall increase in EEG abnormality could possibly be attributed to a previous neurophysiological dysfunction antedating the depression, or to a lesion that may produce both EEG abnormality and subsequent depression, e.g. brain trauma.

The role of cerebral hemisphere dysfunction in the causation of depression has been discussed before. The EEG is a valuable tool in the investigation of epilepsy-related depression. Perris (1980) notes that most authors have pointed out that temporal lobe abnormalities occur more frequently in the left hemisphere than on the right. As we have seen, there is support for right hemisphere involvement in depression. If one regards these depressions as not necessarily secondary depressive reactions, then one may suggest that the EEG abnormality from the temporal lobe reflects both the epilepsy and the depression.

74

Photic stimulation leads to an alpha-blocking response (ABR). It is possible to quantify this, and studies have been undertaken on depressed patients. Perris (1980) shows that the results of most of these investigations are fairly consistent and have shown that the duration of the ABR is longer in patients with retarded depression compared to normal controls, and becomes shorter with successful treatment of the depression. The explanation for this phenomenon is unclear. It has been suggested that the extent of blocking or attenuation of alpha rhythm is a measure of cortical arousal and is determined by the level of activity in the reticular activating system. Thus an explanation of the longer ABR in depression may be related to an increased level of arousal. However, as Perris notes, the results may also be explained in terms of the decreased level of activity in the RAS. Thus, although it can be postulated that subcortical cerebral systems are affected in some way in depression, it is still not clear what the nature of the abnormality and the consequences of this are.

Hendrickson *et al.* (1979) studied the cortical evoked responses to auditory and somatosensory stimuli in elderly depressed patients. This followed the work of Levy *et al.* (1971) who had shown that senile dements had a delay in the appearance of the average evoked response (AER) to somatosensory stimuli. Hendrickson *et al.* (1979) found that this delay was greatest in dements, less so in depressives and least with normal controls. This, of course, accords with the CAT scan findings this group of workers later found with senile depressives, which was discussed in the previous section. The authors made a case for a 'subclinical organic change' in senile depression, and argued for the facilitation of depression in old age by these changes.

Perris (1980) has also discussed the quantitative measure, the mean integrated amplitude (MIA) and its within-patient variance (WPV). This appears to be a fruitful approach both to the objective study of the severity of the clinical state and the changes after treatment. Attention has been paid to integrating the electrical activity of homologous areas of both hemispheres. Results seem to indicate that significant changes in the shape, modality and organization of the distribution of EEG amplitudes accords with the degree of severity of the psychopathology. Instead of studying each hemisphere singly, the differential activity of both hemispheres is taken into account. In depression there appears to be an inter-hemispheric difference in the MIA with a significant bilateral increase in MIA following treatment. The variations of the MIA and WPV appear to be one of the most consistent neurophysiological correlates of depression.

The EEG is discussed again in a further section on sleep disorders in depression. This has been a key neurophysiological investigatory tool in seeking objective evidence of the sleep disorder manifested in depression. The sleep disturbance in depression concerns the excess of time spent awake and in 'sub-sleep' and reduction in stages 1 and 4 and in REM sleep. There is also a reduction in total time asleep as well as a broken sleep pattern. These indices all improve as the depression lifts, and clinicians have long considered an improvement in sleep patterns to be an early indication of improvement in depression. Shortened REM latency, i.e. the time interval to the first appearance of the REM rhythm has been consistently found in depression. It has been claimed (see Perris, 1980) that this shortening in the REM latency is seen in primary, and not in secondary, depression, hence being a possible biological marker for the former condition. It has also been noted that sharp, spike patterns are seen in the sleeping EEG of manic-depressive patients. Perris also notes that a significantly higher incidence of paroxysmal features (mainly positive spikes, paroxysmal slow, focal spikes and small, sharp spikes) were reported in the waking or sleeping EEG of the patients with suicidal symptoms and assaultive behaviour. Some biological aspects of violent behaviour are taken up further in Chapter 7.

Thus the evidence from neuropsychological testing, neuroradiology and EEG leads one to suspect that 'organic' factors are present in, at least, some forms of depression. The changes to be noted by these investigations are far less marked than in cases of discrete brain pathology. However, that has never been in dispute. The point at issue is whether depression is qualitatively different from those disorders that demonstrate an obvious brain pathology. The answer appears to be the difference is quantitative, and this enables us to challenge the concept of 'functional' disorder which has been the basis of the classification of depression. In as much as 'organic' pathology continues to be revealed by secular, technical advance, the concept of functional illness is called further into question.

NEUROCHEMISTRY

The important substances in the neurochemistry of depression appear to be, in the present state of knowledge, the catecholamines, noradrenaline and dopamine, serotonin (5-hydroxytryptamine, 5-HT) and, to a lesser extent, acetylcholine.

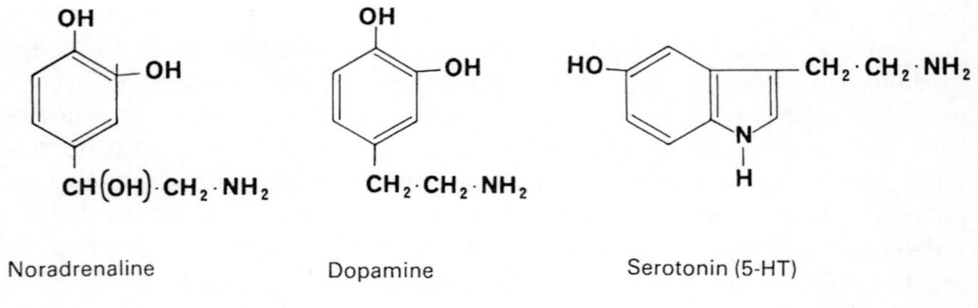

Noradrenaline   Dopamine   Serotonin (5-HT)

Figure 3 The major neurotransmitters

The cell bodies for the catecholamines and 5-HT are situated mainly in the tegmentum of the midbrain, the pons and the medulla oblongata, i.e. in the brainstem. The fibres, therefore, project from the lower centres to those higher up.

Noradrenaline (NA)

The noradrenergic neurones are located in the *locus coeruleus*, and fibres project to both the cerebral and the cerebellar cortex, and the nuclei of the hypothalamus.

There appear to be two 'systems'. In the first, fibres project from cells in the medulla and pons to terminations in the lower brainstem, the midbrain and diencephalon. The fibres from the locus coeruleus project to the lower brainstem, the cerebral and cerebellar cortex and the hippocampus. This system is behaviourally probably the more important is that it appears to have effects on arousal as well as sleep.

The synthesis of both noradrenaline and dopamine starts with the amino acid, tyrosine.

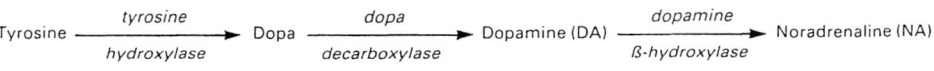

Figure 4   The synthesis of dopamine and noradrenaline

The tyrosine hydroxylase in the normal state is saturated with tyrosine, hence it is thought it is not possible to increase catecholamine synthesis by increasing the supply of tyrosine in the brain (*cf* 5-HT synthesis from tryptophan). This has, however, been questioned by Van Praag (1982).

Noradrenaline is water soluble and does not readily breach the blood–brain barrier. It is metabolized by methylation and oxidative deamination, catalysed by catechol-3-O-methyltransferase (COMT) and oxidative deamination by monoamine oxidase (MAO), to produce 3-methoxy-4-hydroxyphenylglycol (MHPG) as the end product. This is excreted in part in the urine, and it has been estimated that up to 60% of urinary MHPG may have a central origin. The levels of MHPG in the urine, when estimated, had a vogue in both the classification and treatment of depression, but it now appears this might have been taking a too simple view of matters. Bipolar depressives were held to show a lower excretion of MHPG than unipolar depressives, and a differential response to imipramine (more effective in those who have low output of urinary MHPG) and amitriptyline (more effective in those with normal or high levels of output of MHPG).

As Van Praag (1982) has discussed, imipramine potentiates NA more strongly than it does 5-HT; the converse applies to amitriptyline, and desipramine potentiates NA selectively. It is thus possible that low MHPG excretors respond well to imipramine and desipramine because they are deficient in NA, while high MHPG excretors respond better to amitriptyline because they are 5-HT deficient.

Maas *et al.* (1972) have shown that MHPG excretion is reduced in depression with 'endogenous' features, especially in those patients with the bipolar form of the illness, and also in the depressive variety of schizoaffective psychoses.

Vanillyl mandelic acid (VMA) is the main peripheral metabolite of noradrenaline. The mono-amine oxidases exist as iso-enzymes. MAO-A metabolizes both NA and 5-HT, whereas types A and B metabolize DA. An example of MAOI-A is clorgyline which may thus elevate the levels of NA, DA and 5-HT. MAOI-B, such as deprenyl, only elevates brain DA levels.

Dopamine (DA)

There are three major brain DA systems:

(1) The nigro—striatal pathway arises from cell bodies in the *substantia nigra* of the midbrain and projects to the *corpus striatum* (made up of the caudate nucleus, globus pallidum and the putamen) and the central amygdaloid nucleus. This pathway is involved in Parkinson's disease.

(2) The meso–limbic pathway arises from cell bodies in the ventral tegmental area and projects to the *nucleus accumbens*, the olfactory tubercle and cerebral cortex. This pathway may be involved in the schizophrenias.

(3) The tubero–infundibular pathway arises from neurones in the arcuate nucleus of the hypothalamus and innervates the median eminence, and is thus above the level of the brainstem. This pathway is concerned with the control and release of a number of pituitary hormones.

Like NA, DA is water-soluble and does not readily cross the blood–brain barrier. The metabolism of DA is similar to that of NA, the chief metabolite being homovanillic acid (HVA).

The role of dopamine in depression is unclear. There is a suspicion that there may be an involvement of the DA system in the motor disturbance of depression rather than with the affective disorder itself. Van Praag and Korf (1971) showed that in depression with marked motor retardation, the accumulation of HVA in the cerebrospinal fluid is diminished to the same extent as in Parkinson's disease. L-Dopa stimulates increased motor activity, but has only indirect effects on the mood.

Serotonin (5-hydroxytryptamine, 5-HT)

5-HT neurones are found in the median and dorsal raphe nuclei in the region of the midline of the pons and midbrain. They project to the diencephalon, the medulla, spinal cord, cerebellum and the forebrain, including the neocortex and the striatum. Neurones in the raphe system thus project upwards as well as downwards.

The 5-HT neurones of the raphe and reticular systems are thought to have an inhibitory effect on the post-synaptic neurones, and are involved in the regulation of a variety of brain functions including sleep, temperature, sexual and aggressive behaviour, responsiveness to pain and other stimuli,

feeding, posture, motor activity and neuroendocrine regulation.
A schematic representation of 5-HT metabolism is given in Figure 5.

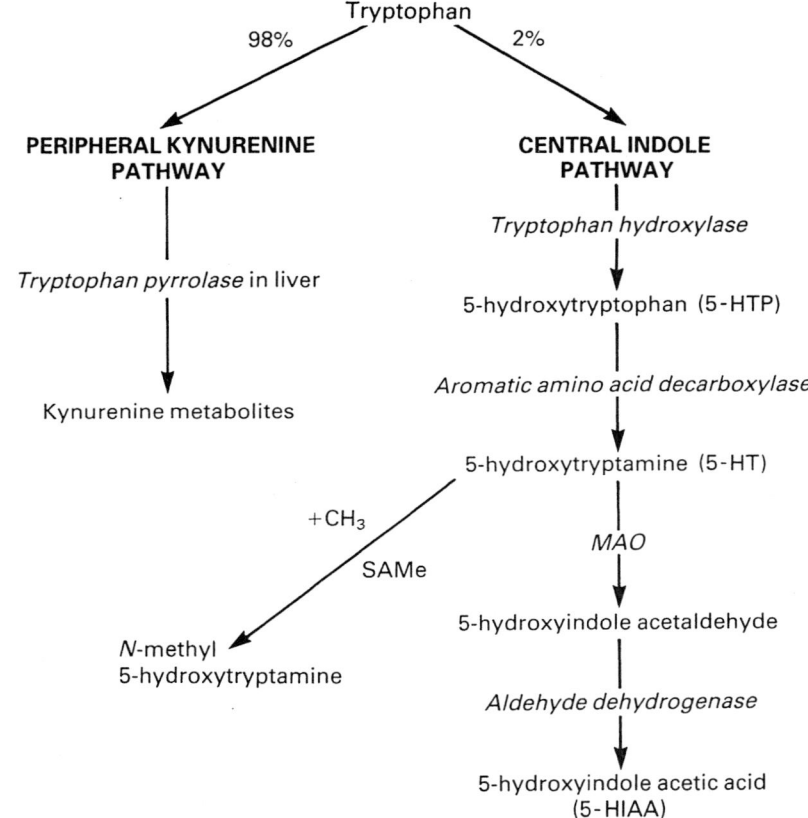

Figure 5 Schematic representation of 5-HT metabolism

As is shown, the synthesis of brain 5-HT is only a minor pathway of tryptophan metabolism, as peripheral metabolism accounts for some 98% of the total. The rate-limiting enzyme for 5-HT synthesis in the brain (tryptophan hydroxylase) is normally not saturated with tryptophan, thus increasing its availability to the brain increases brain 5-HT synthesis. The supply of the precursor, tryptophan, depends largely on the level of free plasma tryptophan. Curzon *et al.* (1980) showed that plasma-free (but not total) tryptophan concentration correlated significantly with both lumbar and ventricular 5-hydroxyindole acetic acid (5-HIAA) concentrations, this being the principal metabolite of 5-HT in the brain.

An important extracerebral pathway of tryptophan metabolism involves the action on it of the liver enzyme, tryptophan pyrrolase, which can be induced by its own substrate tryptophan. Increased pyrrolase activity would divert tryptophan from 5-HT formation, and also lead to the formation of pyrrolase pathway metabolites such as kynurenine which may reduce transport of tryptophan into the brain. Thus the optimum clinical dose of L-tryptophan, when used to treat depression, is considered to be about 3–4 g/day (Binnie, 1982). Higher doses are believed to induce tryptophan pyrrolase, and are associated with a poor therapeutic outcome.

An increase or decrease in 5-HT concentration and turnover is reflected in the levels of brain 5-HIAA which in turn is reflected in the concentration of lumbar CSF 5-HIAA to the extent of about 70%.

5-HT neurones lie in close functional relationship to both NA and DA neurones. Stimulation of the raphe nuclei produces depression of neuronal firing in areas of dense 5-HT innervation such as the substantia nigra where there are many DA cell bodies (Eccleston, 1982). Experiments in animals suggest a local feedback inhibitory mechanism, whereby when DA is released during the activity of the system, adjacent 5-HT neurones are stimulated to release 5-HT which then causes inhibition of further DA release (Figure 6).

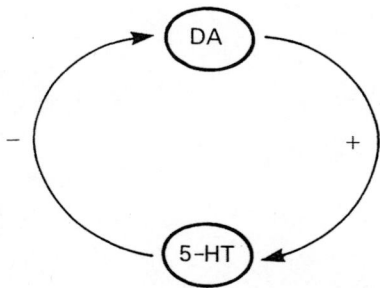

Figure 6 Local feedback inhibition of DA

If DA neurones are under the tonic control of the 5-HT system, then chemically 'switching off' (for example, by the inhibitor, p-chloro-phenylalanine) the 5-HT neurones will release DA cells from the inhibition. Eccleston and Nicolaou (1978) have shown that when tryptophan plus a MAO inhibitor is given to rats, both DA and NA turnover is increased (consequent upon post-synaptic 5-HT receptor blockade), suggesting that 5-HT exhibits an inhibitory control of the NA system as well as the DA system. Jenner et al. (1983) have also reviewed the inhibitory role of 5-HT on cerebral DA mechanisms. L-Dopa administered to man and rat also reduce brain tryptophan and 5-HT content. Also, animal behavioural experimental work has suggested that enhancing 5-HT action in the brain may diminish DA-mediated effects.

Maj (1981) has suggested that 5-HT antagonists may release a 'serotonergic' brake on neurones leading to an increased NA turnover and availability. Gerson and Baldessarini (1980), summarizing the motor effects of 5-HT in the CNS, have pointed out that increase or decrease of brain 5-HT generally tends to respectively decrease and increase responses to catecholamine agonists such as amphetamines, and suggest some effects of 5-HT may be mediated through catecholaminergic systems.

The level of 5-HT activity as a trait characteristic will be discussed in relation to the role of 5-HT function in violent behaviour in Chapter 7.

It has also been shown that stress produces a larger fall in plasma tryptophan levels in depressed patients than in control subjects (Shaw et al., 1980). As has been indicated, the 5-HT neurones need tryptophan mainly for manufacturing protein, but also for the relatively small, but vital, sideline of synthesizing 5-HT. It has been argued that if 5-HT production falters, the post-synaptic 5-HT neurones may become more excitable, leading to a decreased activity in times of stress, and, conversely, overactivity when there is a rise in tryptophan levels, e.g. with diurnal variation.

5-HT is also synthesized in the neurones in the pineal gland and is also a precursor of melatonin. The relationship of melatonin to depression is unclear, and will be taken up in a later section. Melatonin administration may lead to increased 5-HT levels (Mullen and Silman, 1977); however, some depressed patients have had a worsening of their clinical state following melatonin administration (Carman et al., 1976).

5-HT may also play a part in the release of various pituitary hormones, and the relation of this to increased cortisol production is taken up in a later section.

OTHER PUTATIVE TRANSMITTERS AND ASSOCIATED AGENTS

Cholinergic fibres of the ascending reticular system are found as dorsal tegmental tracts which terminate in the tectal, pretectal, geniculate and thalamic areas, and ventral tegmental tracts which project to the hypothalamus and the basal forebrain area. Cholinergic mechanisms are found in the regions of the brainstem, the basal forebrain areas and in the forebrain–limbic–midbrain circuit of the limbic system. It is now thought that these subcortical cholinergic mechanisms which project to the cortex are of major importance in the pathogenesis of Alzheimer's disease and are discussed in detail in Mahendra (1984a).

Somatostatin is a peptide which was originally thought to reside in the hypothalamus and inhibit growth hormone (GH) but is now known to have an extensive distribution elsewhere in the body. It is also now known to influence the release and turnover of both aminergic (NA, DA, 5-HT) and cholinergic (acetylcholine) neurotransmitters which, in turn, modulate somatostatin release (Rubinow et al., 1983). There is evidence that some of the symptoms of depression may be produced by somatostatin, e.g. alteration in motor activity, decrease in REM and total sleep, increase or decrease in eating behaviour and diminished response to painful stimuli. Although depressed patients show significantly lower levels of CSF somatostatin than controls, the severity of depression does not correlate with the level of CSF somatostatin.

Another putative transmitter is vasopressin which is found in high concentration in the hypothalamus as well as the *locus coeruleus*, which is also the site of much NA activity. The role of vasopressin in memory function has been referred to in relation to dementia (Mahendra, 1984a) and Gold *et al.* (1978) have suggested that the memory disorder commonly seen in depression may have a basis also in terms of vasopressin activity. Vasopressin also influences pain thresholds, the synchronization of biological rhythms, REM sleep, and the regulation of fluid and electrolyte balance.

The role of sodium retention has attracted considerable interest. There is known to be a positive sodium balance in depression, and depressed patients appear to show an inhibition of aldosterone secretion. The sodium retention has, therefore, been attributed to a primary deficiency in the aldosterone–angiotensin–renin system. Cells, including neurones, maintain potassium within the cell and sodium outside by an active process involving the enzyme $NA^+K^+ATPase$. In depression, this active process appears to become impaired. Naylor *et al.* (1973) have suggested that in depression $Na^+K^+ATPase$ may be working less efficiently.

Matters were taken further after it was found that vanadium is a natural inhibitor of $Na^+K^+ATPase$. Dick *et al.* (1981) have found higher than normal levels of vanadium in both depressed and manic patients. In an effort to reduce levels of vanadium, Naylor *et al.* (1981) gave low vanadium diets, vitamin E (a reducing agent) and the chelating agent EDTA to depressed patients, and found there was an improvement in the mood state.

There is indirect evidence for a role for both calcium and magnesium in depression. As is shown in Chapter 6, in connection with the hypercalcaemia of malignancy, there appears to be a relationship between high serum calcium and depression. The high serum calcium levels associated with parathyroid tumours are associated with depression, and a reduction of calcium levels following surgery produces an improvement in mood (Jimerson *et al.*, 1979). ECT has been shown to produce a fall in both serum and CSF calcium (Carman *et al.*, 1977). A similar fall in magnesium after ECT has been reported by Frizel *et al.* (1969). It appears that calcium is essential for the release of hypothalamic and pituitary hormones, whose functioning may be impaired by abnormal calcium levels (Fink and Ottoson, 1980). A fall in extracellular calcium may well lead to a rise in intracellular levels and normal control activity may be resumed.

The effects on the immune system of depression are fascinating. Its role in bereavement has already been touched upon in Chapter 2, and the relationship between malignancy and depression will be considered in Chapter 6. There may be a suppression of the immune system in depressed patients (Kronfol *et al.*, 1983). De Lisi *et al.* (1984) reported on serum immunoglobulin concentrations in psychiatric patients. They were uncertain whether this was a primary phenomenon associated with an infectious or auto-immune basis to the disorders, or secondary to the primary disease process, to long-term drug treatment, or a result of an unrecognized systemic disease occurring at the same time as the depression. The authors commented on the low serum IgM levels that were found in depressed patients and on trends for patients with low, but normal serum IgA levels to be associated with greater clinical improvement on discharge. As low levels of circulating immunoglobulins may indicate an inability to mount a response to infections, or to the proliferation of cancer cells, follow-up of depressed patients with low IgM with a view to ascertaining whether they fell prey to increased infections, cancer or other systemic disease may prove instructive.

Possible modes of transmitter action

Early speculation on the possible modes of action of the amines and other putative transmitters and associated agents was influenced largely by what was known about the actions of several drugs, some psychotropic and others only accidentally so. Reserpine, an antihypertensive agent, is known to deplete neurones of catecholamines. This, as has been referred to in a previous section, is now thought to involve a genetic mechanism in susceptible individuals, and about 20% of patients given reserpine become depressed. In the opposite direction, antituberculosis agents such as iproniazid and isoniazid were seen to have euphoriant actions which were later attributed to their monoamine oxidase inhibiting properties. Some years later when the tricyclic antidepressant drugs were found to inhibit the re-uptake of catecholamine, the amine hypothesis of depression was formulated in its simplest form (Figure 7).

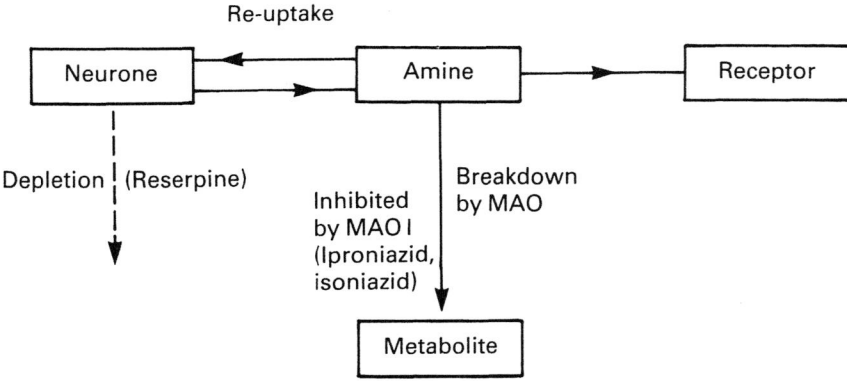

Figure 7 The simplest forms of biogenic amine action

Depression was thought to be due to the unavailability of the amine, which might have been the result of depleted storage and therefore release. Conversely, an increase in availability to the receptor by the accumulation of the amine, whether by inhibition of its breakdown or its re-uptake into the neurone, led to a dispersal of the depression.

As for 5-HT, interest in its role as a psychotropic agent extends from the time its chemical relationship to lysergic acid diethylamide (LSD) became known. Thus, it was suggested, depression may be due to a deficiency of NA (Schildkraut, 1965) or 5-HT (Coppen, 1967). In many ways involvement of 5-HT mechanisms is the more comprehensible and wide-ranging of the two, and it will be taken up first.

A feature very familiar to psychiatrists is the symptomatology that is common to depression and mania, conditions otherwise regarded as 'polar' opposites. Insomnia, poor appetite and weight loss, increased libido, physical overactivity, irritability and aggression, anxiety and agitation are some of the features that may be seen in both conditions, leading to the suspicion that a common mechanism underlies these symptoms. Many of these features are also linked to reduced 5-HT activity which has been noted in both depression and mania. Moreover, the effectiveness of lithium – which has a potent 5-HT agonist activity – as an antidepressive and antimanic agent is established. In an effort to understand this feature, a 'permissive' role has been postulated for 5-HT (Prange et al., 1974). It would appear that inadequate 5-HT function permits instability in the CNS making it more vulnerable. Thus a deficit in central indoleaminergic transmission permits affective disorder but is insufficient for its cause; it is argued that it is the changes in central catecholaminergic transmission, when they occur in the context of a deficit in indoleaminergic transmission, that cause the affective disorders and determine their nature, catecholaminergic transmission being elevated in mania and diminished in depression.

About half the studies have linked low 5-HIAA levels with depression. Asberg et al. (1976) found 'bimodal' sets of high and low values of a distribution of CSF 5-HIAA among depressed patients. Coppen et al. (1972) and Van Praag (1980) found no increase in CSF 5-HIAA following improvement in depression, which would argue for stability of 5-HT metabolism in a given individual. Van Praag (1980) has also reported that depressed patients with low 5-HIAA levels have responded more favourably than those with higher levels to the 5-HT precursor, 5-HTP, to clomipramine and the two in combination. 5-HTP increases the amount of 5-HT, and clomipramine is known to inhibit its re-uptake.

Lithium carbonate stabilizes the 5-HT system in the brain, partly by increasing the uptake of tryptophan into the nerve endings and partly by inhibiting the enzyme tryptophan hydroxylase. It may also enhance 5-HT receptor sensitivity (Goodwin and Post, 1983; Meltzer et al. 1984). Meltzer et al., (1981) confirmed that 5-HT uptake by platelets is significantly reduced among patients with a certain type of affective, especially bipolar, illness. Increased 5-HT uptake in platelets of depressed patients following treatment correlated positively with clinical improvement. Interest has been sustained in the hypothalamo–pituitary–adrenal (HPA) axis in primary depressive illness, as will be discussed in the next section. Orally administered 5-HTP has been shown to produce greater cortisol responses in depressed and manic patients than in normal controls. Meltzer et al. (1984) have argued that this might be additional evidence for the abnormality of the HPA axis and of the 5-HT system in depression and mania. The enhanced response to 5-HTP in these patients is thought to result from stimulation of hypersensitive 5-HT receptors, which results from decreased 5-HT activity.

The features of aggressive behaviour in terms of 5-HT activity are considered in Chapter 7. Both alcoholism and sleep disturbance are important features of depression, and both have relationships with 5-HT activity. Ballenger et al. (1979) showed that the level of CSF 5-HIAA of alcoholics in the abstinent phase was significantly lower than in both non-alcoholic controls and alcoholics in the immediate post-intoxication phase. Animal studies suggest that alcohol depletes cells of 5-HT and that alcoholic preference of genetic strains of rats that prefer alcohol to water is dependent on low central 5-HT levels. It is postulated that alcoholism might involve pre-existing low brain 5-HT levels which are transiently elevated by alcohol consumption, but that brain 5-HT levels gradually undergo further depletion as a consequence of repeated drinking. This alcohol-produced depletion would aggravate the postulated pre-existing 5-HT deficit, setting up a 'vicious circle' in which the alcoholic repeatedly seeks to modify by pharmacological means a central indoleamine defect.

Increased 5-HT activity appears to promote sleep. Narcolepsy is helped by the 5-HT receptor blocking agent, methysergide, and the treatment of choice in cataplexy, which is found in association with narcolepsy, is clomipramine. Two series of experiments provide the basis of support for the hypothesis that central 5-HT has a role in the process of sleep (Jouvet, 1969). Inhibition of the synthesis of 5-HT at the level of tryptophan hydroxylase by PCPA leads to total insomnia. A three-way correlation appears to exist between the extent of destruction of the raphe, the decrease in cerebral 5-HT and the resulting insomnia. There is also evidence that paradoxical sleep appears to depend upon 'priming' 5-HT mechanisms located in the caudal raphe system and upon 'triggering' mechanisms located in the locus coeruleus, once again illustrating the close functional relationship between 5-HT and NA activity.

If the early speculations concentrated on depression as being due to diminished monoaminergic function, the current alternative hypothesis suggests the diminished function may be a secondary effect due to the increase in monoaminergic function which results from increased sensitivity in post-synaptic monoamine receptors. The modification of this view of depression follows the realization that post-synaptic receptors are found to show diminished sensitivity or reduction in numbers following chronic administration of antidepressant drugs. This reduction is limited to the β-adrenergic system, whereas the α-adrenergic system may show an increase. Chronic antidepressant treatment leads to the 'up regulation' of the α_2-adrenergic receptors and desensitization of β-adrenergic receptors.

Leonard (1981) has discussed the modified view of amine function in depression. The noradrenergic neurone, for reasons which are still unclear, begins to show diminished activity. This may be due to hypersensitivity of the presynaptic α_2 receptor. When the patient becomes depressed, he is subjected to antidepressant drugs which restore the equilibrium in several ways. Initially, the drug may block re-uptake and thus allow the amines to accumulate in the synaptic cleft and work upon the post-synaptic receptor. The amines may also accumulate when a MAO inhibitor interferes with the MAO which catabolizes the amine. The post-synaptic receptor is of the β or α_1-noradrenergic type. The antidepressant drug is able to block the presynaptic α_2-receptor, which allows the neurone to resume functioning. It then blocks the re-uptake mechanism of the amines. With sustained drug therapy the number of post-synaptic β-receptors is reduced. The neurone is thus restored to its normal level of activity. There appears to be a delicate balance in normal health, regulated not merely by the absolute amounts of the amine but by their functional action which is determined by the finely-tuned sensitivity of pre-synaptic and post-synaptic receptors.

Changes in receptor sensitivity are not due to a specific group of antidepressants but may be seen with all forms of physical antidepressant treatment. Their effects include reduction of β-adrenergic sensitivity and enhancement of 5-HT and α-adrenergic stimulation. Tricyclic antidepressants, 'second generation' antidepressants (e.g. mianserin), MAO inhibitors and ECT may also show this effect.

As depression, and its resolution, seems to depend on the balance of forces determined by these factors, it is possible for a variety of modes of action to produce a common end result. Thus, a drug such as amitryptyline may give rise to its effects preferentially by post-synaptic receptor blockade, whereas the imipramine metabolite, desipramine, alters pre-synaptic receptor sensitivity. Drugs which block the re-uptake of NA predominantly include desipramine and nortryptline, whereas imipramine, amitriptyline and clomipramine block the re-uptake of both 5-HT and NA. Mianserin blocks neither.

Thus, the more refined view of amine function in depression focuses attention on the 'final common pathway', the end result of activity in the receptors and the synapse. The evidence for specific amine dysfunction is so far limited.

The binding of imipramine to various tissues has been suggested as a measure of 5-HT uptake. In depression there appear to be reduced numbers of imipramine binding sites. Reduced imipramine binding has been shown in the platelets of depressed patients (Paul et al., 1981), in the frontal cortex of cases of suicide (Stanley et al., 1982) and in the hippocampus and occipital cortex of depressed patients (Perry et al., 1983).

The sleep disturbance in depression is taken up in a later section, but it may be mentioned here that depressed patients show diminished stage 4, deep, or slow wave, sleep and have abnormality in the REM latency period. These are in part mediated by 5-HT mechanisms. Slow wave sleep appears to be under the control of 5-HT mechanisms in the brainstem and hypothalamus.

As our knowledge of the amine mechanisms in depression has been obtained from the modes of action of antidepressant drugs and other physical treatment, it is recommended that this section be read in conjunction with Chapter 5.

NEUROENDOCRINOLOGY

Several neuroendocrine disturbances have been noted in depression. Quite apart from any intrinsic interest in the neuroendocrine abnormality in itself, there is in almost every case underlying neurotransmitter involvement implicated that adds further to our understanding of neurobiological dysfunction in depression.

The abnormality studied most intensively is that involving the hypothalamo–pituitary–adreno–cortical (HPA) function with an elevation in plasma, urinary and CSF cortisol levels. This may be schematically represented as in Figure 8.

In normal subjects there appears to be a circadian (see below) variation in plasma cortisol concentration, with a result that late evening and night time values are lower than those obtained in the early morning. There are also 'peaks' in the plasma cortisol levels corresponding to the pulsatile release of adreno-corticotrophic hormone (ACTH). As Sachar *et al.* (1973) point out, in depressed patients, there is an increased number of 'peaks' and an increase in the total cortisol secretion. Also, cortisal secretion occurs during the late evening and early morning – the opposite of the events in normal subjects. Further, there is abnormality of suppression of cortisol production when challenged by dexamethasone, a subject taken up in detail shortly.

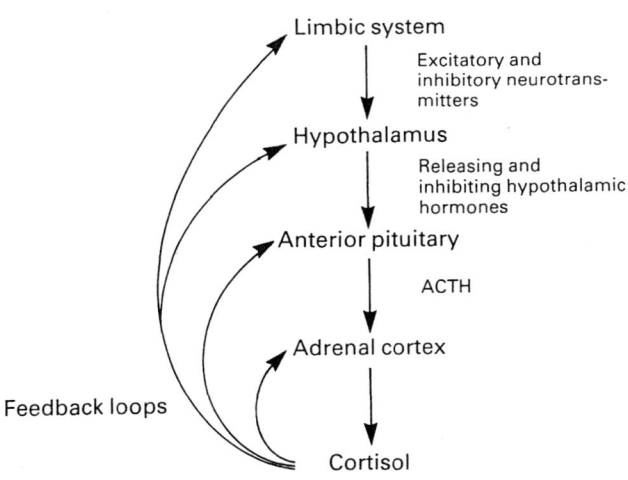

Figure 8 The neuroendocrinology of cortisol (after Sachar, 1982, see text)

Sachar (1982) has noted that about half the patients with 'major' depression have significantly increased cortisol secretion, an abnormality that is made normal with clinical recovery. This cortisol secretion is secondary to increased ACTH secretion. There are other abnormal features of the cortisol hypersecretion in depression – a flattening of the circadian cortisol curve with disproportionate secretion of excess cortisol in the afternoon, evening and early morning, when in normal subjects cortisol secretion is minimal.

The dexamethasone suppression test (DST) was mooted as a specific biological marker of the more severe forms of depression, although its specificity has been constantly undermined by abnormalities shown in patients with a wide variety of psychiatric conditions. Carroll (1982), the major apologist for the diagnostic use of the DST, has reviewed the test and its assumptions. Essentially, extraneous steroid leads to the suppression of intrinsic cortisol production in normal subjects; a proportion of patients with 'major' or 'endogenous' or severe depression fail to demonstrate this suppression. Neuroendocrine function appears to be regulated by the limbic system and the hypothalamus. As the same areas of the brain are postulated to be the site of the pathology in depression, there has been considerable interest in seeking the relationship between neuroendocrine disturbance and depressive disorder. The abnormality in DST cannot be explained in terms of stress alone. While normal subjects suppress their intrinsic cortisol production for at least 24 hours after an overnight dose of dexamethasone many depressed patients may normally suppress plasma cortisol concentrations in the early morning only to escape from suppression later in the day.

It could have been asked if the abnormal DST might be employed to predict therapeutic outcome. Carroll (1982) maintained that if an abnormal DST response remitted to normal early, even before clinical improvement, and after treatment, the response to treatment could be predicted as likely to be successful. Conversely, if after clinical improvement and in follow-up, the abnormal DST persisted, the patients could have been considered to be at risk for relapse, as it might have been argued that the underlying depressive process lay unresolved under these circumstances. It was also claimed that depressed patients with an abnormal DST were more likely to have a positive family history and were more likely to be at risk from suicide.

Carroll et al. (1976) demonstrated that depressed patients with delusions had the highest CSF cortisol concentrations. This appeared to be confirmed by Nelson et al. (1984). Deakin et al. (1983) could not, however, confirm this finding.

The specificity of the abnormal dexamethasone test has been challenged by several workers including Coppen et al. (1983). They found 70% of depressed patients gave an abnormal response against 11% of controls, but so also did 43% of those with 'neurotic' depression, 44% of other neurotics, 22% of schizophrenics, 47% of senile dements and 28% of abstinent alcoholics. They found that though treatment could produce clinical improvement and remission, it had little effect on the DST. They suggested that the abnormal DST is a feature of many psychiatric illnesses and the mechanisms that underlie it are independent of those giving rise to the clinical manifestations of the illness.

Whatever might be the specificity of the abnormal DST in depression there is little doubt that it has given an impetus to the study of neurotransmitter dysfunction in depression. Carroll (1982) has discussed the importance of the limbic system nuclei above the median eminence of the hypothalamus. The cortical and subcortical regions of the limbic system (such as the hippocampus, amygdala, frontal cortex, temporal cortex, parts of the midbrain and septal nuclei) have synaptic links with the hypothalamus. The response to stress and the circadian rhythms is mediated through these inputs. The neurones in the hypothalamus secrete the releasing and inhibitory hormones into the pituitary portal system, by which means they reach the anterior pituitary. The hypothalamic hormones then stimulate or inhibit the synthesis and release of pituitary hormones into the circulation. Next, peripheral hormones, such as cortisol, are released by ACTH. Each of these hormones has feedback effects at every level of the axis.

Carroll (1982) argues for a cholinergic basis to the abnormality reflected by the DST. The evidence for this comes from experimental studies. Physostigmine, a reversible inhibitor of acetylcholinesterase, causes normal subjects to escape from suppression. This effect of physostigmine may be blocked by atropine. These results indicate that a central muscarinic cholinergic mechanism is responsible for the drug-induced HPA escape from dexamethasone suppression. The most likely site of action of physostigmine in producing this effect is at a level in the limbic system above the hypothalamus. Physostigmine also causes psychomotor retardation and anhedonia in normal subjects. It may make existing depression worse, and reduces manic behaviour.

In a recent report, Keshavan et al. (1985) reported a case following benzhexol withdrawal with relapse of his schizoaffective illness. They also showed a reduced REM latency, along with depressive symptoms and an abnormal DST, which lends further support to the hypothesis that depression may be caused by increased cholinergic activity.

There have been rival hypotheses. Jones et al. (1976) suggested that 5-HT and acetylcholine are stimulatory and gamma aminobutyric acid (GABA) and noradrenaline are inhibitory to corticotrophin releasing factor secretion. Sachar (1982) suggested that NA deficiency may disinhibit corticotrophin releasing factor and thus ACTH and cortisol secretion. They infused small quantities of amphetamine, a NA agent, to depressed patients and recorded within 90 minutes a fall to normal cortisol levels in the plasma.

Further evidence for a cholinergic mechanism in depression comes from the work of Mendlewicz et al. (1984) who showed that depressed patients with an abnormal DST have significantly shorter REM latencies. REM sleep disturbances and the abnormal DST response may also be related to chronobiological dysregulation, resulting in circadian disturbances of brain neurotransmitters and of hypothalamic pituitary adrenal activity in some depressed patients.

NA is thought to exert a tonic-inhibitory action on ACTH secretion which may be inhibited in depression with NA deficit (McEwen, 1980). Levy and Davis (1983) have suggested that 5-HT and NA may contribute to the maintenance of the diurnal variation of corticosteroid release. Cortisol levels are increased by elevated 5-HT activity, probably through stimulation of ACTH release. The 5-HT precursor, 5-hydroxytryptophan, has a similar effect.

Checkley (1980) discussed findings which tended to favour the overactivity of cholinergic and defect of α-adrenoceptor functions in patients with depression.

It is said that major or psychotropic drugs, including tricyclic and other antidepressants, neuroleptics, monoamine oxidase inhibitors, lithium and benzodiazepines do not interfere with the test.

Thyroid function

In depressed patients a deficient TSH response to an infusion of the hypothalamic releasing hormone (TRH) may be seen (Sachar, 1982). After clinical recovery, TSH response may be enhanced, but some patients continue to have a subnormal response, and it is suspected that this may be associated with a subsequent relapse. About a third of depressed patients have a reduced TSH response to TRH.

TSH has a synergistic effect with antidepressant medication and it is possible that this is brought about by actions on NA and 5-HT neurotransmission. In turn, NA stimulates TSH release. 5-HT probably inhibits TSH release, which is seen when TSH levels are reduced by 5-HT administration.

Growth hormone (GH)

Human growth hormone response to insulin-induced hypoglycaemia may be diminished in depression (Carroll, 1978). Both NA and 5-HT may mediate this response.

Carroll and Mendels (1976) also showed that depressed patients secrete less GH to a variety of stimuli, such as amphetamine, clonidine and desipramine administration.

Following insulin-induced hypoglycaemia, GH is released into the peripheral circulation. Adrenergic blockers such as phentolamine may diminish such insulin-induced release. Garver and Davis (1979) note that the parallel findings of diminished GH response to insulin-hypoglycaemia and diminished urinary MHPG in depressed patients suggests that a functional deficit of NA neurotransmission occurs in the same patients who show evidence of diminished NA turnover. Furthermore, such 'NA depressions' appear to respond better to drugs such as imipramine or desipramine which cause an increase in synaptic NA. They argue that patients with '5-HT depression' appear to have a normal GH response in addition to lower CSF 5-HIAA and normal or elevated urinary MHPG. These depressions respond better to tricyclic agents such as amitryptyline, which cause an increase in synaptic 5-HT, or following administration of the 5-HT precursor, 5-HTP.

In normal subjects, GH release may occur after administration of L-dopa, which argues also for a dopaminergic mechanism. There is suggestion also of α-adrenergic stimulation and β-adrenergic inhibition of GH release in humans.

The inhibition of GH response may be related to the high levels of cortisol in depression, a picture which may also be seen in patients with Cushing's disease.

Drugs such as clonidine which stimulate α-adrenoceptors stimulate the release of GH. Conversely, drugs such as phenoxybenzamine inhibit the release of GH. Checkley (1979) and Checkley et al. (1981) found that amphetamine and clonidine-induced responses in GH were impaired in depressed patients.

CIRCADIAN RHYTHMS IN DEPRESSION

Circadian rhythms involve the sleep–wake cycle as well as the rhythms of temperature, REM sleep, cortisol production, melatonin activity, urinary electrolytes and volume, and some autonomic functions (Thompson, 1984).

The well-known symptoms of depression such as early morning awakening and the diurnal variation in mood have evoked interest and suggested that the sleep–wake cycle might have been advanced ('phase advanced'). It is also suggested that REM sleep in depression is found in the early part of the night and not later as in normals. Also the phase advancement due to an abnormally short intrinsic period of the circadian system in depression brings about the abnormalities found in REM sleep, cortisol production and in temperature as well as the symptoms noted above.

The cortisol level, for instance, may be mirrored in a daily rhythm in hypothalamic NA, lowest in the morning and highest at midnight, which is consistent with the idea that a varying level of brain NA inhibition modulates the circadian pattern of corticotrophin releasing hormone, ACTH and cortisol secretion (Sachar, 1982).

SEASONAL VARIATIONS

Rosenthal et al. (1984) referred to Seasonal Affective Disorder (SAD) which is characterized by annually occurring winter depressions associated with increased sleep, fatigue, weight gain and a craving for carbohydrate. These individuals show a reversal of symptoms in spring and summer when a hypomanic picture may be seen.

These seasonal rhythms are widely seen in the rest of the animal kingdom and appear to be influenced by environmental cues such as the length of the day and the availability of light. James et al. (1985) experimentally modified day-length by exposing patients with SAD to bright full-spectrum lights before dawn and after dusk. They found that patients improved during bright light treatment and relapsed when the light was withdrawn. In a subsequent study, they administered bright light only in the evening and also examined whether sleep deprivation was an important variable in light treatment. They found that the use of lights only in the evening, about 5 hours' treatment, was sufficient to reverse depressive symptoms. The symptoms reverse within 3 days and are held at bay as long as the light treatment is given; relapse occurring within 3 days of suspension of the light. Thus the mode of action appears to differ from the effects of sleep deprivation, which occurs within a day, and antidepressant drug treatment which takes 10–14 days to show a response.

In animals these effects appear to be mediated by the retinohypothalamic tract (RHT), which links the retina to the supra-chiasmatic nucleus (SCN). In animals the RHT is also involved in the suppression of melatonin and the entrainment of circadian rhythms. Other work has shown that the intensity of the light as used by James *et al.* (1985) is sufficient to suppress melatonin and entrain human circadian rhythms. They speculate the antidepressant effect of bright light may involve these mechanisms including the secretion of melatonin, which is an important mediary in seasonal influences on animal behaviour.

Thompson *et al.* (1985) showed that desipramine treatment did not reduce melatonin secretion. Melatonin secretion was significantly increased after 3 weeks of treatment in depressed subjects, but no increase was found in normal subjects.

In man, as well as in animals, melatonin appears to have a circadian rhythm, with peak levels at night and low levels during the day. It has been suggested that the mechanism of action of antidepressants depends upon their ability to slow and delay the phase position of circadian rhythms.

It may well be that depressed patients have an underlying disorder of circadian rhythms which involve 5-HT metabolism, melatonin production and sleep rhythm (Wehr *et al.*, 1979). Tricyclic antidepressants advance circadian rhythms and increase cyclic time in manic depressive patients (Wehr and Goodwin, 1979). Lithium, which interacts with 5-HT receptors, lengthens endogenous rhythms and decreases the severity of manic-depressive episodes (Johnson *et al.*, 1979). Both tricyclic antidepressants and lithium may alter circadian patterns and depression by modulating central 5-HT neurotransmission.

SLEEP

Sleep disturbance is a cardinal feature of depression. Wide variation in both quantity and quality of sleep is possible (Chen, 1979). She notes that agitated behaviour has been related to insomnia or hyposomnia and early morning awakening, whereas retarded behaviour has been associated with hypersomnia and may be associated with increased appetite and body weight. Thus, the cycle of sleep–wakefulness may be influenced by other biological variables such as mood, activity, appetite and body weight.

REM sleep activity may be reduced in the early phase of illness and there may be a rebound during recovery. The reduction in REM has prognostic significance. Good response to antidepressant treatment is seen with reduced REM sleep and activity and in increase in REM latency.

There are also neuroendocrine correlates of the sleep disorder in depression. Krieger (1979) showed that in normal subjects ACTH and cortisol showed a rhythm with peak concentration about the normal waking time, and a trough in the early hours of the morning soon after onset of sleep.

Prolactin levels rise during the period of sleep and fall on waking (Sassin *et al.*, 1972). Growth hormone secretion shows a relationship to slow wave

92

sleep, a nocturnal surge occurring with the onset of slow wave sleep. NA production may fall during sleep (Mullen, 1983). ACTH reaches a maximum about the time of awakening.

Sleep progresses from wakefulness through stages 1 and 4. Stages 1 and 4 are called deep or slow wave sleep. This sleep is interrupted periodically by REM sleep, in which dreams are prominent and objective neuro-physiological findings may be recorded by EEG and EMG. REM sleep is followed by stages 1–4 of non-REM sleep until the next REM cycle occurs. The cycles come on every 90 minutes or so. In adult life, REM sleep accounts for 25% of all sleep. Slow wave sleep occurs early in sleep, and REM sleep is found before awakening.

REM sleep may be decreased by reduced levels of central 5-HT or increased levels of catecholamines; decreasing brain catecholamines increases REM sleep.

In depression the smooth transition from one stage to another is disturbed (Hawkins, 1980). There is an increase in amount of stage 1 and, particularly, stage 2 sleep. Stages 3 and 4 sleep are reduced, which may account for the unsatisfying nature of the sleep in the condition. With recovery, normal levels of stage 4 sleep are restored more slowly than the rest.

REM sleep in depression occurs much earlier after sleep onset than in the normal state. The more severe the depression, the shorter is the REM latency. In normal individuals the initial REM phase is short, increasing in length and then falling off with later cycles. In depression, the opposite pattern may be seen. When studied early in treatment, good responders to amitriptyline show a significant increase in REM latency as well as a decrease in REM sleep and activity.

All effective antidepressants, except lithium, have REM-suppressant properties. It is possible to improve a depressed state, even if transiently, by both total sleep deprivation and by selective REM deprivation. Kupfer et al. (1976) have shown that early reversal of REM latency abnormality predicted tricyclic antidepressant responsiveness.

Sitaram et al. (1980) have found that shortened REM latency resembled that caused by cholinomimetics.

Slow-wave sleep is under the control of 5-HT mechanisms in the brainstem and hypothalamus. It also regulates REM sleep. However, there appears to be a complex balance in the sleep–wake cycle mediated by all the more important neurotransmitters. Thus brainstem lesions cause insomnia presumably through 5-HT depletion; this may be reversed by agents which block catecholamine function.

DELUSIONAL DEPRESSION

As has been indicated, delusional depressives appear to have a high frequency of HPA dysfunction as measured by the DST.

Abnormality in the HPA axis is also in keeping with disordered catecholamine function in delusional depression. Sweeney et al. (1978) showed diminished urinary MHPG and increased CSF HVA levels in deluded depressives. It has been suggested that the enzyme dopamine-ßhydroxylase (DBH), which converts DA to NA, and which is presumably deficient, may be under genetic control and be a trait which predisposes to delusional depression.

Nelson *et al.* (1984) suggest that the delusional depressive syndrome appears to be a discrete clinical subtype of depression at the severe end of the spectrum. Vulnerability factors for developing this delusional syndrome would include, they argue, a strong genetic loading for depression, HPA axis abnormality, decreased activity of the enzyme DBH, and previous history of delusions when depressed.

Deakin *et al.* (1983) could not confirm high cortisol levels in a group of depressed patients. However, they found that cortisol responses to real or simulated ECT were much reduced in deluded depressives. They refer to the study by Elithorn *et al.* (1969) who found diminished cortisol reponse to ECT in schizophrenics, and wonder if there might be a mechanism common to both schizophrenia and depression for delusion formation. The transmitter mechanism involved may be α-receptor subsensitivity. The mode of treatment of this class of depressed patients is taken up in Chapter 5.

4
Depressed mind, disordered brain – II: The neuropsychiatry of depression

The logical consequence of the argument of Chapter 3 is that depression, when conceptualized as a brain syndrome, will be seen to have affinities with other conditions which, in part, could be considered to be neuropsychiatric syndromes.

SCHIZOPHRENIA

The problem of the overlap between affective illness and schizophrenia is an old one which continues to exercise the minds and efforts of a large number of psychiatrists. In the 1960s, several studies (e.g. Kendell, et al., 1971) drew attention to the broader concept of schizophrenia which appeared to prevail until the advent of research criteria such as the Research Diagnostic Criteria (Spitzer et al., 1978) and administrative manuals such as DSM-III (American Psychiatric Association, 1980). These narrowed the criteria of schizophrenia and depression which, in truth, are greyer concepts than is popularly written in textbooks. All clinicians are, of course, aware of the forms of phenomena such as delusions and hallucinations which are common to both conditions, and which occasionally lead to diagnostic confusion. But it is the presence of affective symptoms that concern us most in this discussion. The sequelae of a schizophrenic syndrome affected by depressive features will be taken up in due course.

Kraepelin observed that affective features can occur early in the course of schizophrenia (Kraepelin, 1919). The relationship between schizophrenia and depression was also referred to by Bleuler (1923). It is known that a 'prodromal' phase of schizophrenia may be a manic-depressive illness. The change from manic-depressive illness to schizophrenia was noted by Lewis and Pietrowski (1954) who found such a change in 50% of cases, but only very rarely did they find a change in the opposite direction. This onset is very reminiscent of the prodromal presentation of Huntington's chorea, a subject taken up in a later section.

The schizo-affective states are examples of a condition which reflects the less than clear-cut boundaries between depression and schizophrenia. Wing et al. (1974) classified schizo-affective disease under the schizophrenias. The Americans have now formally introduced the condition as belonging to a third category of illness. Once again most clinicians will be able to recall cases that tended towards the 'schizophrenic' picture and others which appeared to have affinities with depressive illness.

The term schizo-affective psychoses was given by Kasanin (1933) to nine cases of psychosis of sudden onset, a duration of a few months, with fantastic delusions and occasionally hallucinations in young individuals who appeared to have become ill after some stressful event. The term was employed to reflect the admixture of schizophrenic and affective symptoms.

Welner et al. (1979) reflect the point of view that holds that schizo-affective illness is a form of schizophrenia showing the expected poor prognosis. Others (e.g. Clayton et al., 1968), on the basis of genetic and follow-up studies, consider the disorder as showing the same pattern as depression, or affective illness. A third view is that it is a mixed group of disorders which may show its true colours according to the circumstances in which it is allowed to emerge. Thus, schizo-affective disorder which has an onset before the age of 40 has an onset similar to schizophrenia, while when the onset appears after 40 years, the disorder is closer in genetic terms to depression (Tsuang, 1979).

Schizo-affective disorders must also to be distinguished from depressive psychosis, i.e. depressions with delusions and/or hallucinations. The distinction is attempted that delusions and/or hallucinations in depression must be congruent, i.e. be in keeping with the mood, whereas the psychotic phenomena in schizo-affective illness cannot be understood in terms of the diminished (or elevated) mood. But as Winokur (1984) has pointed out, we have no real reason to believe that mood-incongruent features, when seen in a person with an unequivocal episodic depression, are meaningfully different from mood-congruent psychotic features.

The genetic evidence for schizo-affective disorder being an autonomous condition is sparse. However, in some studies of schizophrenic siblings and twins concordant for schizophrenia, there also appeared to be a strong concordance for affective features (Slater, 1947; Slater, 1953). Tsuang (1965) also found a number of pairs of schizophrenic siblings who had prominent affective symptoms early in the course of their disorder. Angst (1973), studying the incidence of affective illness in the relatives of schizo-affective disorder patients, found almost equally increased frequencies of schizophrenia, manic-depressive illness and schizo-affective disorder in first degree relatives, which indicates that schizo-affective disorder is intermediate to schizophrenic and manic-depressive disorder. Certainly, the prognosis appears to be intermediate to that for schizophrenia and manic-depressive illness.

The view has also been expressed, in the Kraepelinian mode, that a recovered schizophrenic was not fit for inclusion in the schizophrenic category, and that a schizo-affective diagnosis was more appropriate (Vaillant, 1963).

Depression as lowered mood may also be found in cases where the diagnosis of schizophrenia is not in dispute. Several hypotheses have been put forward for this phenomenon, and each commands some degree of support, so much so that 'schools of thought' have infested the debate. The first of these hypotheses is that depression in schizophrenia is not an intrinsic part of the syndrome but due to neuroleptic medication given as part of the management of schizophrenia. Hirsch et al. (1973) and Wistedt (1981) investigated this hypothesis and found it could not be upheld when they withdrew depot neuroleptics from chronic schizophrenic patients. On the contrary, they found that patients who had been switched from neuroleptics to a placebo became more depressed.

The study of drug-induced depressive features is confused by the presence of extrapyramidal and parkinsonian features that result, not uncommonly, from the exhibition of these drugs. It is possible, at least in theory, to distinguish the extrapyramidal features from depression by using oral or parenteral antiparkinsonian medication, but it is believed that depressive symptoms are as common in schizophrenics treated with neuroleptic agents and anticholinergic drugs as in those who are treated with neuroleptics alone (Knights and Hirsch, 1981).

Galdi (1983) showed that schizophrenics with first degree relatives were significantly more depressed after 4–6 weeks of neuroleptic therapy than when they were treated with placebo. His studies also revealed more severe demonstrations of extrapyramidal symptoms in schizophrenic patients who had depressed first degree relatives. He argues that not only do these findings implicate neuroleptics in the causation of depression, but that there might be support for pharmacogenetically induced depression. These findings would suggest that severe 'pseudo-parkinsonism' and related depression may result from the interaction of neuroleptic drugs with a genetic defect affecting the nigro–striatal dopaminergic system of patients. The depression may represent an extrapyramidal component of a dopaminergic disorder which induced a secondary subjective dysphoria. In the treatment of this depression and extrapyramidal features, anticholinergic medication may be more potent agents than tricyclic drugs which have relatively little anticholinergic action. Galdi adduces further support for his argument by referring to studies which associate depression in schizophrenia with increased risks for tardive dyskinesia.

The features of akinetic depression include mild akinesia, with anergia, emotional withdrawal and association with drowsiness (Van Putten and May, 1978). These patients improve rapidly with anticholinergic drugs. However, Moller and Zerssen (1981) have shown that depressive symptoms are as common in schizophrenics on anticholinergics as in those who are not. Furthermore, Johnson (1981) has pointed out that anticholinergic drugs are no more effective than placebo in the treatment of depression in schizophrenia.

Johnson (1981) found depression in half of untreated new acute schizophrenics and in about a third of chronic schizophrenics who had relapsed after being on depot drugs or not having been on them. Depression was commoner in those on higher doses of depot neuroleptics and those who showed extrapyramidal side-effects, which suggests drugs may play a part in inducing depressive features. He found that those patients in remission and on moderate doses of depot drug had the lowest prevalence of depression.

Depression is a significant feature of schizophrenia. The suicidal risk in schizophrenia is some 50 times that of the normal population (Markowe et al., 1967), which is perhaps half of that seen in a depressive population.

Apart from initial presentation, depression may be found during relapse and whilst being on maintenance therapy. For patients on regular maintenance depot injections, there is three times as great a risk of depression as there is of a schizophrenic relapse (Johnson, 1981).

The 'prodromal' depression of schizophrenia is susceptible to two explanations, which in reality are not mutually exclusive. The first is that it is merely non-specific; the second that such patients have a genetic predisposition to both affective illness and schizophrenia. Kendler and Tsuang (1982) believe that the evidence indicates that patients who progress from an apparently typical affective syndrome to schizophrenia are more common than would be expected if this disorder was due to the inheritance of a predisposition to both schizophrenia and affective illness.

Another hypothesis is that the depression in schizophrenia follows as a psychological reaction as the psychosis remits and the patient regains insight. This hypothesis for its support will require there to be an increase in depression following remission of the schizophrenia. Knights and Hirsch (1981) have pointed out that there is actually a decrease in the incidence of depression following the remission of the acute phase of schizophrenia, as several studies show.

Roy et al. (1983) tested the hypothesis that chronic schizophrenic outpatients who developed a depressive episode would have more risk factors for depression, and would have experienced more life events in the 6 months prior to the onset of depression. They found that the depressed schizophrenics had had significantly more psychiatric admissions, past depressive episodes, past treatment for depression, significantly more had attempted suicide, lived alone, had low self-esteem, had early parental loss and had more life events in the 6 months before the onset of depression. However, depression could occur when these risk factors were absent in well remitted schizophrenics or neuroleptics. The results of this study suggest that depressive disorder occurring in chronic schizophrenic outpatients may be reactive, as it occurred in patients who were at risk of developing depressive disorder and who had experienced an excess of life events. In their study there were no significant differences between the depressed group and the non-depressed controls for either the number of patients receiving neuroleptics, the mean chlorpromazine daily dosage equivalents, or the number receiving neuroleptics by injection.

A third hypothesis that has been put forward suggests that depression is a part of the schizophrenic process, both reflecting some underlying neurobiological abnormality (cf depressive dementia). In the florid state of acute schizophrenia, the depression is concealed from, or missed by, clinicians. This hypothesis would require that the depressive and schizophrenic features ran in parallel. Knights and Hirsch (1981) showed a significant decrease in depression after 3 months of admission for acute schizophrenics, as well as at the time of discharge. When depot neuroleptics had been introduced, they found the incidence of depression was still further reduced after 6 months. They employ the term 'revealed depression' to indicate the features of depression which become apparent with the remission of acute schizophrenia.

Depressive features may become apparent or more prominent prior to relapse or an exacerbation of the psychosis. The symptoms seen include depressed mood, insomnia, withdrawal, agitation and anger. An increase in neuroleptic medication may help reverse some of these features.

The rational treatment of depression in a patient with schizophrenia is to increase or re-introduce a neuroleptic agent. A trial of anticholinergic medication may be tried if parkinsonism is suspected. Severe depression in this situation also responds to ECT (Koehler and Sauer, 1983), who also showed that those schizophrenics who were free of first rank symptoms had a significantly better response to ECT.

It has been known for some time that there is an irreducible number of manic-depressive patients who become chronically ill and severely disabled. Johnstone et al. (1985) showed that these chronic in-patients resembled schizophrenic in-patients in terms of disordered cognitive functioning, which they attributed to the effects of institutionalization.

The possibility that depression may influence the course of neuropsychiatric illness is considered in some detail in later sections. It has been taught for several generations that depression in schizophrenia indicates a better prognosis. Kolakowska et al. (1985) confirmed that affective symptoms were associated with good outcome in schizophrenia. They also showed that none of their patients with schizo-affective psychosis had a poor outcome. Thus, the general impression of the ameliorative effect of depression, or at least its underlying neurobiological abnormality, appears to be confirmed in a condition which can only tangentially be described as a brain syndrome.

The mutability of disease has continued to intrigue observers. Some of it is due to changes in management of conditions and others are due to changes in diagnostic fashion. Schizophrenia appears to have changed in character this century and the changes can be shown to precede phenothiazine medication in the 1950s and the diagnostic changes of the 1970s (Hare, 1974). It has now become a milder illness, with a better prognosis, and there appears now to be a larger affective component to the condition. Sheldrick (1984) commented that the change from schizophrenia to affective disorder, considered very rare 30 years ago, now not only occurs in a sizeable minority of schizophrenics but also seems to be occurring over a shorter period of time.

It may well be that the changes that occur in schizophrenia by whatever environmental means also lead to the substrate that induces depression; alternatively, the changes may, by giving rise primarily to depression, alter the course and prognosis of the schizophrenia, as has been suggested in a later section in relation to some degenerative brain conditions. It also has important implications for considering the biological advantages of depression, a subject which will be dealt with in Chapter 9.

MANIA

The relationship with mania is an integral part of a substantial number of depressive disorders. Various aspects of this relationship are discussed in several chapters, most especially in relation to the genetic aspects of manic-depressive illness. It is a relationship steeped in antiquity, as can be seen by reference to Chapter 1.

This is an intriguing connection as depression, taking all degrees and varieties of it, is the commonest mental disorder; whereas mania is an uncommon psychotic illness.

The evidence for the genetic distinction between the unipolar and bipolar depressive illness has been reviewed in Chapter 2. Bipolar illness is characterized by alternating mania and depression. Unipolar illness refers to unipolar depression, unipolar mania being unquestionably rare.

Mania has its onset earlier than depression, so that bipolar illness usually presents with mania. However, the ages of highest risk are taken as being the same for mania and depression.

Like depression, mania may be subdivided into primary and secondary disorders. The causes of the latter condition are reviewed by Krauthammer and Klerman (1978). Commonest of the precipitants nowadays is anti-depressant treatment, including ECT. Historically, the precipitant isoniazid, an antituberculosis drug, is important as it led to the use of MAO inhibitor drugs as antidepressant agents. The antiparkinsonian agent L-dopa may induce mania, and a variety of cerebral conditions, including multiple sclerosis, may produce mania, as can cerebral tumours; neurosyphilis was a well-known association in the past.

Reactive psychosis and the related cycloid psychosis have been discussed in Chapter 2, and maniform symptoms may be found in both. Intriguingly, depression is associated in the clinical picture, which lends further support to the idea that the underlying neurobiology in mania and depression might be closely related. Mania may also be found as the affective component of schizo-affective illness, though considerably less common than the depressive component.

The clinical features of mania are popularly believed to be the mirror image of those seen in depression. This is less than the truth and, as has been pointed out in Chapter 3, several symptoms may be common to both conditions. Insomnia, diminished appetite, weight loss, menstrual irregularities, increased libido, restlessness, irritability, anger, poor attention and concentration, distractability and agitation may be seen in both conditions. The form and content of psychotic features are distinctive, however, and there is usually little clinical difficulty in separating manic psychosis from depression.

The central feature of mania, and from which all other features are derived in the conventional teaching on these matters, is an elevated mood. Although in a substantial number of cases there is elation, aggression is not uncommon, when a hard-pressed clinician at the receiving end of well-directed abuse may well wonder where the textbook description of infectious jollity might be. Anger is commonly seen when the excessive and often outrageous demands of manic patients are not met or they are thwarted in their pursuits. There is disinhibition which may be seen in relation to amorous dallyings or in financial profligacy. The fact that they do no more harm than they do is more a result of their distractability and poor persistence rather than any tribute to their management, which is often associated with the assumption of compulsory powers. Their inability to persist in anything is reflected in their speech (flight of ideas), behaviour (flight of interests) or actions (just plain flight).

The diagnosis in the typical case is the easiest in psychiatry. Problems of a diagnostic kind arise when there is an admixture of other symptoms, depressive or other psychotic illness. Management is straightforward – tranquillize the patient and eliminate a physical basis as a precipitant. The availability of lithium carbonate has revolutionized the management of both mania and recurrent depression, and will be considered in Chapter 5.

ANXIETY

The relationship between anxiety and depression has been known for as long as the relationship between mania and depression. Certainly, Hippocrates was aware of the connection. To the practising clinician the question has always been whether a distinction between anxiety and depression can, or needs to, be made. Most forms of depression present with some anxiety. Clinicians have treated the depression when it was more marked than the anxiety and have worried when the anxiety was the more prominent symptom. This has become a practical point of some importance as the benzodiazepines are in disgrace and the clinician has little other than ß-blocking agents at his disposal. There are also important theoretical considerations which may well throw light on the pathogenesis of depression.

Roth in Newcastle and Cambridge has been instrumental in making the case for the separation of distinct syndromes of anxiety and depression. Anxiety states and 'neurotic' depression, it is argued, fall into separate groups, and commonly used rating scales such as the Hamilton Scale are able to differentiate the clinical syndrome in some 90% of cases (Roth and Mountjoy, 1982). The presence of prominent anxiety reduces the chances that there is a depressive syndrome as well, and such an anxiety syndrome group will consist of patients with poor previous adjustment, whereas depressive patients would have stable personalities with better adjustment (Roth et al., 1972). Prognosis would depend on the presence of anxiety, when it would be poor, or depression, when it would be better (Kerr et al., 1972).

This view is contrary to the experience of most clinicians who are able to observe a considerable overlap in practice. Several authors including Goldberg (1982) have shown that the available evidence did not justify a separation into entities. The general view would be, if there was significant depression, the diagnosis is depression, anxiety being an ancillary feature.

Some 95% of depressed patients have features of psychological and/or physiological manifestations of anxiety. These include feelings of apprehension, tension, tension-related pain, an inability to relax, poor memory, related poor attention and concentration, irritability, insomnia, loss of appetite and so on.

Paykel (1972) showed that a multivariate cluster analysis gave rise to four groups: psychotic depressives, anxious depressives, hostile depressives and young depressives with personality disorders. This typology had treatment implications. Whereas a distinction into 'psychotic' and 'neurotic' had little effect on treatment response to amitriptyline, Paykel found his typology indicated the group which responded poorly (anxious depressives) and those that responded well (the other three groups).

Russell and de Silva (1983) found that anxiety and depressive symptoms persisted in parallel. They argue that the mode of action of antidepressant drugs on affective disorder is more general and fundamental and is not merely on a symptom, or a set of related symptoms, pointing to the easing of both anxiety and depressive features with antidepressant medication, or the failure to relieve both.

Anxiety, like depression, appears to be a product of an interaction between biological or constitutional factors and environmental factors. The influence of environmental factors is generally taken to be marked, especially when depression admixed with anxiety is considered. However, the rare 'pure anxiety' syndrome may have a more considerable constitutional element. Torgerson (1985) differentiated anxiety neurotic and neurotic depressive twin probands into three groups, pure anxiety neurosis, mixed anxiety–depression, and pure neurotic depression. The high concordance for 'pure anxiety neurosis' seemed to indicate an important hereditary basis. He suggests that the aetiology of pure anxiety states is different to that of other affective neurotic states, and that the high monozygotic twin concordance argues for an important genetic element in the genesis of anxiety neurosis. Conversely, there was little evidence for hereditary factors in the development of mixed anxiety—depression or pure neurotic depression.

The practical implication of studies such as this is that there is little evidence for making a valid distinction between depression and anxiety. Except in the rare instances when one encounters a pure anxiety neurosis syndrome, one treats as if for depression.

PARKINSON'S DISEASE

It is clear from Sir James Parkinson's essay on the shaking palsy that an association was known to exist between the condition and depression.

Depression is now known to be frequently found in Parkinson's disease and the reported prevalence ranges between 20% and 90%. The discrepancy in the reports of the incidence and prevalence of depression most likely relates to the methodology employed as well as the populations of patients investigated.

Early reports concentrated on the reactive nature of the depression to be found in Parkinson's disease, and Patrick and Levy (1922) concluded that depression was most likely reactive to the disabling nature of the disease since they found it tended to run in parallel with severity. However, it soon became clear that the incidence of depression in Parkinson's disease was greater than with other chronic, disabling conditions. A consistent relationship cannot now be shown between depression and the severity of the motor disability. The depression also appears not to be correlated with age, sex, degree of disability or the drug regime.

As with conditions as disparate as schizophrenia and Huntington's chorea, depression may be found as a prodromal feature of Parkinson's disease. Patrick and Levy (1922) reported that 34% of their patients had depression prior to the development of Parkinson's disease and Mayeux et al. (1981) noted this feature in 43% of their cases. This, of course, lends some support for the view that both depression and Parkinson's disease are manifestations of some underlying cerebral process, as it is difficult to explain this feature in terms of reaction to disability alone. However, as with schizophrenia or other neuropsychiatric illness, depression may also follow the onset of overt parkinsonian features, and it may well be that there are different mechanisms in operation in these cases of depression.

The treatment of Parkinson's disease by drug therapy complicates the picture as regards depression still further. The role of L-dopa is not yet clear. The initial reports, often sensationally published, was that this drug had an euphoriant action. This was later explained in terms of the improvement in the neurological picture, and the alleviation of the depression secondarily. This view has now been modified somewhat. L-Dopa is now not considered to have any antidepressant properties, and it has indeed been suggested that in susceptible cases, e.g. those with a previous history, there could be a precipitation of a depression. Mindham et al. (1976) remarked that L-dopa was able to cause a re-emergence of pre-existing affective symptoms rather than produce an affective illness ab initio. Thus the psychotropic properties of L-dopa appear to be incidental and with other drugs used in physical illness (e.g. reserpine in hypertension) the emergence of depression is due to the action of the drug on prior susceptibility.

Anticholinergic medication has more established stimulant properties which probably cause both physical and psychological dependence which may lead to its abuse. Its rapid withdrawal may lead to a relapse in depressive symptomatology with several biological indices of the condition being observed (see Keshavan et al., 1985). The role of anticholinergic medication which may confound the picture of depression in schizophrenia has been considered in the previous section. Thus, a case cannot be made for the onset of depression following their use.

The relationship between disability of neurological function and intellectual impairment in Parkinson's disease is more validly suggested. Celesia and Wanamaker (1972) noted that the frequency and severity of the dementia in Parkinson's disease were related to the extent of motor disability. Even when a global dementia is not present, neuropsychological deficit may be related to neurological severity (Mayeux et al., 1981).

103

Age, duration of illness and its severity may possibly be related to the onset of dementia. Parkinson's disease patients with dementia are older, have a later onset of symptoms, have a shorter duration of illness and have a less favourable response to L-dopa (Lieberman *et al.*, 1979). Thus two varieties of Parkinson's disease may be postulated (*cf* Alzheimer's disease) – younger patients with predominantly motor disability, a relatively benign course and a good response to treatment, and older patients with a more malignant course, poor response to treatment and dementia in addition to neurological features associated with Parkinson's disease. This is a mirror image of the picture seen in Alzheimer's disease.

The discussion of dementia in Parkinson's disease is important inasmuch as it throws light on the dementias associated with depression. The mechanisms of dementia in Parkinson's disease are still not clear, but certainly in the older cases, a parallel Alzheimer type degeneration must be considered (see Mahendra, 1984a). The second possibility is that depression, which is present in substantial numbers of cases, induces the dementia, as is discussed in a later section. The third possibility is that the origin of the dementia is in the subcortical structures giving rise to the Parkinson's disease, i.e. the basal ganglia. The last two explanations are not mutually exclusive, as will become clear in a later discussion.

The development of the concept of subcortical dementia and the move away from considering intellectual behaviour as being an exclusively cortical activity has helped the intellectual impairment in Parkinson's disease to be understood. The argument that the dementia in Parkinson's disease may have in some instances a subcortical origin is supported by the finding that the more severe is the parkinsonian disability the more likely is there to be intellectual decline. Subcortical dementia, as was discussed in the critique of the concept of functional disorder in Chapter 3, is characterized by the presence of classical dementia but with the absence of cortical dysfunction such as aphasia, apraxia and agnosia. It can be shown that language function is preserved in Parkinson's disease, although memory and visuo–spatial function decline. Mayeux *et al.* (1981) showed that a distinction could be made between Alzheimer's disease and the dementia of Parkinson's disease on this basis.

Although the dementia of Parkinson's disease may be due to one cause at one stage in the illness, it is possible that subsequent explanations may well be due to another. Thus, when treatment with L-dopa is commenced, there may be an improvement in intellectual function in parallel with improvement in motor function, only for there to be a subsequent decline even when motor function is largely preserved. This may be due to 'cortical' involvement, as was suggested by Loranger *et al.* (1972). As a general rule, therefore, where the dementia appears to be related to neurological disability and there is sparing of cortical function, a subcortical basis to the dementia may be suspected; where, however, the dementia is excessively severe in relation to the degree of neurological symptomatology and there is involvement of cortical function as well, an additional cortical involvement may have to be considered.

The relationship between dementia and depression in Parkinson's disease is further discussed in Mahendra (1985a).

HUNTINGTON'S CHOREA

Another example of a condition with subcortical pathology which gives rise to depression and dementia, with abnormal movements, is Huntington's chorea. There is often a dissociation between the abnormal movements and the psychiatric symptomatology, and a familial basis to this may be noted. Depression is a common prodromal feature and although it may be explained in part as a reaction to the realization that one has chosen the genetic short straw in a condition that is still widely regarded as a tragic misfortune, the depression may precede any other manifestation of the illness and may indeed be found in the minority of cases who do not give a family history of the condition. It is thus hard to avoid the neurobiological basis to some at least of these cases of depression. It is also a feature which was noted by Huntington (1872) who referred to the 'insanity with a tendency to suicide' which is now well accepted with Huntington's chorea.

The depression is often a severe one, and is indistinguishable from depression seen in relation to any other condition or those that are deemed to be of 'functional' onset. Psychotic features are not uncommon, as are psychomotor retardation. They may remit spontaneously over time, and they also respond to conventional antidepressant drugs and ECT. Depression is usually unipolar but bipolar disorders, with a typical mania, may also be seen. It is difficult to separate these 'illness' manifestations from the transient or short lived bouts of misery and distress associated with this appalling condition, but a figure of 50% of patients having some of the features of depression will not be an exaggeration.

As with Alzheimer's disease, the early features of depression tend to be overshadowed by the dementia and the chorea, and in the later stages a progressive apathy takes over and terminally one finds an akinetic and mute picture.

As with Parkinson's disease, cognitive impairment produces a picture of dementia with cortical sparing, hence the dementia of Huntington's chorea is an example of subcortical dementia (see Chapter 3). The dementia is progressive but runs a benign course, lasting up to 15 years (see later discussion). Overlying the dementia is the quite marked apathy which adds to the disability. Aphasia, agnosia, alexia and apraxia are not seen in the dementia of Huntington's chorea, although function may be difficult to elicit on account of the patient's apathy and uncooperativeness.

The early presentation of depression is reflected in the suicidal behaviour, which has been noted by Oltman and Friedman (1961). The cause of death in 7% of cases has been attributed to suicide (Reed and Chandler, 1958). The high level of violence, especially in a domestic setting, seen in families of patients with Huntington's chorea may in part be traced to the depression with its associated psychopathology.

The neurobiological explanations for the depression and other features of Huntington's chorea are far from clear. There seems to be a reduction of

γ-aminobutyric acid in the basal ganglia and substantia nigra (Perry *et al.*, 1973), which is not a transmitter implicated in depression. There also appears to be a decline in cholinergic activity, which is the opposite of that found in some cases of depression. There is also hypersensitivity at dopaminergic receptors in the basal ganglia, so that depleting the amine by drugs such as tetrabenazine will yield a symptomatic improvement of the chorea but at the risk of precipitating depression.

ALZHEIMER'S DISEASE

The true incidence of depression in Alzheimer's Disease (AD) is not known for certain, but Kral (1983) has suggested that depression might have been present in 15% of patients in a series of cases in which AD was clinically diagnosed. Depression is known to be a symptom of the early stages of the disease. It may be fleeting and not well differentiated. Response to treatment may be poor, but the depressive features disappear as the AD progresses and may not be seen at all in the severe form of the illness.

This is an appropriate point at which to refer to the clinical diagnosis of AD. Obviously, the influence of depression on AD can only be usefully studied on long-term follow-up of cases of dementia. For practical purposes, it is equally clear that a clinical diagnosis will have to suffice. There are a few research diagnostic criteria being made available in the USA (e.g. Report of the NINCDS-ADRDA Work Group, 1984). In practice the effect of using them to establish AD results in 'middle of the road' cases being included. Focal lesions are usually an exclusion criterion. Another is depression, and depression at the time of presentation leads to exclusion. Thus, there was no depression in 30 cases of dementia, as Knesevich *et al.* (1983) showed.

In one year in Cornwall, 23 well-documented cases of patients who had been admitted for long-stay care were found. Twenty-two of the patients involved were dead. The record was a retrospective one, and insofar as it pertains to patients in an institution in a far-flung rural county, is also obviously selective. Diagnosis was established on the basis of a progressive dementing condition which had as its onset the gradual impairment of short term memory followed by intellectual decline. The duration of the disorder was deemed to be from the first recording of these symptoms to deaths in all but the one case. Any other neurological or psychiatric disorder at the time of onset led to the exclusion of those cases. The investigations were surprisingly extensive and assisted in this process of exclusion. This and the fact that the course of the condition was known led one to make a clinical diagnosis of AD with fair confidence.

As depression at presentation was an exclusion criterion, the only depressive symptoms considered were those found in the course of the dementing illness.

Of the 23 patients, 14 were female and 9 male. 16 patients had no depression during their dementing illness; 7 patients did have depression. The mean duration of the dementing illness in the group as a whole was 5.7 years. However, when depression was present in the course of the dementia, the mean duration was 10.2 years, almost double the duration of the group as a whole.

It may be argued that there might have been a preponderance of older dements, in whom the illness might have run a relatively benign course with depression a possible feature (see Mahendra, 1984a for discussion). The mean age for the whole sample was 69.3 years and the mean age for the depressed patients was 68.7 years. Therefore the argument that the longer duration might have been due to an older age of onset of the dementia, and therefore with a more benign course, does not hold.

Kral (1983) also took the opportunity of studying 22 so-called 'pseudodements' on follow-up, and found that 20 of them had developed progressive dementia, the clinical appearances being that of AD, and that 11 of these had died. These are surprisingly large numbers of patients with AD presenting with depression. The follow-up, however, was for a mean of 8 years, once again beyond the usual range allowed for survival in the condition. There does seem to be support for the hypothesis that depression in the course of a dementing illness helps modify it in a less malignant direction.

An apparently important consideration when depression emerges in the course of AD is whether it is part of the AD or whether a parallel depressive neurobiology is being facilitated to emerge by the dementing process. There is no clinical distinction available in practice, though it is often said that the depression of AD is less clear-cut than ordinary depressive illness. A past history of depression may be helpful but clearly those who have never shown affective symptoms may be enabled to do so when the brain is otherwise involved in pathological change. The depression in AD is an early feature, subsiding as the disease progresses, as will any ordinary depression with the passage of time. Past and family history are no help in any case in the individual patient; nor are radiology or indices such as the dexamethasone suppression test.

But it could be argued that this distinction is academic. What may be important is that depression or its neurobiological state exists to influence the course of dementing illness. Here we run into another complication. As we have seen, depression is a heterogeneous condition with a multiplicity of permutations being possible in neurobiological terms. Could increased cholinergic activity be as salutary a state of affairs as diminished noradrenergic or serotonergic or peptide activity? It may not be so.

A possible explanation for the early presence of depression and its association with a relatively good prognosis is considered in the section on depressive dementia.

DEMENTIA ASSOCIATED WITH DEPRESSION

Although the relationship between depression and dementia has been known for several centuries, it still appears complex. This topic has been discussed in detail by Mahendra (1985a), and has also been referred to in the introductory section of this chapter.

Cognitive change is part of the symptomatology of depression and is the cardinal feature of dementia. Depression is found predominantly as a condition of the middle-aged and the elderly; 90% of the dementias are

107

found in the senium, i.e. beyond the age of 65. Hence, an association at the very least between depression and dementia is to be expected.

It has been argued (Mahendra, 1985a) that depression could produce cognitive changes which may be reversed with the successful treatment of the depression, even leading to a full resolution of the dementia. As we have seen already, a dementing illness may induce depression of a fleeting and ill-defined nature, as with Alzheimer's disease, or induce a substantial component of the syndrome associated with Parkinson's disease and Huntington's chorea; a depressive illness, like any other condition, may be superimposed upon and aggravate the cognitive state due to a chronic, degenerative condition giving rise to a dementia. And the possibility exists, that dementia and depression may be two limbs of a brain dysfunction which may be reversible to a greater or lesser degree.

Dementia induced by depression was considered to be a 'functional' disorder, hence the dementia was a 'pseudodementia'. This concept has been critically considered in the introductory section and shown to be logically suspect.

Parallel developments in the conceptualization of the dementias has helped us to reconsider the cognitive changes associated with depression. Firstly, the requirement for an irreversible, progressive course for dementia and with it the inevitable criterion for 'organic' causation for the syndrome, ceased to exist. Progression and irreversibility are no longer conditions that need to be satisfied for the diagnosis of dementia; neither is there any consideration of any aetiological factors in the diagnosis. Dementia may result from gross organic disease; it can progress to a fatal termination with no question of reversal. On the other hand, dementia, even perhaps as serious a clinical entity as an 'organically-determined' dementia may reverse and subside with the effective resolution of the 'functional' psychiatric illness responsible for it.

Both states are dementia because they both satisfy the criteria for the diagnosis of dementia—progression, irreversibility and aetiology now being irrelevant factors. As the dementia of depression satisfies all these criteria, depression may now take its place as a cause of dementia and, given its prevalence, it is probably comparable to vascular dementia in the incidence of dementia.

There is another factor which has implications for the understanding of depression-induced dementia. This second new factor in the modified conceptualization of dementia is that the tacit assumption that dementia is a cortical phenomenon can no longer be held to be a central, or even essential, feature of the syndrome. It is now suggested that a category of 'subcortical' dementia exists, and this concept has been discussed in the introductory section in Chapter 3.

In the past one point of distinction between depressive 'pseudodementia' and 'true dementia' used to be the relatively small or no cerebral changes found in the former and the rather gross cerebral changes in the latter. With the advent of the concept of 'subcortical' dementia, this distinction became blurred. Depressive and other 'pseudodementias' are distinguished by the lack of cortical features; but so are the subcortical dementias. Caine

(1981) has shown that psychological testing in 'pseudodementia' reveals a subcortical pattern of cognitive deficit. As we have further seen in Chapter 3, the whole thrust of neuropsychological testing has been to reveal such changes in depression.

Chapter 3 was devoted to the study of the neurobiological basis of depression, which is a chapter-long challenge to the concept of 'functional' illness. There are subtle and not so subtle changes in depression, and there is no qualitative distinction from 'organic' change. Thus depressive dementia, if one insisted, could really be perceived as an organic illness.

On closer scrutiny the features of cases of depressive dementia make revealing reading. While anecdotal and single case reports imply that it is the elderly who present with depression-related dementia, the evidence from reported series of cases seems to suggest a wider age range. Wells (1979) gave an age range between 33 and 69, and 7 of his 10 patients were in their 50s or 60s. Smith and Kiloh (1981), reporting a series of demented patients of all ages, showed that 'pseudodementia' accounted for 10% of all dementias under 45 years and for 13.6% of dementias between the ages of 45 and 64 years, but only for 1.8% of dementias over 65 years. McAllister's (1983) pooled series of cases yielded a mean age of 60.5 years, with a range between 22 and 85 years. Marsden and Harrison (1972), Nott and Fleminger (1975) and Ron et al. (1979) all paid attention to pre-senile cases of dementia with significant numbers of 'pseudodements'. Ron et al. (1979) commented that 'pseudodementia' was under-emphasized in the younger age groups (the latter two studies, indeed, sought to draw attention to the problems posed by 'pseudodementia' in the diagnosis of pre-senile dementia, circumstances which might have reflected the ease of case finding in this age group). Thus, the prevalence of depressive 'pseudodementia' in relatively young patients when by prediction it should have been found with increasing frequency in the older patient, needs to be explained. Also, while it is true, as Tomlinson et al. (1968) have shown, that structural brain changes in non-demented old people increase with age – in effect producing a closer approximation to Alzheimer-like pathology than in the younger subject – there is no significant difference between the changes in the brain between such non-dementing conditions as physical illness, confusional states, depressive illness and paraphrenia. Thus, there is no especially susceptible brain for depressive illness to lead beyond a threshold into dementia. The fact that depressive 'pseudodementia' occurs in middle-age and not necessarily, or preferentially, in the senium when the age changes make the brain most vulnerable suggests that there is more to 'pseudodementia' than the fortuitous association between depressive illness and the ageing brain.

Furthermore, if depressive 'pseudodementia' were indeed induced simply by depression, it would be expected that the depressed affect would precede cognitive change, and that there might be a time interval between the onset of depression and the onset of dementia. However, this does not seem to occur invariably. Clinical experience bears out that depression and dementia often have a simultaneous onset. The lack of consistent temporal relationship between affective and cognitive change is matched by an inconsistent quantitative relationship. Very often, memory difficulties are seen to be as prominent as, if not greater than, the depressive features. McAllister and Price (1982) noted a profound degree of cognitive impairment which appeared to be greatly out of proportion to the degree of depressive symptoms. They go on to say that, 'Referral had been for further evaluation and management of a presumed irreversible dementing illness and a diagnosis of depression and/or depressive pseudodementia had not been considered'. In fact, with the modern management of depressive illness, it is unlikely that depression will be allowed to reach a late stage at which dementia might emerge. Progression of depression in any case is towards increasing psychomotor retardation, through semi-stupor to stupor, which are circumstances of altering consciousness in which the diagnosis of dementia becomes untenable. The evidence from the recent literature, on the other hand, is that, if anything, 'pseudodementia', perhaps because of our awareness of the condition, is being reported more frequently, the prompt modern-day treatment of depression notwithstanding.

This body of evidence must throw considerable doubt in any simple notion of depressive 'pseudodementia' arising out of a depressive illness in an elderly patient, giving rise to cognitive change which progresses to dementia and may then be reversed when the depression is successfully treated. The facts suggest that at least in some cases there is unlikely to be a fortuitous association between depressive illness and a brain with no other complicating factor than the vulnerability wrought by the changes of age. The wide range of the ages of the patients concerned, the mode of onset and presentation, the suspicion of predisposing brain lesions, the evidence of a greater degree of structural and functional brain impairment than would be expected with depressive or other 'functional' illness alone, and the often independent course of the dementia and depression suggest that some cases of 'pseudodementia', at least, may deserve consideration as a discrete entity.

If depression and dementia are related in the way we have discussed in this and previous sections it is only natural to ask if any index pertaining to one had an effect on the other. The DST may be one. As we have seen in Chapter 3, the DST was first mooted as a specific, episode-related biological marker of melancholia. As a measure of limbic-neurendocrine dysfunction in 'endogenous' depression, and potentially reversible with antidepressant therapy, it claimed to bring a significant form of depressive illness, and the underlying neurotransmitter dysfunction, into the realm of laboratory investigation.

It was not too long before the DST was being proposed as a reliable laboratory distinction between 'pseudodementia' of depressive origin and 'true' dementia. Rudorfer and Clayton (1981) reported a case of 'pseudodementia' in which an abnormal DST normalized after treatment of the underlying depressive illness. McAllister et al. (1982) described two patients with severe depressive 'pseudodementia' in whom an abnormal DST seemed to point to depressive rather than 'progressive degenerative' aetiology of the dementia. One of these patients reverted to a normal DST following treatment with ECT. Carnes et al. (1983) also claimed that dementia by itself did not give rise to an abnormal DST, but dementia with depression could do so. None of their 18 patients with dementia alone had an abnormal DST. However, of 15 depressed, demented patients, 40% had abnormal DST.

At the time there appeared to be evidence for the claim that the biological phenomenon of the abnormal DST being related to or associated with melancholia, would be found in depression, absent in dementia, and hence the contentious business of 'pseudodementia' would at last be susceptible to resolution in the laboratory. Reports soon emerged, however, of significant numbers of patients showing an abnormal DST in 'senile' and 'parenchymal' dementia, in whom depression had been carefully excluded, and caution was soon enjoined against premature claims for the specificity of the abnormal DST of depressive illness *vis a vis* dementia. Does this 'little bit of depression' in dementia have any prognostic significance, as might be hypothesized? There is some slight, very slight, evidence for the prognostic significance of the abnormal DST. It was observed (Mahendra, 1984d) that the duration of illness in cases of senile dementia showing an abnormal DST appeared to be greater than in those successfully suppressing in the face of the dexamethasone challenge. The eight non-suppressors investigated by Spar and Gerner (1982) had a mean duration of illness of 4.75 years; the seven suppressors a mean duration of 3.5 years, a figure considerably exaggerated by a freak survival of 15 years. If this were excluded, the normal DST cases had a mean duration of symptoms of 1.66 years, over 3 years shorter than the non-suppressors. Much more work is needed, of course, to see if this is a valid hypothesis.

The mechanisms underlying the DST were discussed in Chapter 3, and the neurochemistry of AD is discussed in Mahendra (1984a). If, as has been supposed, the normal DST is a reflection of the integrity of the hypothalamo–hypophyseal–adrenal axis, mediated by cholinergically active neurones, the abnormal DST may be due to hyperactivity in the muscarinic cholinergic transmitter system. How does one square that with the known neurochemistry of AD? One must suppose that in slowly progressing AD there is a transient, relatively high cholinergic activity at the outset which gives rise to the abnormal DST. As the disease progresses, with diminution of cholinergic activity, there is less scope for an abnormal DST – which, if it occurs, must have another explanation. This relatively normal or high cholinergic activity may be one possible reason for the predisposition to depressive symptoms in the early stages of AD. An analogous finding in Parkinson's disease may yield a clue. Barbeau (1983) has suggested that as dopaminergic neurones are depleted in that condition, in the earliest phases the surviving neurones increase catecholamine synthesis as a homeostatic mechanism to preserve function. Similarly, it may be argued that cholinergic activity may be affected in dementing illness. As everything turns on the gradual loss of cholinergic neurones the slower progressing forms of dementia are more likely to produce depression, a prediction in keeping with the inverse relationship to be suggested shortly between dementia and depression.

Depression and dementia are also features of Parkinson's disease and

111

Huntington's chorea. These two conditions are characterized by a subcortical, slowly progressing dementia and a substantial incidence of depression. They too have a cholinergic function involvement, which may be the common thread tying them to depressive illness on the one hand and one form of AD on the other. The relative increase in cholinergic function in PD is well known, and is the basis for the therapeutic management of the condition.

Thus we have a variety of conditions in which dementia, depression and an aberrant cholinergic transmitter system are common features. It may be permissible to postulate a spectrum of brain dysfunction with a reversible or benign dementia associated with clearly defined depressive features at one end and a malignant dementia with little or no depression at the other. Perhaps conditions such as Parkinson's disease and Huntington's chorea with slower progressing dementias and a substantial depressive component lie in between. Similarly it is also possible to put forward the idea that an inverse relationship exists between depression and dementia. The more severe the dementia, one may speculate, the less prominent or marked is the depression and vice versa.

Depression in schizophrenia has long been known to modify that condition in a more benign direction. The transmitter mechanism there is likely to be a different one. However, the ameliorative role of depression, and its neurobiological substrate, is evident. These matters may have some other biological connotations which are discussed in relation to the biological advantages of depression in Chapter 9.

DEPRESSION IN RELATION TO SOME OTHER CEREBRAL DISORDERS

The incidence of psychiatric disturbance in neurological disease is high, and De Paulo and Folstein (1978) showed that 67% of patients with neurological disease showed some mental disturbance. When one considers the incidence of depression in brain disorder, one has to be able to make a distinction between the depression which may result from a reaction to a serious disease from that where the disease itself supplies the pathological basis for the depression. There appears to be a much higher incidence of psychiatric disturbance in cerebral disease than with peripheral neurological disorder, so that one is entitled to suspect a contributory cerebral factor in depression in cerebral neurological disease.

The generalized cerebral disorders are exemplified by conditions such as the dementias, both cortical and subcortical, and such disorders as multiple sclerosis. In these conditions attributing a specific structural lesion to the depression is a difficult undertaking, as has been previously discussed. The focal disorders are more promising in that their location and extent of lesion can be assessed with marginally greater accuracy. As will be discussed in the section on cerebrovascular disease, a crude anatomico–pathological correlation may be attempted.

Other, related emotional reactions seen in cerebral disorders are emotional lability which, in part, may be traced to a basal lesion, pathological

112

laughing and crying, which may be related to cortico–bulbar tract injury and catastrophic reactions more often seen with generalized cerebral disorders. These are short lived and transient reactions as opposed to a sustained depressive state. In all there is excessive emotional expression over which the patient appears to have little voluntary control ('emotional incontinence'), and in all three the actual volume of expressed emotion may bear little relationship to the emotion experienced, which often leads, in those patients with insight, to some degree of embarrassment.

Normal pressure hydrocephalus (NPH) has been discussed from the point of view of its presentation as a dementia in Mahendra (1984a). The neurological disability takes the form of a prominent gait disturbance. The dementia is not unlike the dementia seen with Parkinson's disease and Huntington's chorea, and is characterized by progressive intellectual impairment, apathy and a sparing of cortical function, i.e. it is a subcortical dementia. The apathy may be indistinguishable from the psychomotor retardation seen in depression, and its similarity to the akinetic syndrome seen in frontal lobe disorders has been commented upon. Whether true depression is seen with NPH is uncertain, but the rapid response of the mental state to surgical intervention makes it likely the mental state and the neurological disability have roots in the same cerebral disorder.

The affective disorder in multiple sclerosis has aroused some interest through the euphoria, which is occasionally seen. However, 27% of patients with multiple sclerosis are seen to be depressed (Surridge, 1969). Euphoria was seen with dementia, and the intensity of the euphoria was correlated with the severity of the intellectual impairment. Surridge believed the depression was reactive and secondary. Thus, he felt, the psychological impact of learning of the diagnosis, living, first, with uncertainty and then with growing disability appear to be more important than any contribution from the neuropathology of the condition. Be that as it may, a severe degree of depression may be noted and suicidal behaviour is not unknown.

Tumours of the brain including meningioma and glioblastoma, especially in the region of the frontal lobe and corpus callosum produce a picture of apathy which may progress to stupor. Tumours of the corpus callosum may also, in a substantial number of cases, produce mental symptoms before the onset of symptoms of space-occupying lesions (Mahendra, 1985b). The rapid onset of stupor may lead to difficulties in the differential diagnosis with depression.

However, tumours in other parts of the brain may also give rise to depression. The psychiatric manifestations of cerebral tumour depend, among other factors, on the type of tumour, its site in the brain, the rate of growth, the presence of raised intracranial pressure and the premorbid personality of the patient (Lishman, 1978) and to these might be added treatment, whether radiotherapy, specific chemotherapy or non-specific chemotherapy, e.g. steroids. Lishman reported a psychiatric incidence of up to three quarters with cerebral tumours. Supratentorial tumours, especially of the frontal and temporal lobes, were more likely to produce mental symptoms, and slow growing tumours were also more likely to present with mental symptoms rather than neurological features. Affective

113

features are found in association with other psychiatric features, and these were partly a reaction to the realization that serious pathology was afoot and partly an independent pathological phenomenon.

Henry (1932) noted that irritability and peevishness could precede clear-cut depression and anger. Suicidal behaviour could be found in 10% of cases and appeared to be related to headache. It was pointed out that in the early cases the premorbid personality of the patient was a major influence in the display of affective symptomatology, but later the pathological features of the tumour itself were more important, implying a more autonomous course in the affective symptomatology.

Tumours with the slowest rate of growth are the least likely to produce symptoms. When mental manifestations including depression arise in relation to slow growing tumours, there is also a likelihood of their overshadowing the features related to the focal location and space occupation. Rapid growth of a tumour presents with a higher degree of psychiatric disturbance but usually in the midst of neurological features. Thus gliomas and other malignant tumours produce more mental symptoms than meningiomas. Rapidly growing tumours invade brain tissue and also give rise to an early increase in intracranial pressure. Also, bilateral tumours e.g. metastases are associated with more mental disturbance than tumours in one hemisphere, even when of large growth (Keschner et al., 1938). Supratentorial tumours are less likely to produce raised intracranial pressure but there is a greater likelihood of psychiatric manifestations. Frontal and temporal lobe tumours are far more likely than tumours in the parietal and occipital lobes to produce depression. In the case of the temporal lobe much of the psychopathology may be attributed to disturbances of a paroxysmal nature that result from lesions in that lobe. Temporal lobe tumours in the dominant hemisphere, especially when associated with dysphasia, are associated with depression and other affective features (Keschner et al., 1936). The role of the dominant hemisphere and its dysfunction has been considered in Chapter 3.

The psychiatric aspects of head injury have been detailed by Lishman (1968, 1978). Affective symptoms were present in 70% of patients with head injury, half of them of a significant degree. Right hemisphere, especially frontal lobe, damage was especially prone to give rise to depression, but Lishman claimed it was not so much the degree of injury but the predisposition of the patient that was responsible for the onset of depression. Lishman also found that the depth of penetration in head injury and the total volume of the brain destroyed were significantly related to mental problems. Overall, he confirmed that left hemisphere injury gave rise to psychiatric disability, especially when left temporal lobe damage had occurred. Disability such as motor and sensory defects, visual field problems, aphasia and epilepsy were all significantly related to psychiatric illness. However, while intellectual and behaviour disorder seemed related to left hemisphere damage, affective syndromes were associated with injury to the right hemisphere.

The indirect effects of systemic disease in relation to the production of depression are beyond the scope of this book, but reference must be made to a few of the depressive syndromes seen with endocrine disorders as they may hold points of aetiological interest. Cohen (1980) showed that 86% of patients with Cushing's syndrome were depressed, but that the severity of the depression was not related to the level of circulating cortisol. However, there was rapid relief of the depression when the tumour or the hyperplastic glands were removed. As medical in-patients have overall only about 20% incidence of depression, there was a substantially increased incidence in Cushing's syndrome. The vulnerability factors already noted for depression were also seen by Cohen, namely a family history of depression or suicide or a history of early bereavement or separation, in nearly half the patients. Depression was especially common in the pituitary-dependent form of Cushing's syndrome and thus, in the absence of psychiatric disturbance, the chances of finding an adrenal tumour was increased. Thus the presence or absence of psychiatric symptoms is a pointer to the aetiology of Cushing's syndrome. What causes the depression in this setting is not clear. As the levels of circulating cortisol had little bearing on the degree of depression, the hormone was clearly not the sole cause of the depression. As the depressive symptoms could be relieved by adrenalectomy, it could have been some other factor secreted by the adrenal glands. On the other hand, it was suggested that the vulnerability and other factors personal to the patient might have determined the onset and depth of depression in the presence of the elevated cortisol.

The depression itself in Cushing's syndrome may be severe and delusional. Auditory hallucinations complete the picture of classical depressive psychosis. Retardation extending to stupor may be seen and the illness may have a fluctuating course.

The depression seen in Cushing's syndrome was confirmed by Kelly *et al.* (1980) who showed that Cushing's syndrome patients with active disease were more depressed than those who had been treated. There had been a suggestion, from animal studies, that an increase in cortisol could lead to tryptophan metabolism being preferentially diverted along the kynurenine pathway (see Chapter 3), with a fall in plasma and brain tryptophan concentrations and 5-HT levels. Kelly *et al.* (1983) could not confirm a fall in either free plasma tryptophan concentrations, and suggested that it was most unlikely this syndrome of depression resulted from a deficiency of tryptophan or a consequent fall in 5-HT.

A more apathetic depression may be seen in hypopituitarism. Mental features are also prominent in hyperparathyroidism, with an apathetic depression the commonest feature. Petersen (1968) found two-thirds of his cases had mental change. Fatiguability, dullness and aspontaneity are characteristic. Unlike the increased cortisol levels and the lack of correlation with the mental state, there is a significant correlation between the raised calcium levels and the psychiatric features (see also the discussion of malignancy in relation to depression in Chapter 6). A quantitative relationship can be found between the severity of psychopathology and the levels of serum calcium. Depression and diminished drive are seen with serum calcium of 12–16mg/100ml, acute organic states between 16–19mg/100ml, and somnolence and coma beyond 19mg/100ml. This implies that personality factors are less important than immediate pathology, and the point has been made that the psychopathology of hyperparathyroidism is less dependent on the dynamics of the personality than other endocrinopathies. Also, it is the level of serum calcium, an intermediary, that is important in the causation of the depression rather than the more immediate parathormone. Thus if serum calcium is even transiently reduced by dialysis, there is an apparent improvement in the mental state.

The question of malignancy in relation to depression is taken up further in Chapter 6. It will suffice here to note that virtually any non-cerebral malignancy may present with depression and the mental features may precede the developments of symptoms and signs pertaining to the organ involved. Nearly half the patients studied by Fras *et al.* (1967) with depression in relation to carcinoma of the pancreas had mental symptoms preceding the physical illness, with an onset on average 6 months before the neoplasm was suspected. Overall, they found mental disturbance could be related to the onset of the carcinoma in nearly three quarters of cases, whereas in the controls with carcinoma of the colon, the figure was less than a fifth. Thus the site of even a primary, non-cerebral malignancy may determine the incidence of psychiatric disturbance.

Epilepsy is a chronic neurological condition, and it would not be surprising if there were an elevated risk of depression in such a condition. Also, until more modern anticonvulsant chemotherapy became available, drugs such as phenytoin, phenobarbitone and primidone were also known to be occasional depressants.

Depression is more often associated with temporal lobe epilepsy rather than with other varieties. Depression may be found in about a third of cases of epilepsy and there is a relationship between a decline in fit frequency and the onset of an episode of depression, almost as if naturally occurring convulsive treatment were keeping the depression at bay. The presence of foci in the non-dominant temporal lobe has been implicated, as has been discussed in Chapter 3. The foci for schizophrenia and confusional states are thought to lie predominantly in the dominant temporal lobe. These observations were made by Flor-Henry (1969), but remain speculative. Other points made were that patients with affective disorder have less frequent seizures than other patients and also have a higher proportion of generalized seizures. They also tend to have less structural brain damage and have more stable previous personalities and better psychosocial adjustment than other groups of patients. The suggestion is that the predisposition to depression is due in large measure to the epileptic focus itself.

Flor-Henry's views have attracted ample criticism, and other workers have found little to suggest that there might be a relationship between epilepsy and the depression. Toone *et al.* (1982), for instance, felt that the affective psychoses which occur in association with epilepsy did not form a distinctive syndrome and might well represent a chance association.

The hemisphere involvement in maintaining mood has been discussed in Chapter 3. In 1979, Flor-Henry developed his ideas of epilepsy further by trying to conceptualize a possible neural substrate for normal and abnormal mood. He believes the primary centre is located in the non-dominant hemisphere but that its regulation is bilateral. A maniform picture results when the dominant centre is no longer inhibited by the non-dominant hemisphere. Conversely, depression results when the activity of the non-dominant is no longer inhibited by the dominant hemisphere.

CEREBROVASCULAR DISEASE

The increased incidence of depression in cerebrovascular disease is beyond dispute and has been commented on at least from the great period of neuropsychiatric study in the last century. Kraepelin noted the predisposition to depression in patients with cerebrovascular disease, along with irritability and emotional lability and Eugen Bleuler confirmed that affective disorder could arise after brain damage.

The degree of disability alone is not sufficient to explain the incidence of depression. When a group of recovered stroke patients are compared to patients with a comparable degree of disability, e.g. orthopaedic patients, substantially greater numbers of stroke patients are found to be depressed.

Robinson and Szetela (1981) compared patients with left hemisphere strokes with traumatic brain injury patients for frequency and severity of depression. Although the two groups had comparable levels of impairment 60% of the stroke patients were depressed compared to about 20% of the trauma patients. CAT scan results showed that the size of the lesions in the two groups was comparable, but that the areas of ischaemic damage were more anteriorly placed. When the lesions were controlled for site, there was no difference between the two groups. The severity of depression was directly related to the proximity of the lesion to the frontal lobe. They suggested that depression following left hemisphere brain injury may not be a non-specific response but may follow damage to specific catecholaminergic pathways as they pass through the frontal cortex.

Speech function is, of course, impaired in dominant hemisphere lesions, but the different varieties of speech disturbance may relate differently to the incidence and severity of depression. Robinson and Benson (1981) showed non-fluent aphasic patients (with expressive deficits) had both greater frequency and severity of depression than either the fluent (receptive) aphasic group or the global aphasic patients. As might be expected, global aphasia showed the most extensive lesions and there was a correlation between brain damage and degree of depression. The patients with receptive dysphasia, however, showed an inverse correlation between the size of the lesion and the depth of depression. Expressive aphasic patients had their pathology close to the anterior pole, and the number of patients with severe depression was greater among those with anterior lesions than posterior lesions.

Robinson et al. (1984) showed that the prevalence of significant depression increases steadily for the first 6 months after a cerebral haemorrhage or ischaemic lesion. Psychopathological lesions were related to the location of the hemispheric lesion. Patients with left hemisphere lesions were more depressed than patients with right hemisphere lesions. Left anterior infarcts produce the greatest severity of depression even when the brain injury is bilateral, whereas right anterior infarcts produce an undue cheerfulness. Although lesion location appeared to be the single most important factor in determining the severity of impairment in activities of daily living, intellectual function as well as the quality of social support were also significantly correlated with the severity of depression following stroke.

Of 30 patients who were depressed at the initial interview, two thirds of those interviewed between 7 and 8 months following the initial interview remained depressed. However, by 10–11 months after the initial evaluation less than 20% of the patients remained depressed and by one year none of the patients remained depressed. Thus, although they are self-limiting disorders, they are responsible for significant psychopathology, and there is little evidence that they are recognized everywhere. Thus they may provide an impediment to the successful rehabilitation of the stroke patient. The available evidence suggests that conventional antidepressant therapy, including ECT, may achieve as good results with these as with what might be called idiopathic depressions.

Several explanations may be offered for presence of depression in stroke. The high incidence in expressive aphasic patients may be attributable to the loss of speech production, an essential component of communication and their subsequent demoralization. The question of insight is important here. It was found that when comprehension difficulties are greatest in those who are receptively aphasic, depression is most severe.

There are neurochemical explanations to which Robinson and Benson (1981) draw attention. Cerebral infarction in the rat leads to extensive changes in biogenic amines in the injured as well as the obviously uninjured parts of the brain. The catecholamine-pathways branch as they pass posteriorly from the frontal lobes, and thus anterior lesions found with expressive dysphasia disrupt more catecholamine pathways than more posterior lesions and hence produce more depression. The fact that small strategically placed lesions can produce more psychopathology than larger lesions may mean that the site involved is more important than the size of the injury.

Other forms of cerebrovascular disease, too, appear to give rise to depressive psychopathology. Subarachnoid haemorrhage is a case in point, and Storey (1970) found that 55% of his patients displayed some form of psychiatric morbidity. However, the degree of brain damage and the ensuing physical disability did not seem always to correspond to the features of depression. Depression was more likely to occur with aneurysms of the posterior communicating artery which has close anatomical and functional links with the hypothalamus.

Haemorrhage into the upper brainstem gives rise to depression (Trimble and Cummings, 1981). Here location of the lesion is important, as lesions in the upper brainstem could disrupt ascending adrenergic and serotonergic fibres which arise in the nuclei of the brainstem and project to diencephalic and forebrain structures.

5
Depressed minds, disputed cures: the management of depression

The logical approach to the management of the depressed patient is by considering those factors that are implicated and correcting them. There may be, on the one hand, the personality of the patient which might have been rendered vulnerable by both his genetic constitution and his subjective experience of his environment. On the other hand, there are stressful life events of different kinds which may impinge on a personality that is vulnerable. There is, as we have seen in a previous chapter, a diverse variety of brain and systemic disease which may predispose to, or even produce in their own right, depression. Depression is the end result and it is convenient to see it as a clinical manifestation of a neurobiological process, even though not every form of depression is liable to such basic change, at least as far as we know today.

The approach to the management of the depressed patient needs to take into account those factors which constitute the diagnostic formulation in the depressed patient. The management will thus include:

(1) Physical treatment to correct the aberrant neurobiological process by such means as antidepressant drugs, electroconvulsive treatment (ECT) and psychosurgery;
(2) The investigation and treatment, where feasible, of cerebral and systemic disease where it contributes to the depression;
(3) The assessment of the psychosocial environment of the patient so that life stresses and vulnerability factors may, where possible, be countered, modified or reduced;
(4) The personality of the patient and his habitual ways of dealing with stress evaluated with the patient so that the current episode may be managed and any in the future forestalled;
(5) We do not have sufficient knowledge to undertake genetic counselling but an awareness of genetic factors is often of help in the patient's understanding of how and why the illness might have come about.

119

This chapter deals with the physical and psychological aspects of treatment of depression. Other aspects of the management of depression are dealt with in the relevant sections of chapters 2, 4, 6, 7 and 8.

PHYSICAL TREATMENT

The tricyclic agents and their successors

These have been separated for convenience into the conventional antidepressant agents, and the monoamine oxidase inhibitors and lithium which are considered separately in the succeeding sections.

Table 5 Some commonly used antidepressants

Antidepressant	Starting daily dose	Full daily dose	Special feature
Amitriptyline	75 mg	300 mg	Marked anticholinergic and sedative actions, caution in elderly
Imipramine	75 mg	225 mg	As above but no sedative action
Clomipramine	10 mg	150 mg	For phobic and obsessional symptoms associated with depression
Dothiepin	75 mg	225 mg	Sedative. Possibly safer in the elderly and those with cardiovascular problems
Doxepin	75 mg	300 mg	As for dothiepin
Lofepramine	70 mg	210 mg	Little sedative action. Safe in elderly and those with cardiovascular problems
Trimipramine	75 mg	300 mg	Marked sedative and hypnotic actions
Mianserin	30 mg	200 mg	Sedative action: safe in the elderly
Phenelzine	15 mg tds	15 mg four or five times	MAO I See text
Isocarboxazid	30 mg	30 mg	
Tranylcypromine	10mg b.d.	10mg tds	
Lithium carbonate	250mg tds tds	up to 2g	Dose given to achieve plasma level of 0.6–1.2 mmol Li^+/l
Lithium carbonate (sustained release)	400 mg	up to 2g	

Modern antidepressant drug treatment has a history of just over a generation. The first of these agents, imipramine, was introduced by Kuhn in 1957, and amitriptyline followed in 1961. A large number of tricyclic, tetracyclic and other agents are now available, and there is a remarkable similarity in the chemical structure of many of these agents, some indeed being metabolites of others.

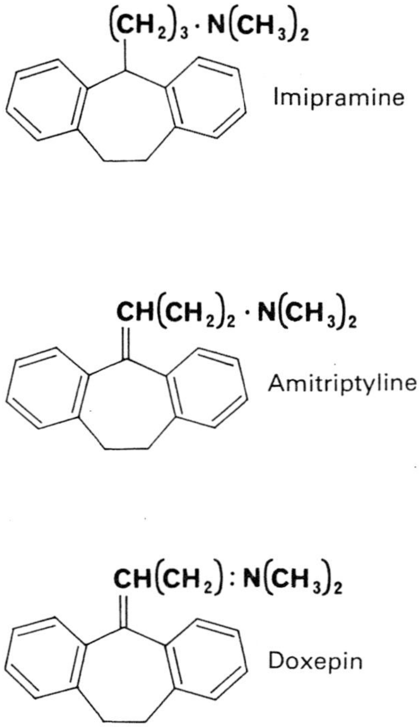

$(CH_2)_3 \cdot N(CH_3)_2$

Imipramine

$CH(CH_2)_2 \cdot N(CH_3)_2$

Amitriptyline

$CH(CH_2) : N(CH_3)_2$

Doxepin

Figure 9 Some commonly used antidepressants

Kuhn (1958) studied imipramine, which is chemically related to chlorpromazine, with a view to its use as a tranquillizing agent. It had no sedative properties but depressed patients responded to it after several weeks of treatment.

Imipramine is metabolized with loss of a methyl group to desipramine, and amitriptyline suffers a similar transformation to nortriptyline. Both metabolites are effective antidepressants in their own right. The newer antidepressant, lofepramine (introduced in 1977), is at least in part metabolized to desipramine.

Clomipramine (introduced in 1968) and lofepramine are similar to imipramine. Desipramine is the metabolic product of both imipramine and lofepramine, but it is not possible to attribute the antidepressant efficacy of the latter to desipramine as its levels in plasma are very low. The advantage of using desipramine is that, at least in theory, it removes a necessary step in the process of its metabolism from imipramine and may thus increase the speed of onset of the antidepressant effect. This is not seen in practice where the efficacy and the speed of onset of the action of all antidepressants in clinical use is comparable. This is no doubt due to the factors which were discussed in Chapter 3 and will be taken up shortly.

Clomipramine, also related to imipramine, was mooted as a drug which might have more specific actions in patients with phobic and obsessive–compulsive symptoms. This is now not thought to be the case, and clomipramine, an established antidepressant, is now believed to exert its effects on those symptoms secondary to improvement in the depression (Marks *et al.*, 1980).

Metabolism

The commonly used antidepressant agents are well absorbed after oral ingestion and there is rapid entry into the plasma. A reversible binding, up to 95%, occurs with plasma albumin and, as with most substances, the unbound part of the drug seems to exert the significant therapeutic actions. The metabolism of the antidepressants takes place in the liver by processes of demethylation and hydroxylation, and excretion is via bile and the urine. Several factors may alter the pharmacokinetic properties of tricyclic agents. The most important of these appears to be the level of activity of the hepatic microsomal enzymes, which are influenced by genetic factors, age and the intake of other drugs. There may be up to a 40-fold variation in blood levels produced by the same dose of drug in different individuals (Peet and Coppen, 1979). However, the use of plasma drug levels has been questioned. They are of obvious value in those patients who do not appear to respond to treatment and where compliance is suspect, and may also be useful in those who display an unusual degree of side-effects or those in whom an associated systemic condition, e.g. cardiac disease, makes the monitoring of drugs essential. However, Kocsis *et al.* (1986) could find little relationship between any plasma measure of amitriptyline or imipramine and any measure of clinical response. They concluded that blood drug level measurement appeared to be of little value in monitoring the clinical response of depressed patients. However, they showed there was a direct relationship between age and tricyclic drug steady-state plasma concentrations, especially when the parent compound was imipramine or amitriptyline. Thus, the elderly, who are prone to suffer more adverse effects of these drugs, may benefit from more cautious administration of these drugs and also from monitoring of plasma levels.

As has been suggested, plasma levels may vary enormously, and part of the variation appears to be genetic (Alexanderson and Borga, 1972). The effects of other drugs are variable. Barbiturates induce the metabolism of tricyclic agents by action on the microsomal enzymes and thereby lower their levels. In the past, at least, a vicious circle was set in motion as tricyclic agent administration, which is said to lower the epileptic threshold, was followed by a prophylactic increase in anti-convulsive medication, which presumably diminished tricyclic drug levels, and compromised their anti-depressant actions. Phenothiazine drugs, on the other hand, inhibit the microsomal enzymes, thereby elevating tricyclic levels and thus probably have a practical bearing on the treatment of severe delusional depression where a combination of phenothiazine and tricyclic drug has significantly greater therapeutic actions than the tricyclic drug alone.

The relationship between the dose ingested and the plasma level is not necessarily linear. For nortriptyline it was suggested (Asberg *et al.*, 1971) that a curvilinear relationship might exist between dose and plasma level, i.e. there was an optimal range of the drug, below or beyond which it exerted less than its most effective actions. Thus where increasing doses of imipramine and amitriptyline might be thought to produce better clinical results, the dosage of nortriptyline which had the best effect was one that produced a range between 50 and 140 ng/ml. At higher plasma levels, especially when the upper limit exceeded 170 ng/ml, there was less effect on the clinical state. This works out to a dosage of about 150 mg nortriptyline daily. Despite a few claims, it has not wholly convincingly shown that nortriptyline, a metabolite of amitriptyline, behaves any differently to other antidepressants.

A parent tertiary amine may give rise to a secondary amine as a metabolite and both may exert effects on the clinical state. With amitriptyline and its metabolite, nortriptyline, both established antidepressants in their own right, the clinical responses to amitriptyline appear to be correlated with the nortriptyline/amitriptyline ratio.

Mode of action

All antidepressants established for use in clinical practice have equal therapeutic effects when used in appropriate doses in a series of patients. However, there is little reason to doubt that their primary modes of action are different, a view that buttresses the argument that their antidepressant actions are due to a 'final common pathway' metabolism.

The tertiary amines, e.g. imipramine, amitriptyline decrease the re-uptake of indoleamines, such as 5-HT, into the nerve endings; secondary amines, e.g. desipramine, nortriptyline exert similar effects on noradrenaline. Clomipramine exerts effects on the re-uptake of 5-HT and some tricyclic agents, presumably because they act as tertiary amines and their secondary amine metabolites, have effects on both noradrenaline and 5-HT.

As has been discussed in Chapter 3, the re-uptake blockade of biogenic amines is of rapid onset, whereas the clinical antidepressant response to nearly all antidepressants takes between 10–14 days. An alternative explanation was sought and this has been dealt with in Chapter 3.

Although several claims have been made for the more rapid onset of action with some antidepressants than others, these cannot be substantiated. The early claims were for desipramine, more recent ones for lofepramine. As we have seen, desipramine, being a metabolite of imipramine, may have been expected theoretically to bring about a quicker response to its antidepressant effects. There is no clinical evidence for this. Some of the claims might have been based on the sedative actions of tricyclic drugs producing a symptomatic improvement in some components of affective disorder, e.g. anxiety, insomnia.

Side-effects and adverse effects

These effects are, of course, relative and depend on many things. Sedation and a hypnotic effect are welcomed in the majority of cases of depression because of the associated symptoms of insomnia and anxiety. Some clearly are always unwelcome, e.g. anticholinergic effects or effects on the heart.

The commonest complained of side effects are those due to anticholinergic activity. These include dryness of the mouth, difficulties with visual accommodation, difficulty in initiating micturition, constipation, excessive sweating, palpitations, postural hypotension, retention of urine, paralytic ileus and cardiac failure. There is also the propensity, especially in the elderly, to toxic confusional states. Although the anticholinergic effects might be considered useful adjuncts in the treatment of Parkinson's disease, there is an occasional worsening of rigidity and tremor. This may be due to the chemical affinities the tricyclic agents have with phenothiazine drugs where a dopamine blocking action overshadows the positive response to the anticholinergic action. Whether the anticholinergic actions might have an antidepressant action by themselves is worthy of consideration in view of the discussion in Chapter 3 and the hypothesis advanced by Janowsky *et al.* (1972) which proposed that depression might result from an imbalance between cholinergic and adrenergic mechanisms. Whatever the merits of that hypothesis and the explanation of cholinergic mechanisms, anticholinergic effects of drugs are now deemed not to have *clinical* antidepressant properties. The evidence for this is that though pioneering agents such as imipramine and amitriptyline have quite marked anticholinergic properties, several of the newer antidepressants lack these effects but are equally efficacious antidepressant agents. For instance, doxepine has only a fraction of the anticholinergic activity of amitriptyline. Conversely, primary anticholinergic drugs such as atropine and hyoscine have no worthwhile antidepressant actions.

The sedative properties of antidepressants are brought to the clinician's notice by direct inquiry rather than complaint, which is more likely with the anticholinergic effects. Amitriptyline, doxepin and trimipramine have sedative and hypnotic actions. Drugs such as protriptyline, nortriptyline and desipramine are better activating agents and may have greater use in those patients with retardation. Imipramine may have mild stimulatory properties. There is also a dissociation between the sedative properties and the antidepressant effects of these agents. The sedative properties are seen early, whereas the antidepressant actions come on after 10–14 days. Also, the relatively long halflife of these agents – 40 hours for amitriptyline – while it means there is no need for more than once daily administration also obviates the need to prescribe an additional hypnotic when a sedative antidepressant such as amitriptyline is used. There may also be a carry over of the anxiolytic properties to the day. The sedative and hypnotic properties may in part be due to an antihistamine action. Histamine is now acknowledged to be a neurotransmitter and acts on H_1 and H_2 receptors. The antihistamine properties of tricyclic antidepressants are expressed by inhibition of H_1 receptors. Doxepin is said to have the most potent histamine-blocking properties of the tricyclic antidepressant drugs (Richelson, 1979) and is followed by amitriptyline, imipramine, nortriptyline, protriptyline and desipramine, and this order accords with the clinically seen sedative properties of the drugs.

The commonly used tricyclic agents exert several effects on the heart, and their actions are usually viewed with concern. The dangers are probably exaggerated. For serious adverse cardiac effects there is a requirement for a prior heart condition and, perhaps, an intervening variable such as stress before effects are seen with therapeutic doses of the drugs. However, some change in heart function, e.g. sinus tachycardia can be explained in terms of the known properties such as anticholinergic activity. There are also effects on myocardial contractility and on atrio–ventricular conduction. The actions of tricyclic drugs on the heart are discussed by Burrows *et al.* (1976). It would appear that at low concentrations, the effects of anticholinergic activity are seen, i.e. tachycardia. At therapeutic concentrations, the concentrations of catecholamines are increased by re-uptake blockade and these exert a direct action on the heart. At higher than therapeutic levels, tricyclic drugs may block the actions of catecholamines, with the result that there is prolongation of the P–R interval and widening of the QRS complex. There is in addition a quinidine-like effect which leads to myocardial contractility being diminished, reduction in the heart rate and a decline in coronary blood flow. Thus in fatal overdose with tricyclic antidepressant drugs, the EEG may show sinus tachycardia, conduction defects, supraventricular tachycardia, ST- and T-wave abnormality, ventricular arrhythmias, bradycardia and asystole.

Table 6 Effects of tricyclic drugs on the heart

Anticholinergic effects ⟶	increased heart rate
Later adrenolytic effect ⟶	decreased heart rate and decreased cardiac output
Quinidine-like effects ⟶	decreased excitability, conduction velocity and myocardial contractions

The actions of tricyclic antidepressant drugs on the heart appear to be dose-related, and thus those patients who are at risk would be those who have taken an accidental or deliberate overdose of the drugs, and those in whom the dosage is being increased as a result of non-response or unexplained, persistent low plasma levels of the drug. Quitkin (1985) suggests that special precautions including regular ECG monitoring must be undertaken. If the heart rate is less than 100, and the QRS complex, QTc and the P–R interval are within normal limits, the dose of tricyclic drugs can be increased in those circumstances to 400–500 mg/day.

Other adverse reactions are considerably less frequent. A lowering of the epileptic threshold is suspected. With more recent antidepressants, blood dyscrasias, skin reactions and fever are more commonly observed. With mianserin, blood dyscrasias and liver dysfunction have been reported; maprotiline has given rise to convulsions; zimeldine had to be withdrawn after reports of the Guillain–Barré syndrome and nomifensine after blood dyscrasias. Lofepramine has had skin reactions, biliary problems and occasional parkinsonian effects attributed to it.

An effect which may be construed as adverse is a switch into mania. There are no pointers to the imminence of this transformation which may occur with those who have had a previous manic illness as well as in those in whom bipolarity of illness has not been recognized.

Tricyclic antidepressant drugs may also provoke sexual disturbances including diminished libido, orgasmic dysfunction and erectile and ejaculatory disturbance. Both the tricyclic group – including amitriptyline, imipramine, clomipramine, desipramine and protiptyline – and mono-amine oxidase inhibitors (MAOI, see below) have been implicated. The effects of antidepressant drugs in sexual function are difficult to evaluate as depression itself has sexual difficulty within its symptomatology. Kowalski *et al.* (1985) have proposed both central and peripheral mechanisms for sexual dysfunction associated with antidepressant medication. The former includes the blocking of 5-HT re-uptake, with increased 5-HT levels centrally, which is known to result in inhibition of sexual functioning. Peripherally the anticholinergic effects may reduce parasympathetic responses. Also, the pre-synaptic α_2 receptor antagonist actions of antidepressants leads to potentiation of adrenergic (noradrenergic) activity. Both amitriptyline and mianserin give rise to adverse effects, even the latter, which is a 5-HT antagonist and which has little effect on central 5-HT re-uptake and turnover. Kowalski *et al.* (1985) felt that the most plausible explanation common to both drugs was the pre-synaptic α_2-adrenoceptor antagonism resulting in increased noradrenaline turnover and the consequent high sympathetic activity leading to sexual dysfunction.

The abnormalities in sleep pattern and rhythm have been discussed in Chapter 3. It is believed that REM sleep has to be suppressed before clinical improvement can occur in depression. It was noted that REM sleep was under cholinergic mechanisms which might be imagined to be influenced by the older antidepressants such as amitriptyline and unaffected by relatively new antidepressants such as mianserin. However, Kowalski *et al.* (1985) found that both amitriptyline and mianserin increase REM sleep latency and significantly decrease REM sleep time. This would argue for central anticholinergic actions, not previously suspected with mianserin.

Increased appetite is a common feature with antidepressants and often confounds the assessment of weight gain which occurs with the improvement in depression.

Some other effects may be briefly noted. Glaucoma is a contra-indication to treatment with tricyclic agents with marked anticholinergic effects. Alcohol may potentiate the sedative and hypnotic effects apart from interfering with the antidepressant action. Tremor may also be seen with these agents.

Administration

The antidepressant drugs are given orally in the vast majority of cases. If there is defective absorption or a refusal to take the drug there may be a case for intramuscular injection in the short term to make the patient more amenable. The initial period of administration of an antidepressant is for a period of at least 6 weeks. The effects, if any, should have become clear by this time and, unless there are exceptional reasons, there is no advantage in changing medication before this time. If there is a lack of response to the drug associated with a worsening in the clinical state, a course of ECT is probably the option of choice rather than a switch to one or more antidepressants in a search for a successful result. As for the length of time the drug needs to be continued, there is no agreement on this point nor on the nature of depression that needs continuation therapy. However, there are pointers of a general nature from the natural history of the illness. As the average phase of illness lasts 6–12 months, it is reasonable to hope to continue with antidepressant drugs at least for this period. As there is no evidence that the longterm effects of antidepressant medication lead to adverse results as do the phenothiazines, the misgivings regarding its longterm use are not of the same order.

One of the less edifying features of antidepressant drug therapy, especially in general practice, is the grossly inadequate doses of drugs that are often exhibited. Quitkin (1985) observed that treatment could not be considered to be satisfactory until patients had received 300 mg of imipramine or equivalent, and a separate trial of 90 mg of phenelzine (an MAOI) or equivalent. Reviewing reports of 'refractory' patients in the literature, he found 30–80% of such 'refractory' patients had appeared to receive inadequate doses of tricyclic agents, but when treated with adequate doses of such drugs, half of them had shown improvement. It also appeared that patients deemed 'refractory' on doses of 150 mg daily of imipramine or its equivalent or less benefit when given a higher dose of tricyclic antidepressants.

This was also a point made by Bridges (1983) who stated that many intractable cases of depression referred for evaluation for psychosurgery had received an inadequate trial of antidepressant medication.

It appears that for a favourable response to be achieved, in general, plasma imipramine levels greater than 200 ng/ml are required. At doses which yield less than this plasma level, the chances of failure are greater.

As has been pointed out, patients given a full or high dosage of drugs may occasionally fail to reach the therapeutically significant plasma range. This is in part due to genetic and individual factors, and the clinician is advised to exceed the 'normal' maximum. As was discussed above, side-effects increase and adverse effects on the heart may become more likely, and careful plasma level and ECG monitoring may be required.

Whether there are biological as opposed to clinical indices of response to tricyclic antidepressants is as yet unclear. Non-suppressors on the dexamethasone suppressed test (DST, see Chapter 3) have been thought to respond better, also responding preferentially to imipramine or desipramine while DST suppressors responded better to amitriptyline or clomipramine (Brown and Shuey, 1980; Brown and Qualls, 1981; see also response in relation to levels of MHPG, Chapter 3). Nelson et al. (1982) noted that higher cortisol levels after dexamethasone administration correlated

127

significantly with greater clinical improvement. This may mean that the more 'biologically' based a depression is, the more likely it is to respond to physical intervention. This view is supported by Coppen *et al.* (1985) who found that in those patients receiving antidepressant therapy, a high post-DST plasma cortisol concentration was associated with greater therapeutic improvement than in patients with a low post-DST plasma cortisol concentration, an effect paralleled though not equalled by ECT.

It has also been shown that normalization on DST response precedes or coincides with a clinical response. This may have pointers for therapy, especially for its continuation. If the DST has normalized, but the clinical response lags, this may well be the signal to continue treatment with the same drug. It has been suggested that if following clinical improvement or remission, the DST remains, or returns to being, abnormal, a clinical relapse will follow. Bowie and Beaini (1985) have found this is not always so, with only 25% of patients relapsing. Whether or not a persistently abnormal DST is indicative of poor prognosis, as was suggested by Greden *et al.* (1983), is not clear.

Relapse may be reduced by giving tricyclic antidepressant drugs for 6 months to one year (Peet and Coppen, 1979). The drug may be reduced gradually after this time. Abrupt cessation incurs the risk of precipitating depression and withdrawal effects, at least in part due to withdrawal from anticholinergic effects – these include malaise, retardation and gastro-intestinal symptoms.

Other non-MAOI antidepressants

Drugs such as imipramine and amitriptyline belong to the first generation of specific antidepressant medication. To extend the scope of antidepressant actions as well as to counter or eliminate the disadvantages of these drugs, especially in vulnerable patient groups such as the elderly, the second generation antidepressants were developed. These lack the tricyclic ring structure and include drugs such as mianserin, maprotiline, viloxazine, trazodone and L-tryptophan which are available for use, and such drugs as zimeldine and nomifensine which have been withdrawn after reports of unacceptable adverse effects.

Mianserin is the most important in clinical practice among these drugs. It has useful sedative properties which aid in the management of anxiety and agitation during the day and is an adjunct to the use of a hypnotic at night. It has a quadricyclic ring structure and has significantly fewer anti-cholinergic effects, which is a desirable property in groups such as the elderly. It is equal in efficacy to any of the commonly used antidepressants, and in a general practice population it was shown to be as effective as imipramine (Murphy *et al.*, 1976). Blood dyscrasias are relatively more common with this drug as is arthralgia. It has minimal effects on cardiac function. As has been seen it exerts its effects not by blocking the re-uptake of noradrenaline or 5-HT but by increasing the turnover of noradrenaline, presumably by blocking the presynaptic adrenoceptors. There is presynaptic α_2-receptor blockade which leads to inhibition of noradrenaline release and a subsequent increase in noradrenaline activity in order to overcome this block. It is readily absorbed, reaching peak levels in the plasma after 2–3 hours and a steady-state after about 2 weeks (Perry et al., 1978). Although plasma levels can be measured they appear to be of little clinical use. The daily dose is between 30–120 mg although the manufacturers claim a higher dose can be used with perfect safety.

Maprotiline is another drug with a quadricyclic structure, and is also an antidepressant with sedative properties. It is as effective as conventional antidepressants and the daily dose is about 150 mg. Adverse reactions include skin conditions.

Nomifensine, now withdrawn, had the property of being a re-uptake blocker of noradrenaline and dopamine rather than 5-HT and might have had some interest in the management of depression associated with Parkinson's disease. It was comparable in its efficacy to the first generation antidepressant agents.

Herrington et al. (1974, 1976), comparing ECT with L-tryptophan, claimed they were equal in efficacy up to about 4 weeks from the commencement of treatment. Patients on ECT, however, had the potential to continue improving while L-tryptophan did not give rise to further changes in depression. There is also a tendency for patients on L-tryptophan to relapse and require further treatment. The later study showed comparable results in relation to amitriptyline. Thus L-tryptophan appears to have some value in the treatment of moderately depressed patients, but the course of drug management after 4 weeks and in longterm follow-up is not clear.

Viloxazine, a bicyclic compound, is a re-uptake blocker of noradrenaline and 5-HT and is a stimulant, while trazodone is more sedative and is promoted for use in the elderly.

Flupenthixol, a thioxanthene-derivative neuroleptic, has been used with success in the drug treatment of the schizophrenias. At a lower dose, it is claimed it has effects on depression. Interestingly, its antidepressant effects are seen in mild to moderate depression with significant anxiety, when a response is expected within a few days. It does not sedate unduly and if it does not act within a few days, there is little effect if treatment is prolonged. For these reasons its mode of action is likely to be different to that of other antidepressants.

Clinical practice

The efficacy of all antidepressants discussed in this section can be confirmed by clinical impressions. However, as was remarked on in the introduction to this chapter, drug treatment is but one approach to the management of the depressed patient. In theory, the best chance for any antidepressant drug to act effectively will be in those depressions where a purely neurochemical aberration might have occurred, which must be very rare indeed considering that even if an exclusively neurochemically mediated situation arose, the consequences of such a depression would have a bearing on the behaviour of the patient with psychosocial implications. There is, therefore, something artificial in evaluating just one limb or another of the management process, though clearly it needs to be done if we are to engage in clinical therapeutics in any meaningful way.

Imipramine was put to the test very early in its career as an antidepressant by Ball and Kiloh (1959) who compared imipramine in a daily dose of 250 mg with a placebo. Imipramine was seen to be significantly superior to placebo in both the 'endogenous' and 'reactive' categories of depression, though results were better in the former. This has been the impression of most workers and in a review of the reports over nearly 20 years, Rogers and Clay (1975) concluded that the drug appeared to have its greatest therapeutic use in 'endogenous' depression of short duration and was less effective in chronic, atypical depressions with neurotic features.

Evaluation of amitriptyline was similarly undertaken following its introduction, and a comparison was made with both placebo and imipramine. Subsequently, we came to find there was no significant difference in the actions of the two drugs, except in their effects on some associated features of depression. Burt et al. (1962) showed that in the first week of treatment amitriptyline appeared to have superior effects when compared to imipramine, but at the end of four weeks of treatment, they were comparable in their effects. The early clinical improvement in the amitriptyline group may well have been due to the anxiolytic sedative properties of the drug which finds clinical use in the management of insomnia, anxiety and agitation which are associated with, and perhaps contribute to, the clinical picture of depression.

The authoritative Medical Research Council trial (MRC, 1965) gave convincing support for the superiority of imipramine and ECT over not only placebo but the MAOI, phenelzine. In a multi-centre trial of 250 depressed patients, ECT was found to be the most effective treatment over 4 weeks. However, over 12 weeks both ECT and imipramine had effective antidepressant actions.

The distinction, if any, between stress-related and other depressions has been critically considered in Chapter 3. There is no doubt stresses of various kinds are important in relation to the onset of depression, but their effects on the course, natural history and the response to treatment appear to be arguable. One could argue that pharmacological and other physical treatments influence the natural history of the depression, and would be predicted not to have important effects on 'stress-free' as opposed to stress-related depression. This has indeed been seen to be the case. Garvey et al. (1984) compared depressed patients whose illness had been preceded by a stressful environmental event with depressives who experienced no stressful life event before illness episodes in their response to pharmacological treatment. There was no difference between the groups in treatment response rates after 4 and 6 weeks of treatment. It would seem success in management of depression depends not on broad diagnostic categories such as 'endogenous', 'reactive', 'situational' and so on, but the precise delineation of the factors contributory to the depression, and hence tailoring the management approaches accordingly.

Since depression, like any other disorder, has a natural history,

130

spontaneous remission of symptoms is likely in a proportion of cases. About a third of untreated subjects are seen to have recovered or improved considerably within a month of entering trials in which they have served as controls (Appleton and Davis, 1980).

There are two situations in which the question of how long the treatment with antidepressant medication needs to be employed in continuing treatment arises. In the first, the depressed patient has been subjected to a course of ECT and a decision has to be taken if a course of antidepressant medication needs to be employed in continuation of treatment. In the second, the patient has responded to tricyclic medication and a decision as to how long to prolong the treatment has to be made. There is convincing evidence now that when the active drug is continued for a period of 6 months, those on it are less likely to relapse. Mindham *et al.* (1973) showed that of those on continuing active medication, 22% relapsed in the course of 6 months, while 50% of those on placebo did so.

This would seem an appropriate point to refer to the drug treatment of delusional depression. An interesting point was made in this context by Abou-Saleh and Coppen (1983) who found that the response of depressed patients to ECT and antidepressant medication showed a curvilinear pattern. Patients with scores in the middle range of the Newcastle Scale showed greater improvement than those who scored low (less likely to be 'endogenous') or those who scored high (most severely 'endogenous'). The explanation for this appears to be that the most severely endogenous group includes the delusional depressives who are reported (Moradi *et al.*, 1979; Nelson *et al.*, 1984) to have a poor response to tricyclic drugs alone and need phenothiazines in addition to antidepressant therapy to provoke a response. At the lower end of the Newcastle Scale, the atypical neurotic depressives congregate and they are traditionally known to respond poorly to tricyclic antidepressants and ECT. On the other hand, and as expected, lithium seemed to have its greatest efficacy in those who were most 'severely endogenous' (see later discussion for properties of lithium salts).

The poor response of delusional depression to antidepressant treatment alone and the need for neuroleptic medication in addition has been the subject of speculation by many authors, including Nelson *et al.* (1984). One possible reason, which has already been touched on, is that plasma levels of antidepressants are elevated when neuroleptic drugs are given at the same time. This may be due to the competitive inhibition of hydroxylation pathways in the liver. Thus, an alternative to high doses of antidepressants would be a moderate dose given together with a neuroleptic agent. However, if the important factor in the therapeutic efficacy of antidepressants is the ratio between the parent antidepressant and its metabolite, then clearly a combination of antidepressant and neuroleptic is preferable to high doses of antidepressants even though the plasma level of the parent antidepressant reached the same level in each case. A third possible explanation requires a more or less specific action on the part of the neuroleptic in modifying the delusion. In this regard, the possible dopaminergic-blocking activity of antipsychotic agents may prove to be the crucial factor.

Many of these clinical trials have been reported with the newer antidepressants and, as has been repeatedly stressed, all commonly used antidepressants have a comparable efficacy. In evaluating the newer antidepressants, it is not enough to show a superiority over placebo; the new agent has to be compared to a representative of the 'first generation' e.g. imipramine or amitriptyline.

Monoamine oxidase inhibitors (MAOI)

The first of this series of drugs, iproniazid, was studied after one of those serendipitous discoveries that have come to be a feature of the history of psychiatry. It was observed, in its capacity as an anti-tuberculous agent, that patients on the drug had a feeling of wellbeing and, indeed, euphoria which was not entirely in keeping with their clinical situation. The first trials were reported by Loomer *et al.* (1958). However, laboratory studies on the effect of iproniazid as a MAO inhibitor had been reported some 6 years earlier (Zeller *et al.*, 1952). But after the initial enthusiasm, several factors contributed to the waning in popularity of this group of drugs. The efficacy of MAO inhibitors in severe 'endogenous' depression with typical features could not be established when the MRC trial (1965) showed that in vigorously controlled, unselected groups of patients the MAO inhibitor, phenelzine, was not significantly superior to placebo. Added to this were the irksome dietary precautions that had to be observed when the drug was used with foods having a high tyramine content, and also with certain other drugs. The latter involved fears for the safety of patients on MAO inhibitors who had to be given an anaesthetic together with a muscle relaxant prior to ECT therapy. Thirdly, a wide range of tricyclic antidepressants and later other, unrelated non-MAOI followed imipramine and amitriptyline onto the market. The efficacy and the relative safety of these agents were favourably compared to the lack of action, inconvenience and potential lethality of drug-induced MAO inhibition.

The MAOI which are in common clinical use are phenelzine, tranylcypromine and isocarboxazid. There are two broad categories of MAOI, the hydrazine, e.g. phenelzine and isocarboxazid and the non-hydrazine groups, e.g. tranylcypromine.

Metabolism

Catecholamines such as noradrenaline, adrenaline and dopamine, and indoleamines such as 5-HT, among the commonly known neurotransmitter agents, undergo oxidative deamination by MAO as the first step in their metabolism.

$$\text{Amine} \xrightarrow[\text{MAO}]{\text{Oxidative deamination}} \text{Aldehyde} \xrightarrow[\text{Aldehyde dehydrogenase}]{\text{Carboxylation}} \text{Acid}$$

The inhibition of MAO by these drugs is irreversible, so that new enzyme has to be formed to replace that which has been lost, a process which takes up to 2 weeks, which is the period of persistence of the drug.

MAO, as was referred to in Chapter 3, can be further divided into MAO-A, which is present in the gut, and MAO-B, which is found in the platelets. Clorgyline and pargyline are inhibitors, of MAO-A and MAO-B, respectively. Worthwhile antidepressant activity is shown only by clorgyline, which suggests that MAO-A inhibition is required for antidepressant action. However, the effects of clorgyline are not different to the standard MAOI drugs (Pare, 1985).

It used to be believed that phenelzine was metabolized by acetylation and that this process was genetically determined. Thus, the rate of acetylation would influence the level of the drug and hence the therapeutic response – slow acetylators tending to show a better clinical response than rapid acetylators. This view has now given way to the idea that acetylation is likely to be a critical factor only in the early stages of treatment and with low levels of the drug (Pare, 1985).

Mode of action

The simple view was that by inhibiting the enzyme, MAO, the biogenic amines which would otherwise have been broken down, would accumulate in the synaptic cleft and allow the concentration of amine to rise and increase the time of contact between amine and post-synaptic receptor. Some MAOI, e.g. tranylcypromine were also believed to have subsidiary actions such as the property of blocking re-uptake, and some induced the release of amines from nerve endings into the synaptic cleft, both actions leading to an increase in amine concentration available for activity at the post-synaptic receptor. However, as with the tricyclic antidepressant drugs, the time lag between MAO inhibition, which can be shown to take only a few days, and the clinical antidepressant actions which take 2 weeks or more to come on had to be explained. As with the tricyclic and other non-MAO agents, emphasis is now placed on the receptors. It is now believed that after the initial increase in amine concentrations, there is adaptive change taking place in α_1, α_2, and β adrenoceptors.

Side-effects and adverse reactions

The direct side-effects of the drugs are relatively trivial, including postural hypotension and possibly insomnia as a result of the activating properties of the drug, increased appetite with weight gain and sexual difficulties.

The major adverse reactions result from the interaction between foods rich in tyramine or with certain drugs. Food containing tyramine, or other pressor amines, include cheeses such as cheddar and camembert, yeast extracts such as marmite and bovril, red wines such as chianti and burgundy, herring, broad beans, chocolate, yoghurt and some game. Drugs which may cause adverse interactions include anti-hypertensive agents such as methyldopa, stimulants such as amphetamines, sympathomimetics such as adrenaline and noradrenaline and related substances found in nasal decongestants, and L-dopa. Tricyclic antidepressants, especially imipramine, are generally contraindicated for simultaneous use, and the effects of general anaesthetics, opiate drugs and insulin may be potentiated.

133

The interaction is clinically manifested by palpitations and the onset of severe throbbing headaches which begin in the back of the head and radiate elsewhere. The associated nausea, vomiting, meningeal irritation and photophobia are indications of an intracranial lesion. Complications include haemorrhage, and death has been reported. The treatment of the hypertensive and intracranial crisis is by the immediate intravenous injection of the α-adrenergic blocker, phentolamine.

Despite the melodramatic picture that can be painted, and reproduced from textbook to textbook, the objective evidence shows that when reasonable precautions are taken, e.g. caution with drug dosage and dietary and simultaneous use of other drugs, the dangers of the MAOI drugs have been much exaggerated. Over a 10-year period only 17, all non-fatal, cases of reaction between phenelzine and food products had been reported (McGilchrist, 1975).

Clinical practice

The discrepancy between the alleged antidepressant properties and their apparent lack of efficacy (as was demonstrated, for instance, in the MRC trial) has been explained on the grounds that the MAOI exert their antidepressant action not on typical depression but in those patients who have atypical features. That the symptomatology of depression might have a bearing on the response to antidepressants has been suspected for a considerable time (e.g. West and Dally, 1959). The symptoms such as diurnal variation of mood, early morning awakening, guilt and other features associated with severe, 'endogenous' depression respond better to ECT and tricyclic and 'second generation' antidepressants, whereas the chronic, atypical, neurotic, 'reactive' depressions are more likely to respond to MAOI. These characteristics are generally seen with out-patient depressives, and Paykel et al. (1979) noted that the vast majority of studies in which MAOI were shown to be effective had been conducted in out-patients.

Pare (1985) has reviewed the current status of MAOI in clinical practice. He considers that low doses might have contributed to the impression that MAOI are weakly effective or ineffective drugs. He quotes Green and Youdim (1976) who, in animal studies, showed that at least 80% of brain MAO had to be inhibited to produce behavioural effects, a level which is probably attained in humans with standard doses of MAOI drugs. Pare comments on how doses of phenelzine sufficient to produce a greater than 80% inhibition of platelet MAO result in a good antidepressant response, but if the inhibition is less than 60%, the antidepressant effect is poor. He believes a dose of 60–75 mg phenelzine or 40–50 mg isocarboxazid a day is usually adequate for an effective antidepressant action. A mild orthostatic hypotensive response occurs after 10–14 days if the dose is an adequate one and may correlate with the clinical response (Murphy, 1981).

This view has been confirmed by others. Tyrer et al. (1980) found that it took 90 mg of phenelzine daily to produce an effective response in 'neurotic' depression, and Ravaris et al. (1976) showed that there was a better response to 60 mg rather than 30 mg of phenelzine daily.

It is possible that even in the elderly there may be a place for MAOI. A good response has been reported in some cases of depression when full doses are employed giving 80% inhibition of platelet MAO (Georgotas *et al.*, 1983). Although the use of MAOI in the elderly is contrary to the practice of most psychogeriatricians, it may well be that their use will avoid some of the adverse effects of non-MAOI antidepressant drugs.

Lithium

The use of lithium salts in clinical practice has a long provenance. In the middle of the last century Garrod advocated lithium carbonate as a treatment for gout and related conditions. Lithium continued to be used for this purpose up to the time of the First World War. After that there was a brief vogue for substituting lithium salts for sodium chloride in the diet of patients with hypertension, heart disease, gout and rheumatic conditions, occasionally in excessive dosage with unfortunate results. It was left to Cade (1949) to show that lithium salts had an effect on mania and behaviour disorders associated with epilepsy. Unlike most psychiatric discoveries, this was less than serendipitous. Cade attempted to find the toxic principle in the urine of manic patients which when injected into guinea pigs produced adverse behavioural responses. These were controlled and the animals sedated by a mixture which contained lithium urate. Realizing this substance might be useful in states of excitement, Cade gave lithium salts to psychiatrically excited patients, and those with mania responded. These patients were free of symptoms as long as the substance was continued. However, its action on depression was uncertain at the time and it was only after a recurrence of interest in the chemical in the 1960s that the value of lithium in both mania and depression came to be known. Further confirmation of the efficacy of lithium salts came from the observations of a handful of workers including Hartigan (1963) who also showed that lithium therapy led to the decline in recurrence of both mania and depression. Thus, the therapeutic actions of lithium were held to extend to the treatment of acute mania and the prophylaxis of manic and depressive illness. Although held with less conviction, it is now the belief that lithium is also of value in the acute phase of depression.

Metabolism

Lithium salts are relatively simple structures. They are absorbed readily, after oral ingestion, from the gastro-intestinal tract, with a peak plasma level reached in 2 hours and a half-life of 18–24 hours. Slow-release preparations are available. Excretion is by the kidneys, and retention may occur with disturbed electrolyte balance as with dehydration following vomiting or diarrhoea, when the retention of lithium parallels the retention of sodium. In practice, diuretic therapy may lead to retention of lithium.

Mode of action

The methods by which lithium appears to exert its effects are not entirely clear. Janowsky (1980) has suggested that lithium might have effects on

135

both adrenergic and cholinergic mechanisms, reducing both hyper-cholinergic as well as hyperadrenergic activity, thereby helping to reduce as well as prevent both depression and mania. Animal studies have shown that lithium helps decrease acetylcholine turnover. The significance of this is not clear as both increased as well as diminished activity may be accounted for by this finding.

Lithium may also increase the availability of 5-HT centrally. The rate of 5-HT uptake by blood platelets is significantly reduced in depression (Coppen et al., 1978). This appears to be a stable trait in that it does not change with clinical recovery and, as with CSF 5-HIAA levels (see Chapters 3 and 7), may indicate a trait that reflects the vulnerability to depression. Coppen et al. (1980) showed that lithium is able to increase the rate of platelet 5-HT transport towards normal levels. This process of accumulation of 5-HT by platelets appears to be an active process which is coupled to Na^+/K^+ adenosine triphosphatase (ATPase) and is dependent on Na^+ concentration. It is said that lithium is able to increase erythrocyte Na^+/K^+ ATPase activity in depressed patients, and thus the effects of lithium may need an intermediary in order to be expressed (see also Chapter 3).

Further evidence of possible 5-HT enhancing effects of lithium come from the important clinical observation that an apparent lack of response to tricyclic antidepressants may be corrected by the introduction of lithium (Heninger et al., 1983). It has been suggested that in this instance lithium acts upon 5-HT neurones which had been sensitized by prior treatment with tricyclic antidepressants. A synergistic action between lithium and clomipramine, a preferential 5-HT re-uptake blocker, has been demonstrated by O'Flanagan (1973). Schrader and Levien (1985) reported a case of treatment-resistant depression responding to a combination of clomipramine and lithium. They suggested that lithium had 5-HT enhancing properties, which, in combination with the 5-HT actions of clomipramine, had powerful synergistic actions on 5-HT function, enough to overcome a refractory depression. De Montigny et al. (1981) showed that when patients suffering from severe depression had failed to respond to treatment for 3 weeks or more with tricyclic antidepressants and had been given lithium there was a remarkable relief of depression within 48 hours.

Animal experiments have shown the possible basis for this synergistic action. Chronic tricyclic drug administration increases the sensitivity to 5-HT of forebrain neurones; short-term lithium treatment enchances the activity of the 5-HT system. Hence, De Montigny et al. (1981) suggest that short-term lithium administration to tricyclic resistant depressive patients might unveil the sensitization of the 5-HT receptors which had been induced by chronic prior tricyclic drug administration.

With lithium, De Montigny et al. (1981) note that short-term administration followed by acute MAO inhibition produces behavioural changes in the rat which are indistinguishable from that obtained with MAO inhibition and L-tryptophan administration. If p-chlorophenylalanine (a 5-HT inhibitor) is given prior, lithium has little effect. Thus, at least on a short-term basis, lithium is able to increase the efficacy of the central 5-HT system. It has no effect on the plasma levels of tricyclic agents, neither does it have any effect on the post-synaptic 5-HT receptor. They suggest that the clinical potentiation of tricyclic agents by lithium might result from their respective post- and pre-synaptic enhancing effects on the 5-HT system.

Adverse reactions

Several organs of the body may be affected by the long-term use of lithium, and some of these effects may be of clinical importance.

Lithium inhibits the release of thyroxine and tri-iodothyronine, with a consequent elevation of thyroid stimulating hormone (TSH). About 15% of patients may have elevated levels of TSH (Bakker, 1977) but a very much smaller proportion become hypothyroid. Replacement thyroxine is required only when the patient is clinically hypothyroid.

It now appears that prior renal damage is necessary before chronic nephropathy can develop in association with long-term maintenance treatment with lithium. Thus in the report of chronic nephropathy by Hestbech et al. (1974), a large number of patients had a history of lithium intoxication. Coppen et al. (1980) showed that there was no significant difference in the renal function of patients with affective illness who had been treated with or without lithium. Probably the only significant abnormality is polyuria (more than 4 litres of urine per 24 hours) and if this occurs, a case may be made for reducing the dose of lithium with a view to lowering the plasma level of lithium to low normal levels or below the normal range altogether. Renal function is routinely assessed in the work-up of patients being considered for lithium therapy and abnormal function is one of the contraindications to lithium. Diuretic therapy, by virtue of its tendency to retain lithium, must also enjoin caution with the use of lithium.

Pregnancy is a contraindication to the use of lithium as there appears to be a small but definite risk of congenital cardiac defects in the newborn.

Lithium is contraindicated in those patients showing cardiac slowing. Heart block has been suspected in some patients but here cautious monitoring rather than immediate cessation of treatment is advised.

As with most antidepressants and some neuroleptics, lithium has a tendency to lower the epileptic threshold. Neurotoxicity is a rare but well recognized unwanted effect which is associated with high serum lithium levels. Neurotoxicity is also possible when neuroleptic drugs, in particular haloperidol, are combined with lithium. Neurotoxicity has also been reported when lithium carbonate has been used in combination with thioridazine even when the serum lithium levels have been within the therapeutic range (Kishimoto et al., 1983). There may also be a tendency to exacerbate extra pyramidal signs when used in conjunction with neuroleptic agents.

As with sodium, there is a tendency to weight gain. Radiological bone changes may be seen. Psoriasis and other chronic skin conditions may be made worse with lithium.

Mild tremor of the fingers, loss of appetite and nausea are common, probably dose-related effects. Longterm treatment leads to lassitude, poor memory (probably due to impaired concentration) and a nephrogenic diabetes insipidus leading to polyuria, weight gain and hypothyroidism.

The adverse reactions of lithium were put into perspective by a survey of the use of the drug in South West Scotland (McCreadie and Morrison, 1985; Morrison and McCreadie, 1985; McCreadie et al., 1985). They found the introduction of lithium as prophylactic therapy was associated with a significant reduction in the number and length of hospital in-patient admissions, as well as in the number of courses and total number of ECTs. They found the principal side-effects of patients receiving lithium were poor memory, weight gain, thirst, diarrhoea, frequent passage of urine, trembling hands, dry mouth, drowsiness, indigestion and constipation. 42% of patients had noticed hair changes which included the thinning and change in texture of the hair, while 7% had either probable or definite diminished thyroid activity.

Symptoms of lithium toxicity include vomiting, diarrhoea, ataxia, cardiac arrhythmias and failure, coma, convulsions and death.

In the assessment of toxicity, clinical evaluation must take precedence over measurement of serum lithium. Where there are clear clinical signs of toxicity, even with serum lithium within the normal range, the drug ought to be reduced or stopped, and recommenced after the symptoms subside.

Despite these (largely theoretical, on the evidence) adverse effects, lithium is probably safer for longterm use than tricyclic antidepressants, especially those with marked anticholinergic actions. And certainly in bipolar illness, lithium has the considerable advantage over tricyclic antidepressants in that it is unlikely to precipitate mania.

Clinical practice

Lithium salts are easily and conveniently prescribed. The nub of the proper clinical use of these drugs is the regular monitoring of plasma levels. Blood for estimation of plasma levels is taken 12 hours after the last dose or in the morning after a sustained release preparation is administered. The measurement of plasma lithium levels is the only example of regular monitoring of drug levels in psychiatry. It is a vital element in the process of management and in situations where there are no facilities for the measurement of this, the use of the drug is contraindicated. Serum levels appear to reflect the levels of lithium in brain tissue and have a direct relationship with the dose ingested, i.e. there is a *pro rata* increase; doubling the dose will double the plasma level, all other factors being unchanged. As with tricyclic antidepressants, the importance of achieving an effective plasma level is stressed. The plasma level required for therapeutic purposes is 0.6–1.2mmol/l, and in general a therapeutic response is expected only when plasma levels are within this range.

However, as with other biologically based treatments, social factors appear to determine the outcome of lithium treatment. The failure rate in longterm lithium therapy is between 20% and 30%, even with rigorous selection of patients and the maintenance of adequate serum levels of lithium (O'Connell et al., 1985). Factors they referred to as being associated with poor outcome included rapidly cycling illness and poor compliance with subsequent low serum levels. They also showed that social support was most strongly correlated with good outcome. Adequate social support may protect against life stresses and adverse circumstances, thus working synergistically with the lithium to protect against relapse. Conversely, adverse social circumstances may well work to undermine the actions of lithium. On the other hand non-compliance may lead to breakdown, which may lead to the rupture of existing social bonds. As O'Connell *et al.* (1985) state, the direction of the causal relationship is not clear, but there appears to be no doubt that both lithium and the patient's psychosocial environment must be taken into account in management.

For the benefits of lithium to be seen one may be required to continue treatment for a year or 18 months. (Srinivasan and Hullin, 1980). The most common reason for discontinuation of lithium treatment appears to be the presence of side-effects, of which tremor is the most frequent.

Thus, there appears to be an irreducible number of patients who do not respond to lithium, and a further number who as a result of adverse responses or contra-indicating medical conditions cannot be given the drug. Interest has been expressed in the anti-convulsant drug carbamazepine as a possible alternative to lithium. It seems it is able to decrease the frequency of episodes but only a few patients show diminished intensity of symptoms (Kishimoto *et al.*, 1983). It also appears that it exerts its actions on the mechanism inducing manic-depressive cycle rather than any mechanism that maintains it. It also appears that carbamazepine was more effective in cases with an onset before the age of 20, and those patients who had a constant pattern of alternating mania and depression showed a better response than those who had a more irregular scatter of depressive and manic episodes. The effects appear sooner than later, as opposed to lithium where 12–18 months may have to pass before significant effects are seen. All in all, there appears to be considerable promise in considering carba-mazepine as a longterm prophylactic agent in manic-depressive illness but, as yet, it is a 'second line' drug.

ELECTROCONVULSIVE THERAPY (ECT)

The induction of convulsions by various means as a mode of treatment of mentally disordered patients has a long history. Olver used camphor as early as 1785. In 1933 Meduna induced convulsions by using a 25% solution of camphor given intramuscularly in schizophrenic patients. The theoretical basis to this therapeutic attempt was the prevailing view that schizophrenia and epilepsy might be mutually antagonistic conditions, i.e. if epilepsy was induced it was hoped the symptoms of schizophrenia would be ameliorated. He later substituted cardiazol for camphor and in 1938 Cerletti and Bini described the process by which convulsions could be induced electrically. As with other treatments for depression – tricyclic drugs, MAOI, lithium and psychosurgery – the discovery that these agents or procedures had their indications specifically or primarily for depression and allied conditions was made incidentally, or serendipitously. This emphasizes the universal nature of depression as any agent which is a substantive antidepressant will act on a condition in which depression is a complaint.

Camphor gave way to metrazol which was unpopular with patients as it gave rise to feelings of acute anxiety on intravenous administration. This became the first physical treatment to be regularly used in psychiatric practice since malarial therapy for general paresis. In the early days, as with most new therapies, it was widely and, as we would now say, indiscriminately used. It had a remarkable effect on the catatonic, who were generally considered then and for several years later as schizophrenic patients. But relatively early on ECT was seen as a treatment for depression (Kalcinowsky and Hippius, 1969).

Unmodified ECT, i.e. unmodified by anaesthetic or muscle relaxant was used in the early days and fractures were not uncommon. Curare derivatives were used as muscle relaxants, but their long duration of action resulted in their being abandoned in favour of succinylcholine which has a shorter duration. As an unanaesthetised paralysed state is an exceedingly unpleasant one, the muscle relaxant is now combined with a general anaesthetic. Anaesthesia is now carried out as a formal procedure by trained anaesthetists, which has not always been the case. A generation ago the operation of all aspects of ECT would have been performed by mental hospital psychiatrists. The recognition that psychiatric patients were an anaesthetic risk like any other patients and the belated recognition by professional bodies that the administration of ECT requires training and skill, even though it might be a treatment for mental illness, has led to ECT being given more appropriately, more effectively and with reduced morbidity.

Mode of action

The mode of action of ECT can be studied in relation to the effect the treatment produces on catecholamine and indoleamine transmission, and on their receptors. An increase in CSF 5-hydroxyindole acetic acid (5-HIAA, the chief metabolite of 5-HT), an increase in the level of dopamine, an increase in the functional activity of 5-HT, dopamine and noradrenaline and an increase in the receptor response to 5-HT, dopamine and noradrenaline have all been noted (Cooper et al., 1968; Kety, 1974; Graham-Smith et al., 1978).

Animal experiments suggest that ECT may decrease both β-adrenoceptor density and the responsiveness of pre-synaptic α_2-adrenoceptors (Cooper et al., 1985). α_2-Adrenoceptors may be studied in platelets and β-adrenoceptor function in lymphocytes. Cooper et al. (1985) examined the hypothesis that ECT may produce changes in adrenoceptor density as reflected by receptors on blood cells that could relate to its antidepressant effect. Their results showed a significant decrease in platelet α_2-adrenoceptor density following ECT, but the relationship between this phenomenon and clinical recovery was a tenuous one, however. Lymphocyte β_2-adrenoceptor density was unaffected by ECT.

Linnoila et al. (1983) had suggested that when ECT was given to

140

depressed patients there might be a reduction in noradrenaline turnover. Cooper *et al.* (1985) found that plasma noradrenaline concentrations were initially high in depression and fell following ECT in a manner which corresponded to clinical recovery. They concluded that plasma noradrenaline studies might be a more useful and valid index of central biogenic amine change during antidepressant treatment than peripheral blood cell receptor densities.

It has been suggested that memory may be impaired, following ECT as a result of increased blood–brain permeability which occurs during ECT. A possible cause might be the elevated blood pressure that might occur during the procedure. Taylor *et al.* (1985) put this to the test, but found they could not support this idea.

Animal studies suggest the possibility of post-synaptic enhancement of action of amine neurotransmitters.

Indications

Wherever depression is found, ECT may be used. It does not seem to matter if depression is the primary or most significant component. Thus schizo-affective disorder responds to ECT and, as will be seen in Chapter 6, the depression associated with malignancy also responds to ECT, if only transiently. The depression of unipolar and bipolar illness responds equally well and, in the latter condition, so well that mania might be precipitated. The treatment of delusional depression is problematical and equivocal results have been noted. Indeed, Sargant and Slater (1969) noted that most forms of 'endogenous' depression responded well with the possible exception of agitated depression with paranoid delusions.

When first used ECT produced dramatic results not merely in melancholics but in manics, puerperal psychotics and acute schizophrenics. It has been used, unmodified, with success in delirious states and the excited phase of reactive depressive psychosis also responds dramatically. Even though many of these conditions can have a depressive component, it is not possible to attribute the efficacy of ECT to its antidepressant actions alone in these situations.

Contraindications

There are few contraindications to ECT, and these are usually as regards matters relating to fitness for anaesthesia. Neither pregnancy nor old age is a contraindication. Indeed, in the former state, short-term ECT may be preferable to the use of antidepressant medication of any kind. As for old age, ECT is by no means a traumatic procedure. The only absolute contraindications to ECT are conditions with raised intracranial pressure (Kalcinowsky and Hippius, 1969), where the sudden further increase in pressure may give rise to compression effects on the brain or may result in herniation of the brain.

ECT is a remarkably safe procedure nowadays, thanks to skilled anaesthetic techniques. The incidence of complications with modified anaesthesia was about 1 in 2–3000 patients (Sargant and Slater, 1969), and

141

is possibly even lower now. It must also be remembered that ECT acts to prevent complications of depression such as suicide that might otherwise have occurred. Avery and Winokur (1978) showed that groups of ECT patients had significantly reduced death rates due to all causes as well as reduced incidence of suicidal attempts.

Complications

The impairment of memory following ECT has been extensively discussed. The memory impairment involves both anterograde and retrograde memory function and may last up to 12 weeks. It has been suggested that there is a failure in both coding and retrieval mechanisms (Stones, 1973), and Squire *et al.* (1976) suggested that the temporal ordering of events rather than the recollection of events themselves might be affected. The most severe impairment of memory function takes place with bilateral ECT. Least impairment occurs after unilateral electrode placement to the non-dominant hemisphere. Visuo-spatial function is affected after placement of electrodes to the non-dominant hemisphere. Accidental placement of unilateral electrode to the dominant hemisphere will result in impairment of verbal ability, but in either case the impairment is less than with bilateral ECT (Squire, 1977).

Squire and Slater (1983) showed that compared to bilateral ECT, right unilateral ECT was associated with only mild memory complaints. At 3 years after treatment, about half the patients who had received bilateral ECT complained of poor memory. They found these reports were influenced by three factors:

(1) Recurrence or persistence of symptoms that were present before ECT,
(2) The experience of amnesia associated with ECT at the time of administration, and a subsequent tendency to question if memory had ever recovered, and
(3) Impaired memory for events that had occurred up to 6 months before treatment and up to 2 months afterwards.

Weeks *et al.* (1980) compared cognitive function in depressed patients who had been given ECT and those who were treated without ECT, and normal controls on admission, at 4 months and 7 months. They found ECT caused little impairment at 4 months and none at 7 months. Severity of depression seemed to have a marked effect on cognition. After one week, bilateral ECT caused more impairment than unilateral ECT, but at 3 months the differences had disappeared. They concluded that ECT does not cause persisting memory impairment and believe that in part, at least, pre-ECT depressive cognitive impairment may account for the finding of post-ECT memory impairment. At follow-up they found both ECT and non-ECT patient groups complained to a comparable extent of memory impairment. Both drugs and ECT can improve cognition by removing depression, but both may induce short-term, reversible memory impairment.

The rarer complications following ECT are cardiac problems such as

142

arrhythmia and arrest, cerebral haemorrhage, subarachnoid haemorrhage, pulmonary embolism and pneumonia. Transient neurological abnormalities are said to be not uncommon. Kriss *et al.* (1978) found neurological abnormality lasting up to 20 minutes. These include asymmetry of reflexes, mild hemiparesis, tactile and visual inattention, homonymous hemianopia and dysphasia, which are all transiently present.

Clinical practice

Unilateral and bilateral modes of ECT administration are available. The techniques of administration and the physical properties of the current are dealt with in books on techniques of physical treatment.

Controversy still smoulders as to whether unilateral or bilateral ECT is the superior procedure, which is perhaps not the question at issue but which is more appropriate. The treatment of choice is generally acknowledged to be unilateral ECT given to the non-dominant hemisphere. Unilateral ECT reduces both the incidence, duration and intensity of post-ictal confusion as well as memory impairment (d'Elia, 1974; Fraser and Glass, 1978). This is of benefit in the treatment of the elderly. Although it has been suggested that unilateral ECT might be marginally less effective than a comparable number of treatments given in the bilateral mode, this is of little practical significance as, the incidence of adverse effects being lower with unilateral treatment, a few more could be given without inconveniencing the patient. Taylor and Abrams (1985) showed that while bilateral ECT induced both retrograde and anterograde amnesia, which were related to the number and frequency of the induced seizures, these effects completely subsided within a month of treatment being completed. They had found that groups of patients undergoing both unilateral and bilateral ECT did not differ significantly in cognitive impairment and concluded that neither form of ECT made cognitive performance other than memory worse, and that both resulted in significant clinical improvement.

Older patients are thought to be at greater risk of complications than younger patients. Stromgren (1973) found that patients over 45 years of age fared significantly better with bilateral treatment than with unilateral treatment. However, Fraser and Glass (1978) showed that when compared with similar times for younger patients, recovery in older patients took on average 5 times as long from unilateral treatment and 9 times as long from bilateral treatment. There were also adverse effects due to the cumulative effects of bilateral ECT, and the time interval between treatments was a material influence. The recovery time for bilateral treatment became significantly greater as each course progressed and bilateral treatments given after a one-day interval led to the patients needing a significantly longer period for recovery than when the treatment was given after an interval of 2 or more days. These authors suggested that in elderly patients unilateral electrode placement in the non-dominant hemisphere is the technique of choice, and that where bilateral ECT is given, it should not be given more often than twice weekly. Also bilateral ECT should be avoided

143

in elderly out-patients as, recovery patterns being unpredictable, there may be an undue degree of confusion in the post-ictal period.

The number of treatments required, given the empirical nature of ECT, is still uncertain. It is usual to give 2–3 treatments a week for 3–4 weeks, assess the response and then give two more treatments for luck and stop the course. This is unscientific but has the sanction of long usage. A practical, if not logical, method of assessment is to note progression with treatment – there is no minimum or maximum but the commonly used range might be 4–16 treatments – and discontinue the treatment, recommencing therapy if it is indicated. However, despite the lack of evidence one way or another, entrenched opinion is firmly against this practice. The patient is not deprived of all antidepressant treatment when ECT has been stopped as an antidepressant drug should have been commenced before or at the time the ECT was begun and its efficacy would be at its optimal as the course of ECT was brought to an end. Relapse following ECT is not uncommon (e.g. Kiloh et al., 1960) and some clinicians have made a case for prophylactic and maintenance ECT but there is no convincing evidence for the efficacy of this. It is possible that depressive illness has a natural history which can be altered by both ECT and drug therapy. The ECT presumably brings about a rapid and relatively short-lived change in the neurobiological substratum giving rise to the symptoms of depression; the drugs do it more gradually and presumably have a more persistent action. In either case, what is required is a neurobiological index – the dexamethasone suppression test (DST) is a possible candidate – which shows the nature of the change with treatment. In the meantime there are few rules, as evidenced by the variety of approaches to the use of ECT.

There is evidence that giving an antidepressant helps maintain the improvement seen with ECT. Seager and Bird (1962) studied patients who had ECT followed by imipramine and placebo, and at follow-up at 6 months found that 17% and 69% of patients, respectively, had relapsed. As was referred to above, there is an appreciable risk of early relapse following ECT, which may be reduced by tricyclic drugs, MAO inhibitors and lithium given for about 6 months (Paykel and Coppen, 1979). Coppen et al. (1981) further demonstrated the value of lithium continuation treatment following ECT in the management of depression. Depressed patients who recovered following ECT and who were well maintained on lithium for one year experienced significantly less affective morbidity than patients who were on placebo. As might have been expected, the prophylactic effects of lithium were seen more clearly in the second 6 months of the trial. This would suggest that the lithium treatment should be initiated early in the course of the depressive episode so as to allow it time to act at its optimal level.

Efficacy

There is now evidence to satisfy all open-minded practitioners of clinical psychiatry that ECT is effective in the treatment of depression. Significant differences can be shown between bilateral and unilateral ECT, and simulated FCT. The precise results may be open to debate. Thus, Heshe *et*

144

al. (1978) noted that bilateral ECT was significantly better than unilateral ECT at one week, a finding confirmed by Gregory *et al.* (1985) who also showed that the unilateral treatments required were some 20% greater in number than a bilateral course of treatment.

We now also have the benefit of double-blind controlled trials. Before this doubts remained as to whether the carefully executed ritual of treatment rather than the treatment itself was sufficient for therapeutic efficacy (*cf* insulin therapy in schizophrenia). However, even before the methodology and results that were needed to convince the sceptics were available, an argument from clinical observation was at hand. A convulsion had to be induced in the patient for there to be an effect on symptoms. A 'sub-convulsive' discharge produced inadvertently for technical reasons has long been known to be insufficient for therapeutic effect.

Discussion of the ethics of giving ECT is beyond the scope of this book, but some of the criticisms levelled against clinicians include that which holds that ECT is a traumatic, brutalizing assault on the dignity of helpless patients. As most of us know, it is not easy to argue with this ideology which is as entrenched as any refractory depression. The argument against trauma does not hold; facts are available and have been discussed in a previous section. As for brutalizing assault, 65% of patients in one large series (Freeman and Kendell, 1980) claimed they would accept ECT again if advised, a figure which one imagines is considerably higher than those opting for most forms of torture.

It is generally stated that the 'endogenous' form of depression is more likely to respond to ECT than the 'reactive' form. This view of the type of depression likely to respond most favourably to ECT has been long known (e.g. Hobson, 1953). He found that favourable features included sudden onset of depression, duration of illness of less than a year, significant retardation, self-reproach, good insight and a premorbid obsessional personality. The unfavourable features included hypochondriasis, depersonalization, emotional lability, neurotic traits, 'hysterical' behaviour, a fluctuating course and a hysterical premorbid personality, all of which indicated a poor response to ECT. It will be seen that several of the features of good and bad prognostic import are those that predict response to non-MAOI antidepressant drugs and are the mirror image of that seen in the response to MAOI drugs. It is generally acknowledged that ECT is contra-indicated in those cases with clear-cut 'neurotic' symptoms. This statement would be unexceptionable if diagnosis were made with the precision that is implied in various studies. Two brief case histories illustrate this point and the presence of 'grey' areas in psychiatric practice which leads to treatment by trial and error rather than scientific precision.

Case 1

This 45-year-old female, in an unhappy marriage to an unsympathetic man, had previous admissions to hospital and been subjected to a variety of treatments with equivocal results. She had on this occasion been thought to have been functioning reasonably well in the community when, following a

145

domestic disagreement, she took an overdose. On psychiatric follow-up after this incident she claimed she was perfectly well – 'as well as I have been since I married' – and wished to discontinue attendance at the out-patients' clinic. She refused all medication. Within a couple of weeks she had become depressed, agitated and showed marked histrionic features. She was put back on an antidepressant with little clinical response and just about managed to survive with help in the community. One day she rang her general practitioner and threatened suicide and was admitted by him as an emergency. In hospital she became very fretful and threatened to leave on several occasions. Her clinical condition remained the same and changes in medication made no difference. She reluctantly agreed to a course of ECT and made a rapid and full recovery, turning into a confident, energetic woman who was full of spirits. However, no-one who had cared for her in hospital or in the community over several years had any doubt her next 'breakdown' was at the mercy of the next domestic argument.

Case 2

A 38-year-old woman with severe peripheral vascular disease was also unhappily married and felt more isolated and miserable since leaving her family in the Midlands. She was depressed and complained of marked somatic features which had been extensively investigated without a 'physical' basis being found, and were held not to be related to arteriopathy. Her husband was a travelling salesman and whilst he was at home there were serious disagreements and even physical violence of which she was the victim. On the other hand, when he was away on business, she felt lonely and even more depressed. She, too, was admitted as an emergency following suicidal threats and complaints of being unbearably depressed. Another change of medication made no difference and she was given a course of ECT. She made a full recovery with resolution of all her physical complaints including those relating to her vascular problem. She was discharged very well but, once again, within a few weeks, with the return of her husband, her symptoms, both mental and physical, had returned in full force and in the same pattern as before.

PSYCHOSURGERY

Aspects of the limbic system of the brain which have a bearing on the surgical treatment of depression have been considered briefly in Chapter 3. Psychosurgery for depression is reserved for chronic, severe, intractable depression which has responded poorly, or not at all, to conventional treatment. Some other aspects of psychosurgery in the treatment of violence are taken up briefly in Chapter 7.

The first modern operation was devised by the Portuguese neurologist, Egas Moniz, in collaboration with the neurosurgeon, Almeida Lima, who were influenced by the account of the effects of frontal lobectomy in chimpanzees. The first human operations were lobotomies, rather radical in their extent, and popularized by Freeman and Watts (1942). They devised the 'standard pre-frontal leucotomy' which effectively separated the frontal

146

lobes from the rest of the brain. The desired results were often overshadowed by gross personality change, convulsions and death. However, between 1940 and 1950, most patients operated on were schizophrenics and the 'success rate' was a not inconsiderable 18% who were able to leave hospital and make a reasonable social adjustment (Tooth and Newton, 1961).

However, as with convulsive therapy, even while the treatment was being undertaken for a medley of psychiatric disorders, results were observed to be better in affective disorder.

Modified techniques

The surgical procedures available in psychosurgery may be broadly classified as 'free hand' and stereotactic methods. The former refers to the crude, radical cutting methods, initially used to perform lobotomy and, later, the marginally more sophisticated leucotomies. Freeman and Watts (1942) described and popularized the standard labotomy which was associated with 6% mortality, neurological complications such as epilepsy and incontinence, and personality change of an adverse kind. The lobotomies gave way to the leucotomies which showed rapid results following surgery. These include the bimedial frontal leucotomy, rostral frontal leucotomy and the orbital undercut. The results of the orbital undercut show recovery in more than 50% of patients with affective disorder (Sykes and Tredgold, 1964) but epilepsy is troublesome (incidence of some 16%) and there is still appreciable mortality.

The operations of choice now are the stereotactic procedures, though they take longer than the modified leucotomies to display their effects. Two stereotactic procedures are available. In the stereotactic subcaudate tractotomy (Knight, 1965), radioactive yttrium is introduced into the ventro-medial parts of the frontal lobe. The results are as good with this procedure as with modified leucotomy. A good response is obtained in 56–68% of depressed patients, with an incidence of fits of less than 2% and only one death following 1000 operations (Strom-Olsen and Carlisle, 1971; Goktepe et al., 1975). The adverse effects on the personality are of the order of 5%. Those who do well remain well and one measure of success is a reduction in the incidence of attempted suicide. This is probably the treatment of choice for patients selected according to the procedure outlined below, when 60% of patients may be expected to show substantial improvement (Bridges and Bartlett, 1977).

Indications and clinical practice

The length of the depressive illness may be variable as it is the consequences of the disorder that leads one to consider the suitability of the patient for the purposes of surgical intervention. The patient is deemed to have intractable or refractory depression before he qualifies for consideration for psychosurgery and thus, unlike other physical treatments, the primary indication for psychosurgery is a negative one. As yet, psychosurgery is not a treatment of first choice.

In cases of refractory depression, it is essential the history be reconsidered and reviewed with the help of additional informants (see Table 7) as it is necessary that a personality disorder be ruled out either as the cause of chronic distress or as a premorbid condition which might militate against surgery. A second psychiatric opinion needs *always* to be sought, even in advance of a formal 'psychosurgery conference', and the second consultant may well be able to review all the points in the formulation.

Table 7 Refractory depression: a check list

(1) Check history – for medical and other psychiatric conditions
  – drug history
  – social situation
(2) Review investigations. Rule out malignancy especially in the elderly.
(3) Check drug treatment – long enough? full dose? given by staff? compliance
  (a) Tricyclic antidepressants
  (b) 'Second generation' antidepressants
  (c) Lithium
  (d) MAOI
  (e) ECT
  (f) L-Tryptophan + MAOI

The social difficulties associated with the depression being considered for psychosurgery should not be neglected or underestimated. If the depression has been a prolonged one, there are consequences which are bound to be evident in relation to employment, marriage, family and social activity in general. Also, once surgery has been carried out the patient will recuperate within the family and the attitudes of the family to the patient, his illness and surgery will determine in large measure the patient's eventual postoperative state. The family needs to be contacted well before surgery and it is essential the spouse or other relative is kept well informed as to what is taking place, the nature of the operation and what might, in the light of previous surgical experience, be reasonable to prophesy. If the patient makes a good recovery from surgery and there is an amelioration in the depressive symptoms, further work may be needed with the family to make them adjust to the improved clinical state which may lead to a change in the roles of the individuals in the family. This is a not uncommon feature in psychiatric practice where any change in the clinical state of a chronic psychiatric condition such as agoraphobia or alcoholism may lead to a change in the dynamics of personal or family relationships which may require intensive work to make the families aware.

The one positive clinical feature which enables one to recommend a patient for leucotomy is associated anxiety or tension. The definite contraindications to psychosurgery are severe personality disorders and their clinical and social manifestations. Alcoholism, drug dependence, violence, self-mutilation and psychopathic features in general in the premorbid personality will constitute contraindications. These patients, as a rule, respond adversely to psychosurgery. However, some of these behaviours may be part of the depressive syndrome, and it is here that the importance of reviewing the history of the condition can be shown in its true light.

Before a depression is deemed to be intractable, it is necessary for a full clinical review to be undertaken. This includes a re-evaluation of the history and the re-examination of the physical and mental status of the patient. Special attention is paid to medical or other psychiatric conditions which may impede an antidepressant response. Intractable or recurring depression is a feature of malignant disease (see Chapter 6) and the commoner malignancies must be ruled out, especially in elderly patients. The role of drugs being given for incidental conditons, e.g. anti-hypertensives must also be re-assessed. As has been referred to already, the social situation of the patient must be re-considered. Additional informants are vital here. The case comes to mind of the 33-year-old patient whose wife was quite certain he was the idle, disinterested and self-neglectful man she had married and lived with for 10 years. A business colleague gave a picture of an energetic and successfully self-employed window cleaner who had lapsed into apathy and depression just 4 years before.

Next, the assessment of whether a full and fair trial of the whole gamut of conventional antidepressant treatment has been given must be made. No antidepressant can be written off until at least 6 weeks' treatment at full dosage has been given. As has been pointed out in an earlier section, the commonest cause for an apparent refractory depression is inadequate dosage of the prescribed drugs. Compliance must be checked by observation, supervision and the estimation of plasma levels. It is a delicate matter, but drugs prescribed by doctors are not always given by nurses, especially in some wards of mental hospitals where an independent or alternative plan of management other than that decided at a ward round may be carried out in a defiant spirit of democracy. It is in situations like this that plasma level measurements may have their greatest value, and these can be carried out without giving offence to conscientious staff. Occasionally, as with other industrial products, a 'dud' supply of drug might have been used. An alternative proprietary preparation or another drug of the same class may be given a trial. The principle of antidepressant drug therapy is that a trial of a tricyclic drug be followed by a 'second generation' antidepressant and then with lithium in combination. At any point in these proceedings a course of ECT may be given. If this does not seem to succeed, after a period of 2 weeks, MAOI may be introduced and later combined with L-tryptophan. A second course of ECT may be attempted. All the while psychotherapeutic and sociotherapeutic techniques will continue and additional knowledge will have been gathered. The description 'refractory depression' cannot be applied, one imagines, until at least a year has passed, so that a natural remission is given a chance to make itself felt.

The full consent of the patient must be obtained and Section 57 of the Mental Health Act of 1983 applies in such instances. This section applies to 'any surgical operation for destroying brain tissue or for destroying the function of brain tissue'. Whether a patient is detained or of informal status, he may not be subjected to psychosurgery, or other irreversible treatments unless:

(1) He has given his consent;

(2) An independent doctor and two other persons have certified in writing that the patient is capable of understanding the nature, purpose and the likely effects of psychosurgery and has consented to it; and

(3) The independent doctor has certified in writing that, having regard to the likelihood of the treatment alleviating or preventing a deterioration of the patient's condition, that the treatment should be given.

Before giving his opinion the independent doctor is required to consult two other persons who have been professionally concerned with the patient's medical treatment. One of these persons must be a nurse and the other neither a nurse nor a doctor.

But whether a patient with a chronic, intractable mental disorder can give full, informed consent is moot. Also, it could be argued that in a climate of controversy and with an irreversible procedure whose results can by no means be guaranteed there is limited scope for obtaining full and informed consent even if serious mental disorder had not been present. These ethical considerations are always important. Much of the controversy is generated not by patients or their relatives but by lobbyists more influenced by ideology, doctrine and emotion. However, this does not invalidate their protest. The situation has some similarities to the one that pertains to administration of ECT or to the procedure for obtaining brain biopsies in dementia (Mahendra, 1984b). All that can be said is that in the longterm the medical profession obtain the best possible results and perfect the safest surgical procedure so that facts and results can be pitted against emotion, and patients and their families be given a clearer choice. The move from structural destruction of brain tissue to precise, stereotactic procedures, the clearer delineation of the type of patient likely to benefit from surgery and the passing away from the psychiatric profession of the more fanatical proponents of psychosurgery have all helped ease the atmosphere in which the clear-headed and open-minded eclectic can work.

PSYCHOLOGICAL APPROACHES

The approach to psychotherapy in relation to depression in this book is an eclectic one and the term psychotherapy is used in its broadest sense. Psychotherapy is an integral part of medicine and every doctor–patient contact is leavened by the psychotherapeutic angle. It must be clear that psychosocial considerations inform the appraisal of problems of every depressed patient. These factors, as we have noted in Chapter 2, may have aetiological and pathogenetic significance. They may also be the consequence of any neurobiological change that has been brought about, so ensuring the disorder persisted with effects that have a bearing on the rest of the patient's life, in his relationship with others and the world at large.

It is unfortunate that teaching of trainee psychiatrists is often undertaken by a variety of specialists with little attempt being made to provide a synthesis of the overall management of the patient. Psychopharmacologists teach about drugs and ECT, (often) a maverick teaches about psychosurgery, some austere psychotherapist does the psychotherapy, a social psychiatrist takes on social, community and rehabilitation aspects and the trainee is left to his own devices to square the circle. Sometimes, if the trainee is sufficiently blessed with an open-minded curiosity, he may succeed in doing so after much trial and error. Yet, this co-ordinated approach to the management of the patient and his disorder which the trainee strives to perfect would be an eminently suitable approach to the practice of every branch of medicine. The narrowness of medical training has been criticized, yet the critics themselves, often from the social sciences, suffer from doctrinaire exiguity themselves, the results of which become evident when clinicians attempt to use, or portray the use of, drugs, ECT or psychosurgery.

There is little to commend an 'either/or' approach. As was shown in the introduction to this chapter, a depressed patient, like any other, requires physical and psychological treatment. The proportions in which one or the other is dispensed may vary from case to case and the wise and informed clinician keeps his options open.

As has been hinted, doctrines are of little value to the average clinician coming to grips with the average depressed patient. This rules out much psychoanalytic theory and practice, for whatever intellectual merit they may have in other contexts their rigid doctrines and arcane body of knowledge have little practical benefit for the average busy doctor working within the resources of a state-funded health service or the average patient who becomes depressed in the context of day to day living.

The practical, eclectic psychotherapeutic relationship begins with the initial contact with the patient. Indeed the experienced and skilled clinician does not even make a deliberate or conscious decision to begin to establish a relationship or effect a psychotherapeutic intervention. It begins when doctor and patient meet. When he is visiting a patient, the doctor must not conceal his identity or his authority, which he may summon to his aid. Whether the doctor calls himself a psychiatrist (if he is entitled to call himself thus) is moot. With more sophisticated patients the call of the psychiatrist or a visit to see him may be reassuring as it implies the availability of specialist help, and that the patient may safely focus on his mental problem, without fear that he might puzzle or embarrass the non-specialist. With simpler patients, the elderly and in rural parts, the term 'psychiatrist' from the local mental hospital may bring back memories of the alienist from the asylum, institutions which invariably seem to have had notorious pasts. A not untruthful introduction as a 'specialist' often eases the introduction.

Contrary to belief expressed in some quarters, the purely medical business of eliciting the features of illness is not unwelcome to either patient or practitioner. Patients appear to obtain comfort and relief when asked about such biological functions as sleep, appetite, bowel function, libido and menstrual history, one or more of which are almost invariably

151

disturbed in depression. Taking a detailed history also spares both the practitioner and patient from embarrassing silences that can engulf them once the introductions have been made. Part of the success in initiating a psychotherapeutic relationship with a patient is in convincing him that one understands his predicament, howsoever it might have been caused. It is here that even the inexperienced or psychotherapeutically unskilled of doctors need have little difficulty in appreciating the intensity of biological change. Once the doctor has established his credentials in this regard he can move on to less tangible features such as personality, family and social relationships. Contrary to received wisdom, it is probably the wisest course in most instances to talk to both patient and informant together at some time as this not only saves time but leaves less to be misunderstood or misconstrued. It is even more important when plans for management are being outlined.

The doctor may construct his formulation aloud, so patient and informant can expand on any factor that the doctor might have neglected or elevated to an unwarranted degree. It is unwise in general to be too specific at this early stage on precise aetiology or pathogenesis. Even if there is a previous history of similar illness, the doctor cannot be certain that additional precipitating factors, especially current physical illness, are not operating. In his approach to treatment, it goes without saying, the doctor must have access, at least in his own mind, to all available interventions. Any drug treatment must be outlined clearly to the patient and relatives, with remarks about onset of action, adverse effects and length of treatment. In out-patient departments and in people's homes, where patients are seen at the invitation of the general practitioner (GP), drugs must not be given without the GP's knowledge or consent except in the most exceptional cases. Psychiatric drugs, as has already been indicated, are not agents which work with absolute precision. An element of trial and error enters into the treatment of any patient and the doses are often prescribed in the most general terms and the day to day management of the patient will be by the GP. There are also considerations such as concurrent physical illness and drug therapy for these may have a material bearing on the treatment of depression. This is an even more relevant consideration in the management of the elderly depressed patient. The psychiatrist who does not consult or communicate with the GP does a disservice to the patient and deprives himself of a valuable ally.

There is no area of the patient's life that cannot or should not be explored, though obviously tact and sensitivity must be exercised all times. More sophisticated patients may well inveigle the doctor into supporting him in his allegations that one or more family members are responsible for his depression. The doctor must guard himself against this. The aetiology of depression is usually multifactorial and the doctor who encourages the patient or family to seek a scapegoat may be wrong as well as foolish.

It is generally accepted that questioning about suicidal ideas, thoughts preoccupation and plans are part of the assessment of every psychiatric patient. Provided the questions are elicited with sympathy and

152

understanding, there is every reason to believe that the patient is afforded relief and the doctor information.

Any hypochondriacal features must, of course, be noted but the doctor must make no attempt to explain these at first contact. The patient may well have a physical basis to these features which may emerge upon further investigation; on the other hand, the somatic symptoms may be part of the depressive syndrome and the doctor, who has no way of knowing for sure at a first meeting, is wise to remain non-committal. At later meetings, features of anxiety may well be clear-cut enough to allow for a ready explanation and most patients are reassured by being told of the physiological basis for symptoms which may well be frightening them.

On second and subsequent meetings, the effects of drug therapy can be evaluated and the psychotherapeutic relationship consolidated. There is uncertainty about how soon after the first meeting, the second ought to be arranged. For psychotherapeutic purposes a week's interval between first and second appointments may be needed. However, the positive effects of drugs cannot be seen for about 2 weeks and, in the meantime, the patient may be even more despondent. A great deal of reassurance may have to be given. Symptomatic treatment of insomnia and anxiety is beneficial in this interval and the sedative side effects of a drug such as amitriptyline are useful in this respect.

Once the depression begins to lift, the patient's awareness of change in his perceptions of the world may be explored. It is important, however sceptical one might be of matters, to project an optimistic view of the patient's condition. A quick run through of the patient's presenting symptoms may reveal improvement in one or other parameters and even the most determinedly negative of patients rarely has any counter to objective evidence which has been gathered from, and presented to, him. An apparent improvement in, say, sleep pattern may be most creatively extrapolated to other areas of the patient's life. It is remarkable how often patients will respond, however reluctantly, to suggestions that as their sleep and appetite have improved, some other aspects of their life too must have improved.

At the second and subsequent meetings, areas of life such as work, marriage and other personal relationships may be explored in greater depth. Reassurance may still be needed for persisting symptoms, most especially loss of attention and concentration which may take several weeks to subside even after the depression has lifted. Loss of confidence, too, persists for a considerable time and in the security of the doctor–patient relationship the patient may take the first tentative steps to re-establish his confidence. The doctor communicates, reassures, encourages and predicts. At every stage it will be noted the doctor does not make facile predictions but those which are based on fact in his experience of depression and its response to treatment. The doctor needs to work at keeping the patient's trust and at subsequent meetings a sensitive query as regards suicidal thoughts may strike a chord in the patient whose depression may appear to be lifting but who is still tormented by suicidal thoughts.

It is the proposition of this chapter that physical treatment and psychotherapy go hand in hand in the management of the depressed patient. There is little doubt that an effective armamentarium of drugs now exists for depression. But doubts have always been cast on the efficacy of formal psychotherapy, especially of the psychoanalytic kind. We are not here concerned with formal psychotherapy but with the relationship every doctor establishes with the patient. This is as much social and personal as technical and professional. It is not scientific in that there is no formal, systematic, quantified observation of phenomena or the rigorously controlled testing of hypotheses. It is not measurable in any meaningful terms and the criteria applicable to the evaluation of drugs are irrelevant in this situation. It is individual, as opposed to the evaluation of treatment on series of patients and the effects are generalizable only in broad terms. It is sometimes called supportive therapy and it complements physical treatment.

Klerman and Schechter (1982) have reviewed studies that combined drugs and psychotherapy and the issues involved in combined therapies of this kind. Weissman (1979) has reviewed the efficacy of formal psychotherapeutic approaches including the behavioural, cognitive, group, interpersonal and marital psychotherapies in relation to depression. Psychotherapy alone appeared to be superior to no treatment. The results of comparison between drug treatment and psychotherapy appeared less clear. Drugs appeared to be superior to psychotherapy in relieving symptoms and preventing relapses, but psychotherapy seemed superior to drugs in bringing about social readjustment.

Klerman and Schechter (1982) have noted the possible drawbacks that drug therapy might have on the psychotherapeutic process. These considerations include what they call the 'negative placebo' effect where the effect of drug prescription has effects other than the non-pharmacological and has possibly deleterious effects on the doctor–patient relationship. The prescription of the drug, they felt, might be construed as an authoritarian act, forcing the patient into being a passive and compliant receiver of treatment, and also initiating or augmenting mechanisms of counter-transference that might hinder the development of insight and thus be ultimately counter-therapeutic.

A certain level of anxiety is necessary to motivate individuals to strive. The effects of drugs may reduce anxiety and related symptoms and thereby reduce the motivation to change, which is the *raison d'etre* of psychotherapy. Lowered anxiety brings reduced motivation; it also reduces the necessity to engage wholeheartedly in the psychotherapeutic process. The sum total of these effects might be that the patient turns away from the concentrated, and at times distressing, work that is necessary to bring about fundamental personality change. A third point they make involves the possible effects on symptom reduction and the substitution of other symptoms. Symptoms are held to maintain a balance between conflict and defences, and the reduction of symptoms such as anxiety or depression could upset this equilibrium and release deeper conflicts which produce new symptoms. Their fourth suggestion is a peculiarly American one in that if the patient felt he was being fobbed off with drugs when he expected psychotherapy, he might feel robbed and his self-esteem, already low, might be subjected to a wounding blow. There are socio-cultural expectations of psychotherapy in the United States which, of course, determine this view. A white, middle class, literate, educated and well-off person has been deemed more likely to receive psychotherapy, and even if drugs are prescribed with the best of motives, the sense of inferiority implied may affect the patient.

There are, of course, positive effects that drugs may have on psychotherapy. By reducing anxiety and other symptoms drugs could make the patient more accessible to psychotherapy. This is well understood in terms of the widely-known model in physiological psychology which shows an optimal level of anxiety enables a subject to behave most effectively. Similar considerations apply to the improvement in attention and concentration, memory and other cognitive functions and verbal skills which facilitate the psychotherapeutic process. Another factor, more applicable to clinical practices in the past, is the abreactive role drugs such as intravenous barbiturate and amphetamine could play. Finally, the placebo as opposed to the pharmacological effects of drugs could enhance the well-being of the patient and lead to greater psychotherapeutic accessibility.

The objection from the point of view of drug therapy is that psychotherapy might prove a turbulent influence, undoing the sympto-matic relief that drugs provide, especially in the early or acute phase of the illness. The positive effects of psychotherapy on drugs might be the facilitation of the doctor–patient relationship; an indirect benefit might well be better compliance in drug taking.

However, the majority of studies (e.g. Luborsky, 1975) appear to show that drugs and psychotherapy together are superior to either approach alone. It seems, as has been suggested before, that different areas of a depressed patient's problems are improved by drugs and psychotherapy, and that their effects do not counter one another but are additive.

Cognitive therapy

It is customary to think of disturbed cognitive function being a consequence of depression. However, it is possible to conceive of the symptoms of depression as following upon disordered cognition. Thus cognitive function may play a part in the causation of depression. It is alleged the individual takes a negative view of himself, of the world and the future, and this is brought about by distortions and biases in his mental scheme leading to inappropriate inferences, abstractions, overgeneralizations, magnifications and minimizations of issues, problems and events. There is a cognitive misinterpretation and then over-reaction to this interpretation which leads to depression, a state in which there is further misinterpretation and distortion and so on, thus compounding a vicious circle.

The essence of the cognitive behavioural approach to treatment is to bring about an awareness in the patient that his negative thoughts have a causal bearing on his feelings and behaviours and consciously teach him manoeuvres that will reduce his capacity for thinking negatively. The patient, in the course of treatment, begins to make an association between

155

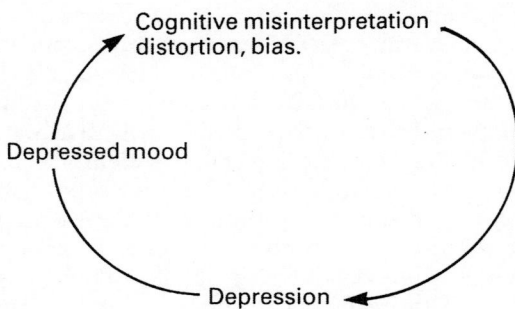

DEPRESSION

Cognitive misinterpretation
distortion, bias.

Depressed mood

Depression

Figure 10 The vicious circle of cognitive dysfunction and depression

his negative thoughts and his feelings. If at the same time he can make an association between positive thoughts and positive feelings, it may well be possible to increase the frequency of the former. The crucial task is to see that there is a carry-over of this change in attitude beyond the period of therapy, and there is no theoretical objection to the use of ancillary behavioural methods such as assertion and relaxation.

Zeiss *et al.* (1979) have listed the critical components of an approach to a successful cognitive–behavioural therapy. There should have been a carefully constructed and well planned scheme of treatment which must assure the patient that, at the end of the course of treatment, he could hope to control his behaviour and thereby his depression. The treatment must involve the teaching of skills to the patient who must find these relevant to his daily life. The patient must become aware that there will be a general need for the skills he has been taught, and learned, outside the context of the immediate treatment setting. If, as his mood improves, he becomes aware that his newly acquired skills, rather than those of the therapists, have contributed to his well-being, his confidence will be enhanced the greater.

The emotional state can, equally clearly, influence thought content, with several studies (e.g. Lloyd and Lishman, 1975) which have shown that unpleasant and pleasant moods are differentially affected by the mood state in their accessibility. The mood state at the time of retrieval of a memory selectively affects the type of cognition; depressed mood increases the accessibility of unpleasant memories and decreases that of pleasant ones.

There may be a reciprocal relationship between cognition and emotion, with emotional states able to selectively increase the like occurrence of cognitions of the type likely to maintain them. As the depressed person appears to have greater access to the negative cognitions, he is more likely to think of himself in relation to past negative experiences which, in turn, may bias in a negative way his current experiences and also his predictions regarding the future. Thus Beck's (1967) idea of a 'cognitive triad', consisting of a person's negative view of his world, a negative concept of himself and a negative appraisal of his future, is sustained.

How effective is cognitive therapy? Blackburn *et al.* (1981) reported a study which compared cognitive therapy, antidepressant drugs and a combination of these two, in depressed patients seen either in general practice or an out-patient department. Patients were randomly assigned to cognitive therapy, antidepressants or a combination of the two. The antidepressant drug group did less well in both hospital and general practice and combination treatment was superior to drug treatment in both hospital and general practice. In general practice, cognitive therapy was superior to drug treatment. The presence of 'endogenous' features did not appear to affect response to treatment. There also did not seem to be a bias in favour of the better educated or more intellectual who might have been expected to respond best.

Social aspects

The important point here is to obtain an objective report on the functioning of the patient in relation to his family, his employment and other social roles. While there can be no dispute that depression is a disabling condition, the patient may well have had difficulties in these areas prior to the development of his disorder.

During treatment, the family may well have to be told explicitly of the patient's improving condition as there is a tendency in some families not to accept change, even for the better, on the part of the depressed patient.

At the time of discharge it becomes important to involve the family in such matters as ensuring that maintenance treatment and prophylactic therapy are continued.

Although finding employment for patients is beyond the purview and control of doctors, the patient must encouraged to seek paid employment as there seems little doubt that work is therapeutic and counters depression (see Chapter 9). All available resources in the health service such as occupational therapy departments, industrial therapy units, the disablement resettlement officer and the hospital social work department must be tapped in helping the patient to seek employment, and the patient supported and encouraged to keep employment.

Rehabilitation

Hospital admission must be considered to be a last resort for the depressed patient nowadays. Severe psychomotor retardation which leads to problems in eating and drinking may require hospital in-patient stay for the correction of nutrition and hydration by trained staff. Another possible reason for admission is suicidal risk. The only other possible indication for hospital admission is where there are doubts about the clinical state, e.g. an unusual degree of cognitive impairment or where there is a discrepancy in accounts of the patient's behaviour furnished by relatives or other informants. Here a period of in-patient stay may become necessary in order to clarify points in the history. Certainly if an irreversible procedure such as leucotomy is being considered it may well be advisable to admit the patient for a period of observation.

157

Admission of patients for 'social reasons' is to be deprecated. The social reasons are likely to be the cause, or consequence, of depression. If the former, it is certainly untherapeutic in the long run to provide the patient with a haven from the cares of the world, and then to discharge him to an unchanged world when he is symptomatically better. It would certainly help the patient more if his symptoms and problems could be tackled in relation to the stresses of the real world.

For these reasons the question of 'rehabilitation' of depressed patients must not arise in anything like substantial numbers. The patient continues to live in his own home and has access to treatment which to as great an extent as possible must be provided for him in the setting in which he lives. He visits the hospital to see his doctor or other therapist – who in an ideal world would have seen him at home – to have treatment which may include out-patient ECT and go back to lead his own life in the midst of having treatment. This calls for coping abilities on the part of the family, spouse, other relatives, friends, colleagues and neighbours. But that is the reality of care in the community which is not simply a case of the state providing, or not providing as the case may be, resources for the care of patients in the settings in which they lead their lives but also makes demands on the tolerance of others who share the same community. With all the resources needed made available there will be no future for community care if the attitudes of the very large majority who are neither patients nor therapists do not change to embrace this reality.

6
Depressed minds, disordered cells: malignancy and depression

The relationship between depression and malignancy has already been alluded to in Chapter 2, in the context of speculation as to how stress and life events may determine the onset and course of depression.

The relationship between malignancy and mental states has been the subject of speculation for 2000 years. Bahnson (1980) and Greer (1983) have made reference to the historical antecedents of the subject. In the second century AD Galen noted that melancholic women were more liable to develop breast cancer than were sanguine women. The fact that emotional distress can precede the diagnosis of cancer has been suspected for at least the past two centuries. In 1759 the surgeon, Richard Guy, described women who were prone to develop cancer as '...of a sedentary, melancholic disposition of mind, (who) meet with such disasters in life as occasion much trouble and grief', and Sir James Paget wrote in 1870 that, 'we can hardly doubt that mental depression is a weighty addition to the other influences favouring the development of a cancerous constitution'. In 1846, Walshe had noted that 'moral emotions' (mental misery, sudden reverses of fortune, habitual gloominess) produced a state which was vulnerable to the formation of cancer. Another writer stated in 1854 that the 'influence of grief appears to be... the most common cause of cancer'.

The last decades of the 19th century were especially productive of ideas regarding the role of mental influences on the formation and spread of cancer. In 1893, Snow had observed that there were too many instances of breast and uterine malignancy following depression for them to be accounted for in terms of chance occurrence alone. Later, the influence of loss, bereavement, grief and melancholy were related to the development of malignancy. In 1926, Evans, reporting on 100 cancer patients who had undergone psychotherapy, found her patients had lost, or had disrupted, a significant relationship prior to the development of cancer. In general, there was more cautious speculation in the 20th century, with the emphasis being on emotional factors as secondary precipitants, factors that influenced the

159

course of a malignant neoplasm that might have another cause. The Frenchman Foque in 1931 ascribed depression as being an 'activating and secondary' cause in certain human malignancies. He noted that in many of the patients who had subsequently developed cancer there had been major life crises, severe depression and profound mourning.

In studying the relationship between depression and malignancy, there are several factors that need to be considered. Firstly, as we have seen, the personality of a patient may predispose to both depression and certain malignant disorders. Readers will be familiar with a not very convincing and, perhaps, slightly tendentious argument that sought to explain bronchial carcinoma in terms of the personality of the patient who was driven to excessive cigarette smoking. However, certain personality factors in the make-up of an individual, especially those related to the expression of emotion, may have an influence on the progression of malignancy, and this subject will be considered shortly. Secondly, there is a possibility that stresses and life events may determine the onset and progression of both depression and malignant disorder. Thirdly, one must take into account the manifestation of psychiatric symptoms of the malignant disease which has not yet become apparent.

DEPRESSION SECONDARY TO CANCER

In purely medical terms, the last of the above points is perhaps the easiest to understand and explain. Depression is well known both to precede, and present with, malignant disease. If there were early spread to the brain, the metastases could manifest themselves as depression before there were clinical features related to the primary carcinoma site, such as features of a space occupying lesion or of focal involvement. This subject was considered in relation to depression in cerebral disease in Chapter 4. Depression could also be a non-metastatic feature of a malignant illness which did not give rise to clinical features attributable to the primary site. Brain and Henson (1958) pointed out that non-metastatic neurological abnormalities could antedate the appearance of a malignant lesion by 3 years. This may present as more obvious neurological or neuropsychiatric phenomena, but there is also a prominent presence of depression. The classic example, referred to in cautionary terms in surgical textbooks ('Cancer somewhere, cancer nowhere, cancer in head of pancreas') is well known to most clinicians as a cause of severe, unremitting, intractable depression which precedes the jaundice and pain. Fras et al. (1967) discovered an incidence of 76% depression in patients with carcinoma of the pancreas and in half their cases the depression had preceded the clinical features due to the malignancy itself. Brain and Henson (1958) found that in 74% of cases with neurological abnormality in similar circumstances, carcinoma of the lung was the implicated malignancy. The third explanation for depression in association with a malignant process is that there are non-metastatic metabolic and endocrine effects due to the malignancy which may give rise to depression in a manner which has been dealt with in Chapter 3. Hypercalcaemia as a cause of depression and the significant correlation between serum calcium and the clinical features of depression have been considered in Chapter 4, and the less certain relationship between increased adrenocortical activity and depression has also been taken up. An interesting hypothesis linking increased blood levels of calcium with depression in malignancy is considered later in this chapter. There is also the possibility that depression and malignant disease may be different ways in which some common genetic element is given expression. The somewhat contentious issue of 'depressive equivalents' was dealt with in Chapter 3, but the consistent finding that the incidence of cancer is increased in depressed patients may arguably be explained in terms that are also employed to explain the increased incidence of alcoholism and some forms of violent behaviour in depression.

There are also commonsense explanations. Depression may also arise as a result of the knowledge that one has a serious condition that may threaten life, and may also have other distressing consequences before eventual death. These include the consequences of bodily malfunction as with bowel or stomach malignancies; the loss of parts of the body such as limbs, breast or uterus; the loss in appearance or an aesthetic loss, e.g. facial disfiguration or mastectomy; pain; the realization that those who are left behind will grieve; the inability to work; the expense and inconvenience of treatment; the treatment itself (surgery, irradiation, chemotherapy).

DEPRESSION PRECEDING CANCER

The follow-up of depressive illness in the expectation that there might be a higher incidence of malignancy has been undertaken by several authors. Varsamis et al. (1972) followed up 24 patients and found a quarter had developed a malignancy on 6 year follow-up. Whitlock and Siskind (1979) followed-up depressed patients and found that deaths due to cancer were significantly higher in their male patients. Interestingly, some of the deaths occurred within 6 months of the diagnosis of depression, which is probably too short a period to ascribe a causal role to the depression, which was presumably an early clinical feature of a latent malignant condition. Kerr et al. (1969) found that 5 of 28 depressed male patients had died on average at 4 years follow-up, which was due to a significantly greater occurrence of malignancy than might have been predicted. The period between the onset of depression and death due to malignancy was again short, a mean of 2.4 years. Those authors also quote the 6 year follow-up of American prisoners of war in Japanese camps. There an increase in mortality for malignant as well as for cardiovascular and gastro-intestinal disease was noted. However, these patients had been subjected to quite obvious and exceptional physical and emotional privation, and it is probably not valid to compare these cases with series of uncomplicated depressed patients.

Sainsbury (1955) showed that in a series of suicides, cancer was 20 times as common as in the general population. Whitlock (1978) compared suicides over the age of 50 with other violent deaths and found that a significantly higher proportion of patients had had cancer and also more benign brain tumours. The point is made by Whitlock that the widely accepted

161

association between alcoholism and malignancies of the larynx, lung and upper gastro-intestinal tract may have an intermediate variable in depression. The idea that alcoholism may in certain circumstances be considered a depressive equivalent has been discussed in Chapter 3.

Whether any of the features of depression as it presented might help predict the later onset of cancer has been considered by several authors. Whitlock and Siskind (1979) concluded that the depressed patient most at risk of developing a later malignancy might be a middle-aged or elderly male patient developing a severe depression for the first time, but in whom the features of depression *did not include* feelings of guilt, suicidal ideas or behaviour, diurnal mood change or psychotic features such as delusions and hallucinations. Kerr *et al.* (1969) had noted that there was no previous history of depression, a stable premorbid personality, an insidious onset of depression with no apparent precipitating factor, an unremitting course and a progressive deterioration in the clinical state. They confirmed the absence of psychomotor retardation and psychotic features, but found early awakening, loss of energy and interest and an absence of diurnal variation and the presence of reactivity of mood. There was no cognitive impairment. In both series a rapid and full response to tricyclic antidepressant therapy and ECT was noted, there being a tendency to early relapse which, however, responded well to further treatment. Interestingly, it has been claimed that the malignancy can regress with the successful treatment of the depression (Goldfarb *et al.*, 1967).

Thus, as Kerr *et al.* (1969) stated, a depressive illness which occurs in middle-aged male patients, with no previous history of depression or vulnerable personality, without apparent precipitating factors, and characterized by a 'mixed bag' of depressive symptomatology may be an early indicator and direct manifestation of malignancy.

Explanations have been offered for some of the features of depression in malignant disease. Brown and Paraskevas (1982) have proposed that some cases of depression in cancer may be caused by immunological interference with the activity of 5-HT. This interference, they propose, could be brought about by two mechanisms. Antibody induced against a protein released from cancer cells could, as a result of cross-reactivity with CNS tissue, bind to receptors for 5-HT and block these. Subsequently, such primary antibodies could themselves stimulate the production of the corresponding antibodies, which would act as alternative receptors for 5-HT and reduce its synaptic availability. They argue that this hypothesis is supported by the evidence that immunological cross-reactivity exists between cancer cells and neurones, and there is also cross-reactivity between a basic protein of cancer cells and myelin basic protein. The following would stem from their hypotheses. Tumour basic protein should be able to induce experimental allergic encephalomyelitis in laboratory animals; tumour basic protein should induce antibodies that will reduce 5-HT activity in experimental tissue; some cancer patients should have an antibody that will reduce 5-HT activity in experimental tissue; and that this antibody should occur more commonly and in higher concentration in depressed cancer patients than in non-depressed cancer patients.

162

Weizman *et al.* (1979) observed a relationship between the hypercalcaemia due to malignancy and mental disorder, including depression. As has been discussed in Chapter 4, they confirmed that the mental disorder subsided with treatment which succeeded in restoring the plasma calcium levels to within their normal range. However, contrary to earlier findings, they found there was no direct relationship between hypercalcaemia and the mental state, and suggested that intermediary variables such as age, pre-morbid personality, type of malignancy, the rate of increase in calcium levels and the psychological reaction to the neoplasm may play a part in inducing the psychiatric symptoms and determining their course and severity.

The biological factors associated with depression which may play a part in inducing a subsequent malignancy are matters for speculation but the immune and endocrine systems have been implicated in the suggested mechanism. There appears to be a diminution of effectiveness in immunological mechanism following bereavement (Bartrop *et al.*, 1977; see also Chapter 2). The suggestion has been made (Burnet, 1976) that when the immune mechanism is compromised by, say, age, malignancy might be induced. Hence, diminished effectiveness of the immune system after emotional stress may play a similar role. However, not all cancers appear to be related to reduced immunocompetence, and those that are, are not necessarily related to depression.

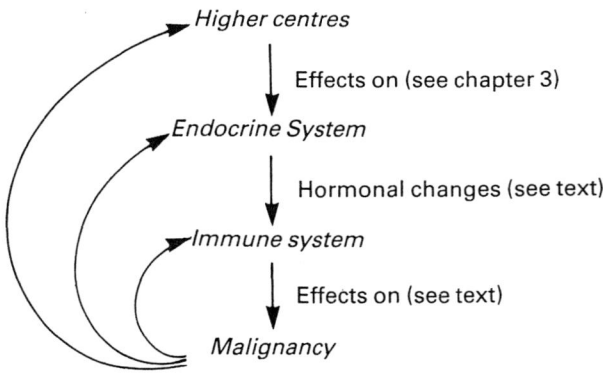

Figure 11 The biological effects of malignancy, and its response

The immune system consists of a mechanism of cell-mediated immunity and antibody-mediated reactions. The former is involved in the delayed hypersensitivity reaction and in the rejection of transplants. The mechanism involves the T-cells which are brought into play by antigens interacting with receptors on the surface. In the latter mechanism, there is an antigen–antibody reaction involving the transformation of some lymphocytes into plasma cells which produce immunoglobulins such as IgA, IgG, IgM or IgE. Both mechanisms may be influenced by hormones such as cortisol and thyroxine. Lymphocyte function may also be influenced by insulin, histamine and catecholamines. In primates, stress can increase the levels of catecholamines as well as pituitary, thyroid and growth hormone (Mason, 1972).

The relationship between stress and tumour growth is likely to be a complex one. It is said that mild stress may be helpful in the resistance to tumour growth, but more excessive stress may lead to increased steroid production which may inhibit the activities of the macrophages, which may then disinhibit tumour growth (Bahnson, 1981).

Most stress reactions appear to lead to an increase in 17-hydroxycortico-steroids (17-OHCS), catecholamines, the thyroid hormones and growth hormone. The lowest levels of 17-OHCS appear to be found with effective ego defences; high levels with failed defences, highest with complete ego breakdown as with psychotic depression. This is a plausible explanation of the association between methods of coping and the endocrine and immune response which may explain the pattern of findings in the next sections.

Of more specific interest in relation to malignancy are the changes which are found in steroid levels in response to psychological events (Mason, 1975). Parents of children with leukaemia have demonstrated individual differences in mean basal urinary 17-OHCS levels and were 'high', 'middle' or 'low' level excretors. When they were subjected to stresses – in relation to the condition of their sick children – those who excreted low levels of the metabolite had even lower levels; high excretors had even higher levels of excretion. It appeared that those who relied on denial as a defence mechanism had low levels which diminished further with further denial. Thus it was suggested that steroid levels may reflect not stress directly but the effectiveness of the defence mechanism. In a similar vein, Rasmussen (1969) suggested that the immune response could have been enhanced by optimal, intermediate steroid levels, and undermined by both low and high levels of steroids.

Other emotions find reflection in the response of the neuroendocrine system. Thus anger directed inwards appears to be associated with increased adrenaline production and anger directed outwards by increased noradrenaline activity (Funkenstein, 1957).

Although these suggestions remain speculative, their consistency has been such that some workers (e.g. Marmorston et al., 1969) have claimed to be able to differentiate between malignancies in the breast, prostate and lung on the basis of specific hormonal profiles. It is also possible to distinguish between malignant and benign tumours on the basis of hormone profiles. In lung cancer adrenaline is increased compared to chronic, non-malignant lung disease (Kissen and Rao, 1969).

Thus there is integrated activity between the nervous system, the endocrine system and the immune system. Changes in the outer environment and from internal psychic events are relayed by the nervous system to the centres for neuroendocrine mechanisms. The ensuing hormonal changes may affect the immune system (Bahnson, 1981). Nucleotides such as cyclic adenosine monophosphate (cAMP) and cyclic guanosine monophosphate (cGMP) appear to liaise between the endocrine and immune systems. α-Adrenergic and β-adrenergic effects inhibit and stimulate cAMP, respectively. Anxiety and depression appear to decrease the capacity of cAMP, and thus the result may be to reduce immunocompetence overall. Interferon can also be affected by stressful events, a response which varies according to stress and between species. Thyroxine may also influence the immune system. When the thymus is damaged in mice, immunocompetence is compromised. This can be restored and the system stimulated by thyroxine. Cortisol, on the other hand, inhibits thymic activity (Bahnson, 1981).

(a) cancer giving rise to depression

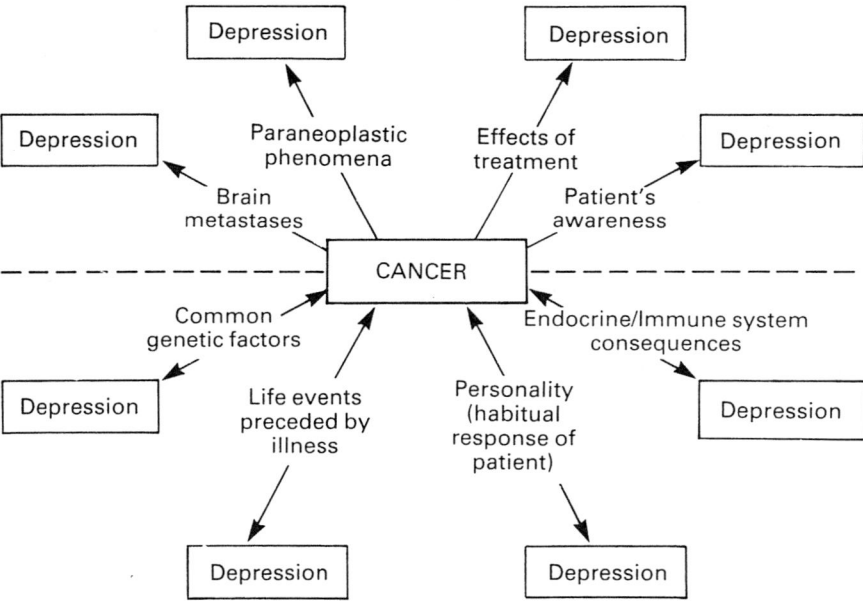

(b) cancer and depression as consequences of one another

Figure 12 The relationships between cancer and depression

DEPRESSION AND CANCER: SOME PSYCHOLOGICAL FACTORS

The primarily psychological influences on the onset and course of malignant illness involve the effects that life events and stresses might have, and also the impact of personality on the course of malignant illness. The subject is, as might be expected, a complex one with enormous methodological pitfalls. Less than rigorous studies up to now may mean some of the conclusions might have been unwarranted. Greer (1983) has set the minimum requirements that are needed before reasonably valid conclusions can be drawn:

(1) Unselected series of patients with documented neoplastic disease need to be compared with control series of patients who are free of neoplastic disease.

165

(2) The investigations must be blind, i.e. the investigators must be ignorant of the diagnosis at the time of the study.

(3) Standardized measurement must be used, i.e. specified clinical ratings or standardized psychological tests must be used.

(4) Appropriate statistical analysis needs to be carried out.

(5) All patients must be aware of the diagnosis.

(6) Full staging of the cancer must have been done.

(7) In the follow-up period there must be full documentation of stressful events and psychological support.

(8) Full documentation must be available about both the duration of the survival as well as the occurrence of the metastases.

(9) Wherever possible, relevant endocrine and immune functions must be measured.

It has been shown that even when genetic and environmental factors were shared, the experience of stress might influence the onset of illness. Thus, Greene and Swisher (1969) showed that in twins discordant for leukaemia the affected twin had suffered significantly more stress than the twin who remained well.

Loss and depression may be causal antecedents of cancer, it has been argued. Several studies, chiefly on the lymphomas, leukaemias and uterine cancer, have suggested that separation or serious loss may precede the development of those malignant conditions. Le Shan and Worthington (1956) reported that patients with cancer had experienced the loss of significant relationships before the onset of the condition. They also lacked the ability to express feelings of hostility and appeared not to have resolved the feelings associated with the death of a parent several years before. A consistent theme in the earlier work on the subject is the presence of these unresolved anxieties involving parents.

As noted in the previous section, several workers have commented on the presence of antecedent depression in malignant disease. This appears to be associated with the loss of a significant figure, or the loss of a goal in life, with consequent hopelessness, despair and 'giving up' prior to the onset of the malignancy. The loss of a significant person might have been in the period 1–2 years before the onset of the symptoms of cancer (Neumann, 1959). Lung cancer patients have been reported as having sustained a significant loss in the preceding 5-year period when compared to control subjects (Horne and Picard, 1979).

Loss is merely one factor. After all, virtually everyone experiences loss at one time or another and not all contract malignant disease. The nature of the loss and its impact on the personality might be thought as worth a more detailed inquiry (Bahnson, 1980). He observes that the effects of the loss gain their significance in cancer patients as a result of what might have gone before. The patient, as a child, seems to have had an ambivalent relationship to the significant person whose loss when experienced in adult life has such repercussions. The relationship might have been dependent, but also might have featured conflict and been unsatisfying, especially in relation to the mother. Some of this is seen in the personality of the grown up patient who grows up bearing the scars of childhood trauma, the loss of childhood figures and the lack of a secure, loving base. The child that becomes the father of the man who gets cancer appears to have grown with an ingrained sense of pessimism and associated feelings of self-blame and guilt (see also Chapter 5). This kind of person also tends to be driven, on anniversaries and similar occasions, in a self-destructive way, even before the onset of malignant conditions.

It might be asked if any particular features of depression could predict the later onset of cancer. It might have been expected on commonsense grounds that psychological features of depression were especially predictive. However, as was shown in Chapter 2, there is no direct relationship between those factors implicated in the onset of depression and the ensuing malignancy, and Bieliauskas *et al.* (1979) suggested that the somatic features of depression rather than self-reported sadness might be more predictive of cancer.

The view that early life experiences may determine the behaviour which may increase the propensity or liability to cancer has been criticized by Crisp (1970) on the grounds that much of the speculation has followed the extrapolation of data from animal experiments, which may not be strictly applicable to the human case.

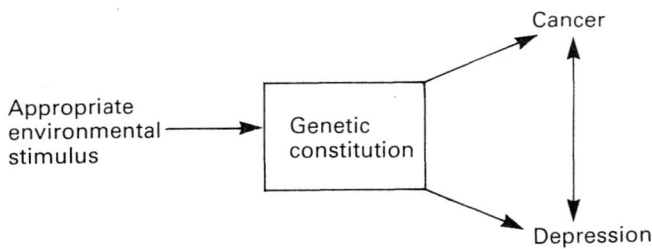

Figure 13 Vulnerability to cancer and depression

DEPRESSION AND THE ONSET OF CANCER

It would be too simplistic to suggest that a depressive personality was likely to predispose to cancer. The speculations are of a somewhat more sophisticated order in that they suggest there are factors which are associated with a depressive personality which may put the patient at risk. These factors include a rigidity of outlook with a rather strong internal control, an unbending view of norms and conventions and the excessive presence of defence mechanisms such as denial and repression. The cancer-prone individual is said to be inhibited, over-controlled and with impaired capacity for expressing strong emotion, especially anger.

This was shown by Abse *et al.* (1974) with reference to the personality of patients with lung cancer. They appear to have harboured denial and repression, were poorly able to discharge hostile feelings, tended to blame themselves, projected an air of self-sacrifice and were predisposed to hopelessness and despair. Their inhibited nature was associated with an inability to examine themselves or introspect. They would, in a simple typology, be called introverted, whereas patients with breast cancer are found to be extraverted. The repression in the latter includes a repressed sexuality.

The simple typologies of introversion and extraversion have some historical interest. As was briefly noted in the introduction to this chapter, it was once put about that the extroverted were more prone to take up smoking anyway, and thus their personalities might have been conducive to lung cancer, rather than some carcinogen in the cigarette. This was examined by Kissen (1964) who compared patients with lung cancer with those with chronic, non-malignant, lung disease and suggested that both a vulnerability in the personality and heavy cigarette smoking were necessary for lung cancer to develop. Repressed emotional expression was found in his patients, too, but seemed unrelated to heavy smoking. (Extroverted persons were also held in those days to be more accident prone, more likely to get pregnant accidentally and were also more predisposed to hysteria, psychopathy and crime: life was simpler 30 years ago).

These findings have more recently been extended to women patients with gynaecological cancers who are alleged to be more inhibited, more conforming and less overtly hostile than controls who had benign disease (Mastrovito et al., 1979).

The work of Kissen in the study of psychological factors associated with heavy cigarette smoking and lung cancer has been reviewed by Crisp (1970). Kissen was concerned to find a difference between those heavy smokers who contracted cancer and those who did not. He compared lung cancer patients with patients who had chronic, but not malignant, pulmonary disease and found early on that patients with lung cancer scored significantly low on measures of neuroticism. Later, he used personality inventories such as the Maudsley Personality Inventory and the Eysenck Personality Inventory to confirm his clinical suspicions that patients with lung cancer had an impaired capacity to release emotion. Also, contrary to expectation, Kissen found lung cancer patients who had developed lung cancer despite taking the advice not to inhale the cigarette fumes appeared to show even more abnormality in their personality make-up. Thus it seemed that although the carcinogens were potentially pathogenic to everybody, their role as a factor might be reduced if there was a personality vulnerability in the smoker.

Hagnell (1966) conducted a prospective study of 2500 individuals in Sweden. A test of Sjobring's personality measures – such as capacity, stability, solidity and validity – had been administered 20 years before. There appeared to be a significant association between female cancer and sub-stability, a measure characterized by warmth, extroversion and sociability. It also has associations with both pyknic body build and with an increased output of 17-OHCS, in other words, indices which have also been associated with depression.

Greer (1983), commenting on studies carried out in his department, noted that earlier observations had linked breast cancer to such personality features as extroversion, denial in the face of stress, inhibited sexuality and intropunitiveness. In their studies, he and his colleagues found there was an association between the diagnosis of breast cancer and a life-long behaviour pattern characterized by the extreme suppression of anger. This association appeared to be significant for women who were under 50 years of age. There was also an association between cancer of the breast and low levels of anxiety. Greer quotes three subsequent studies of women patients with breast cancer. In one, patients with cancer were reported as showing less anxiety, more suppression of emotion, more optimism and a greater tendency to avoid conflict than controls with benign tumours. In both other studies expression of anger was less common among cancer patients than controls, but was again significant only in women aged under 50. In one of these studies, patients with cancer were found to have been more depressed and less demonstrative than controls.

A wide variety of factors may be implicated in the development of cancer. These are known to include environmental factors such as carcinogens, impaired immunity due to some of the factors discussed in an earlier section, ageing and genetic factors. Where does personality fit in? Reports of studies such as those discussed above indicate that patients under the age of 50 may have their personalities playing a more substantial role in the onset of cancer than in those who are much younger, or older. Certainly, ageing in the elderly would appear to have an impact on the immune system and the more prolonged exposure to carcinogens as more important factors in the pathogenesis of malignant disease; young children, on the other hand, have a proportionately greater contribution from genetic factors in some tumours of very early life. Psychological factors may contribute most in middle life. In this interactionist model some of the comments made in Chapter 2 in the causation of depression are not without relevance.

For lung cancer, Kissen (1963) attempted to set out the psychological factors which would have some pathogenic significance in men aged between 55 and 64 years. These included:

(1) Before the age of 15, where the key factor might be an effective separation from the parents, i.e. death of parent, an unhappy home due to parental friction or, to a lesser extent, prolonged parental absence from home;

(2) In adult life, the main adverse effects relate to work and to interpersonal difficulties, especially marital problems. As might be expected, chronic difficulties of 10 years' duration or greater appeared to have a greater impact than those of a briefer duration.

It might be argued that the personality factors allegedly influencing the onset and course might have a similar effect on non-malignant 'psychosomatic' disease. Kissen (1963) concedes that in contrast to 'non-psychosomatic' patients, lung cancer and 'psychosomatic' patients have similar psychosocial histories. However, lung cancer patients were typically unable to discharge emotions, a feature that stood out.

Noting that several investigators had reported that feelings of

169

hopelessness, high scores on the MMPI depression scale and the loss of close personal relationships were associated with the occurrence of cancer. Shekelle *et al.* (1981) set out to test the hypothesis that 'depression' as measured by the MMPI would be associated with an increased risk of death from cancer over a 17-year follow-up period. They found that depression thus measured in middle-aged men was associated with increased risk of death from a variety of cancers and was independent of such other contributory factors as age, cigarette smoking, alcohol consumption, family history of cancer and occupational record. The strength of the association persisted over 17 years of follow-up and allied with the duration argued against the interpretation having been an early manifestation of malignancy. The question of an intermediary between life events and 'organic' illness has been considered in Chapter 2. The prime suspect here was thought to be depression and its associated features. Similarly, with life events, the response to the life event may be the significant variable. Schmale and Iker (1966) showed that women who had reacted to a life event 6 months previously with feelings of hopelessness were more likely to have developed cervical cancer. The life event itself was not considered as important as the feelings of hopelessness.

A modest transcultural contribution was offered several years ago (Mahendra, 1977b, c). A personality inventory was put together from items that were thought to be of significance from a study of the literature. It was given to 71 patients with neoplasm and 34 control patients in surgical and medical wards of a general hospital in Ceylon. The patients were unaware of the diagnosis of malignancy and, things being what they were, of any other diagnosis. The idea was to inquire retrospectively what the premorbid personality of the patients might have been, and to see if any constellation of personality traits might be associated with the malignancy. It was found that patients with a neoplasm were significantly more inhibited regarding the opposite sex, given to brooding, had disturbed sleep, were sensitive, ambitious, hypochondriacal, held firmer astrological beliefs and were more religious, while controls were troubled by guilt and were more likely to be upset by trivialities. Comparison between patients with malignant and benign neoplasm revealed that the former were significantly more likely to be meticulous at work, dissatisfied with their life, preferred action to thought, were more moralistic and more religious. No significant differences could be found between type of malignancy or the organ in which it was found. The neoplastic patient gave the impression of being an insecure but ambitious, probably depressive individual who presented a 'facade of benign goodness', a consistent finding in the literature up to the time. All the criticisms detailed on previous pages of this chapter are as applicable to this study as to anything else. Moreover, as the responses to the questions showed, there was a considerable cultural influence and the fact the inventory was put together empirically from significant items alluded to in the literature added its own bias. Yet, allowing for all this, the 'core' personality of the potentially neoplastic patient emerges.

It is a matter for argument whether the stresses experienced in the 6 months prior to the onset or relapse of malignancy are to be considered independent life events. If denial, suppression of anger and hostility lead to a neurotic distortion of the personality the possibility arises that the individual possessing these qualities may be drawn to stressful life experiences with biopsychological consequences. Similarly, it is possible that an individual is drawn to experiencing some environmental carcinogen, e.g. cigarette smoking or food or engaging in behaviour e.g. breast feeding or not so doing by virtue of his or her personality make-up. There is a determinism in the logic of this argument that may not be welcomed by everyone. Cancer, to them, may appear to be a moral problem, no mere accidental result of a vulnerable body meeting a chance carcinogen.

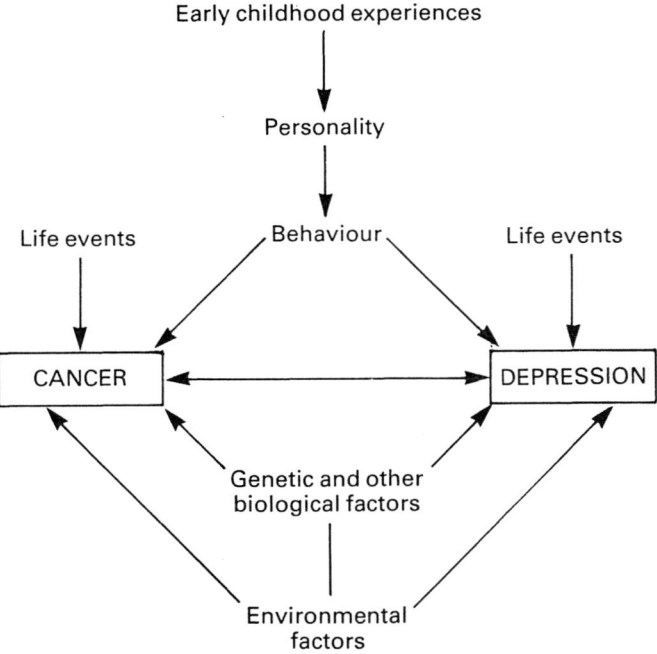

Figure 14 The mind–cancer problem

DEPRESSION AND THE COURSE OF CANCER

Interest in whether the course of a malignant disease can be influenced by psychological factors stems from the observations of clinicians that there are some patients who despite the inexorable clinical and pathological progression of the disease are able to survive. There is usually no other explanation except those that are couched in such vague terms as the 'will to live'. There are also patients whose clinical state appears to suffer a relapse from a previously apparently dormant state, following some stressful event.

Personality and emotional states may influence the course of the cancer. It has been suggested that those who are more anxious, depressed or passive are likely to have a rapidly progressing cancer (Blumberg *et al.*, 1954). Those who appear to be aggressive and hostile and exhibit a 'fighting spirit' are likely to show the most favourable outcome to their illness. With breast cancer patients, Stavraky *et al.* (1968) showed that the patients with the best prognosis had the most hostile drives, albeit with the preservation of emotional control, when subject to severe stress. The sequelae of malignancy including early death may, therefore, be associated with those who give up rather than those who fight on. Greer *et al.* (1979) showed that survival without recurrence of the malignancy in breast cancer was associated with denial.

More recent studies on a variety of cancers have produced conflicting results. On the one hand, poor prognosis has been characterized by the acceptance of one's fate and passivity; better prognosis with adjustment and more adaptive coping abilities. On the other hand, it has been found that those who have fared best have shown evidence of emotional distress and poor adjustment. It is perhaps possible to understand these conflicting reports in terms of the less than precise use of terms used in describing mental states and psychological mechanisms. What is adjustment in the face of a disease very likely to significantly shorten life? One could argue that the person who accepts his fate with stoicism and lives out the rest of his life in peace and with minimal disruption of others' lives and schedules is the better adjusted to the inevitable. The one who noisily protests against the manifest injustice to his life and work is perhaps the more natural response. Until objective methods of assessing adjustment and mental equanimity are available, one is reduced to judging inner mental state – probably the crucial influence on the neurobiological effects on malignancy – by the altogether insufficient indices of overt behavioural response.

DEPRESSION AND CANCER: MANAGEMENT

The subject of depression which arises following diagnosis of depression and in the course of anti-cancer treatment is a relatively neglected one. Relatively few patients are referred for a psychiatric assessment of even overt depression, which therefore lies untreated. The commonest cause is undeniably the attitudes of non-psychiatric doctors and nurses, and the majority of relatives, who understand too much in terms of the patient's life situation. This is curiously the obverse of the situation that obtains with bereavement reactions (see Chapter 2) where, commonly, relatively more patients are exhorted to get treated, even though physical treatment may well be less desirable in that state. As has been discussed before, the response of depression to cancer is a good one, though the therapeutic effects may be transient. Even then, a relapse may be expected to respond reasonably well to antidepressant drugs and ECT.

The features of depression and its management following the diagnosis and treatment of cancer have been reviewed by Maguire (1981). His comments apply to cancer of the breast, but the general principles remain valid for most cancers. He notes that at least 25% of those undergoing mastectomy develop depression or anxiety within 12–18 months, and a third of these require active psychiatric intervention. Guilt may be prominently associated with depression and suicidal ideas are common. Psychotic features such as delusions and hallucinations are uncommon, as is retardation. Indeed the features of depression following the diagnosis of malignancy may be remarkably similar to the depressive symptomatology due to latent malignancy discussed in an earlier section. A similar proportion of patients with ano–rectal carcinoma with a subsequent colostomy develop affective disorder.

As has been mentioned, the treatment of malignancy may lead to depression. Both irradiation and chemotherapy have been implicated. A pointer to subsequent mental symptoms with chemotherapy is the incidence of adverse effects immediately seen on commencement of anti-cancer drugs. Drugs such as cyclophosphamide, methotrexate, 5-fluorouracil and the steroids have all been known to produce depression.

As psychiatrists only see cancer patients through referral by other doctors, it is important to establish a service by which patients may be referred. The single biggest influence is the interest shown by a psychiatrist in liaison work with his medical and surgical colleagues. The psychiatrist must be accessible and referrals taken up with minimal delay. Where the patients are seen is important. Medical and surgical wards are in general grossly inadequate places for psychiatric assessment of patients and an out-patient room, or an office in the psychiatric department are far more suitable places. The patient might as well learn that depressions are dealt with by psychiatrists. Privacy is assured and the psychiatrist can get on with his work uninterrupted.

The educational task of the liaison psychiatrist is an important component of his duties. There seems little doubt that some professionals are temperamentally incapable of understanding the nature of mental disturbance. The inculcation of knowledge and exposure to training make little difference. Even personal experience of a condition such as depression seems insufficient to make some doctors and nurses appreciate the condition in their patients, especially when those patients have a primary condition of any severity. This is, very briefly, due to an inability to comprehend the 'grey' areas of life and disease. There are those who require evidence in 'black' and 'white', however unsatisfactory that evidence might be. This temperament is an authoritarian one, impatient with ambiguities and ambivalencies, which still characterize psychiatric assessment. They want 'clean' certainties, not the 'messy' uncertainties of mental function and dysfunction. However, among the ward staff treating cancer patients there are those lacking only the knowledge, and it may be satisfying and rewarding to ensure they are given some training. Nurses in particular may be valuable aides in this respect.

Some cancer patients are at greater risk of developing depression than others. Those with a past history of depression, a family history of depression, and those who are vulnerable in the sense described in Chapter 2 may fall into this category. A preventive assessment before anti-cancer treatment is undertaken in these patients may reduce the incidence of depression, or its intensity.

There are no contraindications to the use of antidepressants or ECT in any cancer patient but the physical state of the patient is obviously a more immediate consideration than in a patient who presents with uncomplicated depression.

It is surprising the number of practical social work issues that are not given thought to in medical and surgical wards. All the psychiatrist may need to do in this respect is alert the ward as to the existence of a hospital social work department.

DEPRESSION AND CANCER: THE COMMON GROUND

Table 8 Properties common to depression and cancer

Depression	Cancer
Role for antecedent life events.	Possible role for antecedent life events.
Genetic element – stronger influence in younger age group.	Genetic element – strongest influence in young.
Individuals suppress anger, hostility and have a tendency to denial.	Individuals suppress anger, hostility and have a tendency to denial.
Qualitative and quantitative change from normal function, also possibly structure.	Qualitative and quantitative change in normal structure and function.
Incidence increases with age, but peak before old age.	Incidence increases with age, peak before old age.
Sex bias towards females.	Sex bias in many individual cancers.
Natural tendency to progress and remit.	Progression, some remission.
Physical treatments effective in inducing remission.	Physical treatment effective in inducing remission.
Reduces life expectancy.	Reduces life expectancy.
Heterogeneous condition.	Heterogeneous condition.

The features common to malignant disease as well as depression include, firstly, a genetic element which is said to be strongest in the earliest years in cancer. Next, both cancer and depression are abnormal states which need to be distinguished from a wide range of possible normal activity. In one there is normal body tissue with a range of growth, degeneration, loss and regeneration. Any excess of this in both qualitative and quantitative terms is recognizable when the structure and function of the tissue in question are altered or compromised. In the other, there is a normal mood state, again defined within the limits of a wide range. Deviation from this and descent into pathological depression is both quantitative and qualitative and, as with abnormal and excessive tissue growth, is accompanied by a large number of ancillary or associated clinical features. Both conditions are found with increasing age but the peak incidence is reached before extreme old age so that ageing is an important but not necessary condition for the development of both cancer and depression. There is a definite sex bias in relation to many individual organ or tissue cancers as well as with depression. Malignant neoplasms may progress and regress as well as can depression, and in both remissions can be effected by physical treatments, and in both natural, and sometimes permanent, remission is known to take place. Both cancer and depression are known to reduce life expectancy, thus satisfying one criterion of true illness. Both are, at least in part, hormone-dependent in the broad sense. To this may be added that what we now know as depression will almost certainly turn out to be a heterogeneous collection of disorders, thus matching malignant disease in the range of pathology which may be involved in the condition, with a corresponding increase in the number of implicated structures. It seems only natural to consider the role of personality, emotion and the place of life events and stresses known to be involved in the aetiology and pathogenesis of depression and to seek a possible role for these factors in the onset, presentation and progression of malignant disease.

7
Depressed minds, dastardly acts: violence and depression

There are biological and social roots to both depression and violent behaviour. Hence it is only reasonable to suppose that any relationship between the two has to be explored in terms of both aspects, and any consideration in exclusively biological or social terms would be invalid and misleading. The study of violence is further complicated by the fact that its public manifestation is limited by legal considerations and can be studied only within the framework of existing social convention. It is of some interest that two of the more public forms of violence to pre-occupy Britain in recent years, violence associated with supporters of football teams and child abuse, both have considerable sociological interest apart from raising obvious legal points. This complexity is unfortunately not always reflected in the literature on violence, where it is sadly rare for a worker to take an overview of the problem in all its legal, psychological, social and biological aspects.

Things do not stand still. Even legal considerations change with amendments in statute, and comparison between even close time periods may be difficult, e.g. when the law relating to attempted suicide was changed. Another point as regards social factors in the study of violence is in regard to secular changes in civic life, e.g. changes in the domestic gas supply which has made it less lethal, and is generally held to have been a major factor in the recent decline in the number of suicides. Also, as will become clearer in a brief while, the act of completed suicide varies so enormously with world changes, these being outside the control of anyone involved in the study of suicide, e.g. unemployment, economic depression, war, that it is impossible to draw firm conclusions from any study over a given period of time.

Violent behaviour is clearly of multifactorial origin. The act of violence involving a person, an animal or property is obviously dependent on the situation existing at the time the violence was perpetrated. Less obvious is that the person committing or participating in an act of violence might have had a mental state influenced by, say, a disorder such as depression or agents such as alcohol or drugs; even less obvious may be the fact that it is not the formal diagnosis of illness which might have determined the violent act or its form but individual symptoms such as anxiety or a low blood sugar level due to diminished appetite. Moreover, the mental state at the time of the act might have been the end result of a process which began some time before, and could well have no direct relation to the act of violence. Underlying all this are socio-cultural factors which may determine the mode of behaviour in any given situation in an individual. Thus, a man might become depressed in ways that have been discussed in Chapter 2. Whilst depressed, he may also suffer from tension and drink heavily. Whilst under the influence, and faced by some provocation, he might have attacked someone or damaged property. It will be seen that the fact he was depressed was just one, and not perhaps even the most important, of a large number of factors associated with, and contributing to, the violent act.

BIOLOGICAL ASPECTS OF DEPRESSIVE VIOLENCE

Amongst the biological factors which may be contributory to violence, the limbic system is an important element. Its structure and function have been discussed briefly in Chapter 3 but, briefly, it may be understood more as a functional network rather than an anatomical entity with a direct relationship to emotion and behaviour. Effects are seen when the component parts are stimulated or have suffered a lesion. It is not possible when dealing with the limbic system to localize lesions in the normal way and all such attempts are merely simplistic efforts to interpret the results of effects on behaviour. The connections of the limbic system are unimaginably intricate, and it is clear that their relationship to such complex behaviours as are involved in aggression and violence will be of great complexity. A brief introductory review of the system and its workings is available in Pincus and Tucker (1978).

Human aggression and violence may be studied in some respects in relation to animal behaviour. Rage reactions in cats may follow lesions in the limbic system as well as with loss of cortical inhibition, as in decortication. In these reactions animals respond excessively and inappropriately to stimuli that do not cause rage in the intact, normal animal. This tends to occur with the decorticate animal, whose habitual personality is preserved but whose response to stimuli is abnormal. If the ventral medial nucleus of the hypothalamus is destroyed, the habitual state is turned into one of aggression. Stimulation of parts of the posterior hypothalamus, amygdala or midbrain may also cause excessive aggression, or abnormal forms of aggression. A lesion in one part of the limbic system may be counterbalanced by stimulation of the remaining intact parts. When the amygdala is removed, animals become placid although lesions of the ventral medial nucleus in such animals may make them aggressive. Lesions in the septal region may also make animals aggresive; these may be pacified by the removal of the amygdala. Thus, stimulation of one part of the limbic system makes animals, including man, aggressive; a stimulation or destruction of other parts neutralizes this aggression, and may even make the animal permanently and unnaturally peaceable.

The amygdala may have more specific effects on violence than other parts of the limbic system. It has, as has been discussed before, significant connections with the rest of the system, in particular with the thalamus, hypothalamus and cortex. It plays a regulatory role on sex and other hormones which may have a more than incidental function in determining aggressive behaviour. Bilateral removal of the amygdala reduces fear and aggression in all species, including the human (Kaada, 1972). The medial part of the amygdala is especially concerned with this behaviour. The possibility suggests itself that some forms of aggressive behaviour may be related to abnormal functioning in the amygdala and that surgical ablation of this structure might prove beneficial. On a similar line of reasoning, surgery has also been proposed on the cingulum and the hypothalamus. How exactly it might have its effects is still unknown. It is possible that the amygdala is the locus, or centre, for aggression; it may only be a conduit for nerve pathways going elsewhere in the limbic system, and these may be interrupted with surgery; its effects on the production of sex hormones, in particular testosterone, may be affected.

Some results are available, though these suffer somewhat in being produced by enthusiasts of the procedure. Heimburger *et al.* (1978), reviewing stereotactic amygdalotomized patients on up to 11 years post-operative follow-up, showed that 33% of patients with severe conduct disorders and 50% with seizures and conduct disorders were improved with surgery, whereas the unoperated controls deteriorated.

It has been suggested that the important function of the amygdala is to modulate hypothalamic activity. There may be anatomically distinct parts in the structure, some facilitating, some suppressing, the activities of the hypothalamus. In the intact animal, it is the net result of facilitatory and suppressant actions which determines the level of activity of hypothalamic function. The anterior cingulate gyrus modulates aggressive impulses from the hypothalamus, as does the septum.

The activity of the frontal lobe – the 'major, although not the only neocortical representative of the limbic system (Nauta, 1971)' – is able to exert considerable effects on the activity of the limbic mechanisms. It probably exerts its effects in two ways. Firstly, it acts in liaison with autonomic, endocrine and motor responses which are essential to homeostatic regulation. Changes in the external environment are conveyed by the frontal lobe and synthesized from the information received from the internal environment of the body. Secondly, the frontal lobe ensures that the visceral components of the emotional reaction act in concert with the motor and behavioural responses.

Lindsley (1970) has elaborated on the specific manifestations of emotion due to each level of arousal. Thus thought and anxiety reflect emotional arousal at the cortical level; weeping, sweating and visceral activity are due to autonomic arousal at the level of cortical, diencephalic and brainstem arousal; facial expression, muscle tension and tremors are manifestations of somatomotor arousal. Mechanisms of arousal are chiefly associated with

179

activity in the reticular formation of the lower brainstem, whereas the upper portions, including the ascending reticular activating systems, are identified with diencephalic and limbic systems which have a more direct involvement with emotional expression.

Eichelman *et al.* (1981) have divided aggressive behaviour in animals into attack behaviour and defensive aggressive behaviour. Attack behaviour is natural predatory behaviour, but it can also be seen following stimulation of the hypothalamus. In defensive aggressive behaviour, there is intense autonomic activity, threatening postures and cries, and can be produced in the natural state by pain, frustration, isolation or restricted space. It can also be simulated by brain lesions.

In man, focal brain lesions may be associated with features of abnormal aggression. Neoplasms of the hypothalamus, the septum pellucidum, of the limbic system, and normal pressure hydrocephalus have all been reported to give rise to abnormal aggression.

In psychological terms, suicide may be conceptualized as aggression directed against the self. Therefore, considerable interest has been evinced in findings of 5-HT deficiency in various studies of aggressive behaviour including suicide. Asberg *et al.* (1976) showed a bimodal distribution of CSF 5-HIAA among depressed patients, with those making violent suicide attempts being found in the lower mode. Since then, Brown *et al.* (1979, 1982) have shown that low 5-HIAA is correlated with suicidal behaviour in enlisted US Navy men with personality disorders and borderline states, and Goodwin and Post (1983) have referred to similar findings among schizophrenic patients. Low 5-HIAA is also correlated with a history of aggression and impulsivity in personality disorder, violent homicides, distinguishes psychopathic murders from paranoid murders and is also found in violent offenders with 47 XYY chromosomal disorder (Goodwin and Post, 1983; Bioulac *et al.*, 1980). It would seem that the relation of the aggressive behaviour is to lowered 5-HT activity rather than to any particular diagnostic category, which lends further support to the idea that 5-HT activity is a trait characteristic. Disinhibition due to diminished 5-HT activity, followed by heightened arousal and increased reaction to stimuli could be an explanation for aggressive behaviour. An indirect piece of evidence implicating diminished 5-HT activity with aggressive behaviour comes from Sheard (1975) who has also shown that lithium reduces the incidence of violence in selected groups of patients, a subject taken up later.

A much simplified conceptualization of the effects of 5-HT deficiency may be as follows. (Figure 15)

The role of 5-HT function in depression has been discussed in Chapter 3. As regards violent behaviour, interest stems from a presumed deficiency in 5-HT following studies on both the hind and forebrains of suicides, and reflected in low 5-HT and low 5-HIAA concentrations. The early view that it was a consequence or an association with depression has been modified to suggest that it might be a trait-characteristic predisposing to violence, whether of a homicidal or suicidal kind, in general.

Brown *et al.* (1979) found that human aggression and suicide were associated with lower levels of CSF 5-HIAA, a metabolite of 5-HT. That

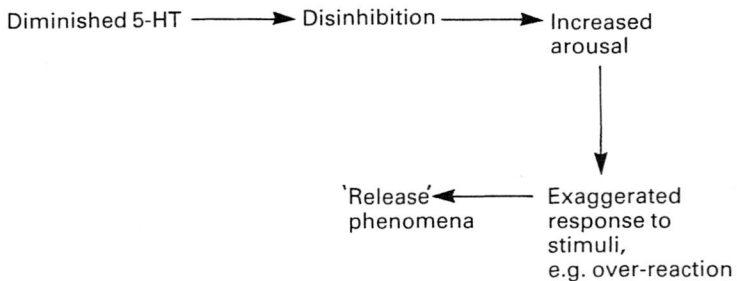

Figure 15 Speculation on effects of lowered 5-HT activity and violence

study took place in patients with personality disorders without affective illness. Brown *et al.* (1982) examined the histories of aggression and suicidal behaviour in subjects with borderline personality disorders without major affective disorder. They found a history of aggression significantly associated with suicidal attempts, and each was significantly associated with lower 5-HIAA levels.

What might be termed clinical studies on suicide have focused on depressive illness, but biochemical studies of brain 5-HT, 5-HIAA and noradrenaline have taken on board various diagnostic categories. Suicidal behaviour seems to be the end result of a process to which impulsive-aggressive traits, depression and low CSF 5-HIAA all contribute. It may be that behaviour, rather than psychiatric diagnosis, is more justifiably correlated with aberrant biochemistry. There is also some suggestion of a genetic factor in suicide (Schulsinger *et al.*, 1979). This in turn is in keeping with the view of Sedvall *et al.* (1980) that a higher concordance exists for CSF 5-HIAA levels among monozygotic twins compared with dizygotic pairs, further strengthening the genetic argument. Even among normal subjects there is three times as much chance for a subject with lower CSF 5-HIAA levels of having a family history of affective illness as in the upper mode.

However, the matter is by no means clear-cut and the complexities of the experimental and methodological problems are immense. Roy-Byrne *et al.* (1984) could find no significant difference in the 5-HIAA levels between those who had and had not attempted suicide, and found 5-HIAA was unrelated to the severity of the attempt.

Traskman *et al.* (1981) have suggested that a low 5-HIAA level may not be associated with psychiatric illness as such, but with an increased vulnerability, possibly genetically determined, to a range of psychiatric disturbance and to suicidal behaviour.

Brown *et al.* (1979) examined the major central metabolites of 5-HT, noradrenaline and dopamine – 5-HIAA, 3-methoxy-4-hydroxyphenyl glycol (MHPG) and homovanillic acid (HVA), respectively – in the CSF of men with a variety of aggressive, violent and impulsive behaviours. They found that there was a significant negative correlation between the history of aggressive behaviour and CSF 5-HIAA, and a significant positive correlation between aggressive behaviour and CSF MHPG. This is in keeping with the hypothesis that in animals aggression is related to 5-HT and catecholamine balance, i.e. decreased 5-HT and/or increased noradrenaline and dopamine levels, rather than simply to the functional level of either system independently. As they note, different animal models of aggression may be related to specific neurotransmitter alterations. Thus muricidal behaviour may be associated with decreased 5-HT metabolism; spontaneous aggression can be induced by stimulation of dopaminergic terminals; stress-facilitated or shock-induced aggression appears to be related to the noradrenergic system.

These authors also suggest that the level of central 5-HT and noradrenergic function in a given individual might contribute to a subject's characteristic level of impulse control and aggressiveness, with the clinical diagnosis being merely an incidental factor. If depression occurred in an individual who had an imbalance of 5-HT and noradrenaline, the combination of depression and predisposition toward increased aggression with lowered impulse control might lead to a higher risk of suicide.

Noradrenergic stimulation may lead to an increase in some forms of aggression (Eichelman, 1977); however, it appears to diminish predatory attack. On the other hand, blockade of 5-HT transmission provokes predatory aggression but prevents some other types of aggression (Malick and Barnett, 1976).

The role of sex hormones is a valid consideration in studies of aggression. There is a correlation between hostility (as reported by the patient) and testosterone levels and a significant relationship between depression and plasma testosterone (Doering et al., 1974). This is a more direct link between a hormone associated with aggression and depression, and understandable in terms of the widespread hormonal disturbance in depression.

An indirect study of depressive aggression and violence comes from the known effects of some of the anti-aggressive properties of antidepressant drugs. The effect most commonly studied in the laboratory is muricidal behaviour, i.e. the spontaneous, predatory, mouse-killing behaviour in rats which happens whether man wants it or not. Several workers, including Goldberg and Horovitz (1978) have shown that drugs such as amitriptyline and imipramine reduced the muricidal tendencies of rats. Neuroleptics and other tranquillizers can do this, too, but only at the cost of impairing motor activity, i.e. the pacifying effects may well be secondary to the sedation, whereas antidepressants may have a specific, sedative action. There is no precise explanation for this effect, but it has been suggested that an increase in availability of noradrenaline at receptor sites may inhibit muricidal activity, the rationale for which is that when noradrenaline is applied directly to parts of the amygdala, muricidal behaviour is inhibited (Leaf et al., 1969). However, as was shown in Chapter 5, the primary effect of antidepressants is not by re-uptake blockade; similarly the re-uptake blockade does not appear to be closely related to antimuricidal effects. The primary antimuricidal effect, like the primary antidepressant effect, may lie in more direct receptor sensitivity change. It is also possible that 5-HT

182

activity, as illustrated by the potency of clomipramine, may enhance inhibition of muricidal behaviour; or, as has been suggested by Goldberg and Horovitz (1978), the anticholinergic effects of antidepressants may be responsible.

However, all antidepressants in common clinical use are able to inhibit muricidal behaviour which, taken in addition to the seemingly common modes of action on depression and muricidal behaviour, leads one to wonder if there are common sites of origin for depression and aggression in the limbic system, perhaps in the amygdala. An interesting series of experiments (Horovitz, 1967) seems to provide some evidence. Destruction of the amygdala and injection of imipramine, but not chlorpromazine, into the structure inhibits muricidal activity, whereas injecting other parts of the system does not produce this effect. However, the relationship between antimuricidal action and antidepressant action is not a simple one. Antimuricidal actions are of rapid onset, while the antidepressant actions are well known to require a period of at least a week or two to appear. Also, while predatory aggression may be inhibited, other forms of aggression may not be affected, or may indeed be facilitated, as case reports of antidepressant-associated increase in violence testify. This is further evidence for the heterogeneous nature of violent behaviour. Paradoxical rage reactions have been noted with several antidepressants, including imipramine and amitriptyline (Rampling, 1978).

The drugs used on depressed patients have a variable effect on aggression. Bond and Lader (1984) have reviewed the literature on the subject. These drugs include the benzodiazepines, still all too commonly used in the symptomatic treatment of anxiety in depression. Whether they can provoke aggression, as has been widely suspected, is not clear. Caution is enjoined in their use with patients with a previous history of aggression or a history of poor impulse control. Much of the evidence for the aggression-inducing effects of benzodiazepines appears to have come from case reports which feature an above therapeutic dose of the benzodiazepine which may well lead to personality change and consequent episodes of aggression. Their use is especially dangerous in prison populations, especially where abuse of one drug is allied to a high incidence of poor impulse control and history of violence. Barbiturates have a similar effect with chronic abuse. The role of alcohol in violence is a complex one, as is well known. The relationship between alcohol abuse and depression has been touched on in Chapter 2. There is no doubt alcohol is an inhibiting agent, but other variables such as alcohol-related brain damage, the associated symptoms and the socio-cultural context may be as, if not more, important as the pharmacological properties of alcohol itself.

In the recovery phase of depression, the 'aggression' that was turned inwards during depression, may be revealed when it is projected outwards, a measure of the efficacy of the antidepressant treatment rather than a specific adverse effect.

The role of lithium in the treatment of aggression has been increasingly studied in the past 10 years. This effect appears to be non-specific in that a wide range of psychiatric disorders and other conditions with no formal psychiatric diagnosis respond to its anti-aggressive properties. Sheard *et al.* (1976) reported a controlled study in male inmates in prison. The men had histories of impulsive, aggressive and anti-social behaviour and had been convicted of violent crimes. Lithium brought about an improvement in their behaviour in prison. The mode of action is uncertain, although an explanation in terms of 5-HT inhibition has been suggested (Sheard, 1975). These were non-depressive cases, although it was suggested that atypical depression with aggression may find itself more commonly in prison.

HOMICIDE AND EXTERNALIZED VIOLENCE

Depressive homicide is considered rare. Only a very small proportion of men awaiting trial for homicide are diagnosed as depressed (Taylor and Gunn, 1984). This is partly because a substantial proportion of those who kill others subsequently kill themselves (West, 1965). In Great Britain, a quarter of homicides are followed by suicide, whereas in the United States the figure is less than 10% (Guze, 1976). As homicide is a relatively uncommon crime, study of convicted criminals or those awaiting trial for indictable offences is not likely to yield many depressive homicides. However, depression plays a more important role in homicide in Britain. Before more profound hypotheses of causation are sought, it is important to remind ourselves of the means of homicide. Where firearms are available freely, say, the death rate is higher and the proportion due to the availability of the firearms is higher, too. Diagnostic practices are crucial influences on statistics in psychiatry, and it will be interesting to find out if the increase in the diagnosis of affective illness is reflected in the number of depression-related violent crimes in the future.

Psychiatric illness is generally weakly represented in the statistics of serious crime. Guze (1976) showed that conditions such as psychopathy, alcoholism and drug dependence – mental disorder rather than illness – were more likely to be associated with serious crime than schizophrenia or primary affective disorder which occurred in about 2% of convicted criminals in his series.

However, even if the numbers are small there are interesting points raised by those who engage in depressive homicide. As has been shown by Hafner and Boker (1973), depressed women perpetrate more homicidal violence than do men. Whereas the figures for schizophrenias in those who had committed homicide were comparable (about 7% of both men and women), the incidence of depressive homicide was 12 times greater in women. For men, Taylor and Gunn (1984) estimate that of the homicidal violence committed in Europe, 5–10% of violence by men is accounted for by schizophrenia, but only 0.5–1% by depression.

It is not clear why the proportion of women who commit homicide should be high. There is obviously no connection with violence by psychiatrically normal persons, where women, as is well known, are considerably under-represented. One explanation may well be there is a disinhibiting factor, facilitating killing by depressed females. Another possible explanation, already referred to in relation to the social aspects of the development of depression in Chapter 2, is that the social and environmental antecedents of vulnerability may also facilitate their killing. Certainly, there is no light thrown by the symptomatology of depression which remains broadly similar in the two sexes. If there are biological factors involved, they appear to be playing a rather selective role as facilitators of homicide than suicide, where women are again under-represented. The difference between homicide and suicide is not as between two different behaviours, but in the direction of the behaviour. It used to be held that an inverse relationship existed between homicide and suicide, and it is possible that in the limited case of depression in women, this may hold true. A further suggestion is based on socio-cultural considerations, and is related to the explanation that depression may be a disinhibiting factor. It may well be that in the normal mood state and under the constraints of social and cultural pressure, women have contained within themselves anger, irritation, hostility and aggression and these are then released by depression. Why this should prefer homicide as a vehicle and not suicide deserves explanation. In the same context, the disinhibiting role of alcohol and such drugs as the benzodiazepines and, in an earlier age, barbiturates must be mentioned. As was discussed in the previous section, it is as well to bear in mind a possible iatrogenic factor.

It is well known that homicide is more likely to be committed when there is a close relationship between perpetrator and victim. It has been shown (Hafner and Boker, 1973) that this relationship holds good when the offender is mentally disordered.

A study of depressive violence including homicide must take into account the depressed patient's previous personality and his propensity to violence. In their premorbid state there is often little evidence of unnatural aggression; in fact, those who are prone to depression may show less than natural aggression. In the division of individuals into over-controlled and under-controlled persons, most of those who are predisposed to depression belong to the former category. The latter have few inhibitions against violence, being provoked by environmental stimuli the average individual would consider trivial, and often lead assaultive, if not dangerous, careers. Most habitual street and bar-room brawlers come under this category. In contrast, the over-controlled person has habitually formidable inhibitions against violence, but it appears that if the provocation is sufficient to overcome these inhibitions, especially if the threshold has been lowered by emotional disturbance, the rush of pent-up forces may lead to a great deal of destructive behaviour including homicide.

As has already been mentioned, the symptoms of the depressive syndrome, such as anxiety and tension, may be implicated in violent behaviour. The symptom of irritability is also well known as featuring in the mental state of a large number of conditions, including depression, mania and schizophrenia, and is associated with physical and verbal outbursts. Recently, Snaith and Taylor (1985) made a convincing case for outwardly expressed irritability being an independent mood disorder, and one not merely symptomatic of other psychiatric states.

185

RELATIONSHIP BETWEEN HOMICIDE AND SUICIDE

This has been briefly alluded to before. Whether a true relationship exists between homicide and suicide is still uncertain. It is certainly true the inverse relationship that has been proposed in the past has many, too many exceptions, for it to be valid. An earlier view was that homicide was suicide turned outwards, perhaps as a 'projected' suicide or an 'acting-out' suicide. Occasionally, it was suggested, an individual contemplating suicide provoked the homicide in another, and thereby resulted a homicide, rather than suicide, statistic (Wolfgang, 1968). The close relationship between victim and perpetrator and the substantial incidence of victim participation in such crimes may be additional evidence that these offences are not simply due to chance. The idea goes back at least to Freud (1917) who noted that all suicidal impulses had been murderous impulses first. West (1965) showed that there was a high incidence of suicide following homicide in countries such as the United Kingdom and Denmark. Further evidence comes from the study of suicide notes which confirm that one of the principal motives in taking one's life is aggression against others (Capstick, 1960). Suicide is, then, internalized aggression whereas homicide is externalized aggression. The 'clinical' features may be common to both conditions, but some epidemiological and personality factors may differ, as was discussed in regard to the relatively high incidence of homicide in depressed women. One may also mention here the biological substrate, far from clear at the time of writing, that may underlie depressive violence, also discussed in the previous section. It becomes quite clear that the issue of the relationship between homicide and suicide is more complex than a mere consideration of suicide and homicide statistics.

Myers and Neal (1978) also found an association between suicide and non-psychotic violence in patients diagnosed as being depressed. They put forward the hypothesis that violence could have been present in previous, undiagnosed bouts of depression. They believed that those who are violent during a depressive illness are particularly prone to harming themselves. Other factors which were associated with violence and which might have contributed to suicide in depressed patients was the previous loss of relationships and alcohol abuse. Alcohol, of course, is associated with both violence and suicide. It was also suggested that the violence that is predictive of future suicide is also predictive of future violence.

West (1965) found that 15 of his homicidal offenders had had preoccupations with suicide in the week of their offence, in some it being considered an option only a few hours before. In a sense, the aggression appears to have been displaced from inside to outside. A third of murders in his study were followed by suicide. These cases of pathological homicide were to be distinguished from uncomplicated homicide in that fewer individuals had previous criminal convictions and more had a past history of suicidal attempts.

Some attempts to explain the relationship between homicide and suicide have taken on board the notion of aggression that may be turned inward or outward, but they have gone further in suggesting the influence of macroeconomic forces (Henry and Short, 1964). It was suggested that economic cycles undergo expansion and depression, peaks and troughs, which may affect the hierarchical position of individuals in their groups in society. A decline in status may cause frustration which leads to aggression which may be directed inwards or outwards. But this fails to account for the individual nature of these acts, and also their lack of cultural specificity. Economic expansion and depression are universal phenomena, yet some societies are persistently violent, and the patterns of homicide and suicide may differ in them.

Pokorny (1965, quoted by Stengel) studied four forms of violence – suicide, attempted suicide, homicide and serious assault – and their incidence in relation to behaviour and socio–demographic indices. The only common feature, on superficial examination, between suicide and homicide was that they were more commonly to be found in men. Suicide and attempted suicide were found to be domestic phenomena, whereas homicide and assault took place elsewhere. Suicide is a behaviour of middle life and beyond, reaching a peak after the age of 50; homicide is an activity of the 20s. Suicide occurs in relation to self, and since there is a deliberate desire to die, it will most usually be in the home. Homicide and assault require a victim and the offence will take place where he is to be found. One is not concerned here with what may be termed 'criminal' or acquisitive violence, but rather with more interpersonal matters in relation to mental disorder. Superficial contrasts may well conceal deeper similarities. The fact that environmentally-induced chronic respiratory problems are considerably more commonly found among the poor, in association with poor housing and in inner city areas is not incompatible with these conditions having a physical basis.

The relationship between homicide and suicide may finally be considered in the light of what is revealed by suicide pacts (Stengel, 1975). Contrary to popular belief, it is not young lovers stymied by events or heartless, uncomprehending parents who die in tandem but married couples who die together. They are physically seriously ill and often childless. In the typical case, a depressed individual may persuade the spouse to join in. There is occasionally evidence of homicidal impulses on the part of the person initiating the suicide, and it is the possibility of this outcome that has led to the retention of legal sanctions in the case of a suicide pact. But the phenomenon of double suicide is by no means common, accounting for less than 1% of all suicides. The well-publicized suicide pact involving an eminent writer and thinker and his wife some years ago led to some claims that as he had been the dominating influence in life, it was likely that he had also dominated the move into death.

SUICIDE

For reasons outlined in an earlier section epidemiology of any form of violence is fraught with difficulty. This applies to suicide as well. Suicide is associated with a large number of social, economic, cultural and environmental factors, some of which will be discussed in due course.

Economic prosperity or decline has been suspected as being a factor for a quite considerable time. Comparing the mortality figures for 20 countries between a period of prosperity in the early 1920s with a period of depression in the early 1930s, Sainsbury (1975) showed there was a dramatic increase in most of them in the latter period. Not merely that but the increase in the rate was most clearly seen among the middle-aged and the elderly, those for whom there was little prospect of work. This is a telling statistic, but does not reveal the presence of an intervening variable that may be common to both unemployment and suicide. Shepherd and Barraclough (1980) inquired into this and showed that suicides had had a high level of occupational loss, were unstable in their work performance and had been in high-risk occupations. Overall, their data seemed to lend support to Durkheim's view that belonging to a work force conferred protection against suicide. The importance of their study, which was conducted on the records of suicides between 1967 and 1969, a period of high employment and prosperity in the south of England is that factors relating to work other than purely socio–economic ones may help account for suicide. There are crucial personal factors, too, as clinicians have long suspected. In time the suicide data for the 1980s, a period of unremittingly high unemployment, will come to be studied. A simple correlation will no doubt be demonstrated to exist between a rising suicide rate and the loss of employment. A somewhat simplistic explanation will, no doubt, be offered, and countered by those of a different ideological persuasion. It is important to keep in mind the notion that it is not merely the lack of work, but the inability to work in a society where a man's (or woman's) ability to work and enjoy the fruits of that work are counted important. Durkheim's thesis was propounded in advance of the economic climate that showed cyclical changes. Considerable concern must, therefore, be expressed as to the lack of education or training that may make substantial numbers of a younger generation unfit for work. Employment and prosperity may return, but a large proportion of a generation may continue to be alienated by not being able to avail themselves of the work on offer.

After some years of decline, the suicide rate in England and Wales has shown an annual increase in the period from 1975 to 1980, and will probably continue to do so. In 1975, Adelstein and Mardon (quoted by McClure, 1984) showed there had been a peak in the incidence of suicide for England and Wales in 1963 and then a decline continuing into the early 1970s. This decrease was largely as a result of a lower number of suicides in the 'traditional', older age groups, whereas the under 35 rate remained unchanged. The decline in the suicide rate is generally acknowledged to be due to the changes in methods used and the diminished lethality of previously commonly used agents, in particular domestic gas which had become detoxified in the period under consideration. There appears to be a correlation between the availability of toxic domestic gas and the suicide rate (Low et al., 1981). This reduced lethality of the domestic gas has been paralleled by the diminished risk of some commonly prescribed drugs. Barbiturates have given way to benzodiazepines as anxiolytic sedatives and hypnotics, and despite their widespread prescription, use, abuse and their role as agents of overdose, they have the merit of having minimal risk to life.

The increase in the suicide rate in the period from 1975 to 1980 has been noted in both sexes, but was greater for men. The decrease in poisoning with drugs and other chemicals has been more than made up by the use of poisoning in the form of vehicle exhaust gas, which contains the lethal agent carbon monoxide. Before a claim is made for the suicidal human being's compulsive desire for carbon monoxide in some form, car exhaust gas if not the gas in the oven, a more prosaic explanation may be proffered – the greater availability of cars. The rise in violent methods such as hanging, strangulation and suffocation is worthy of comment. It was discussed in a previous section of this chapter that violent suicide may reflect certain biological features which may be a trait characteristic, i.e. part of the personality rather than a feature of illness. It is extremely unlikely that such trait characteristics can substantially increase in the infinitesimally (in terms of genetics) small period of time in which methods of suicide by violent means have increased. An alternative explanation, assuming the validity of the biological argument in at least a proportion of cases, is that such factors might have been brought into play by some selective, socio-cultural events. What these might be are almost entirely unknown (one might argue that society has grown more competitive, and the aggressive have come forward). But the anxiety that has been expressed as to the nature and form of violence in general in society, and the role such influences as television, newspapers and films may play as well as the impact they may have on susceptible individuals may be worthy of consideration in this debate.

The rate itself is related to social and demographic change. The role of women has changed, unemployment began rising in the early years of this decade, divorce rates have risen, and MacClure (1984) notes an increase in consumption of alcohol.

The seasonal variation in suicide has long aroused interest. Originally, it was suggested that most suicides occurred in autumn, when the dull weather precipitated a melancholic mood. Nayha (1982) relates this to the climate theory of Montesquieu as presented in his book *De L'esprit des Lois* in 1748. This view held till well into the middle of the last century, and it is claimed that when Esquirol showed, in 1820, that hospital admissions for melancholia and suicidal attempts had a summer peak, he was aware of the paradox. Durkheim, in his turn, suggested that the increased daylight produced an increasing intensity in social life and that those who were not able to cope killed themselves. Changing times have brought developments – increased mobility, round the clock heating and light – which have made social contact possible irrespective of the season and the state of the weather. The most intense social contact nowadays is arguably over Christmas, yet even if there is evidence of increased distress and, perhaps, even relapse in conditions such as schizophrenia, there is no evidence for an increase in suicide. In fact, the contrary is reported. Apart from biological factors (e.g. seasonal variation due to intensity of light, see Chapter 3), such factors as seasonal variation in employment are probably still more important.

189

Swinscow (1951) found a peak for suicide in the spring and summer months for England and Wales, with a corresponding peak for the spring and summer in the southern hemisphere, in Australia. Parker and Walter (1982) studied the seasonal variation in depression and suicide in New South Wales, Australia and found that peak incidence of depression was in the spring months. There was a significant associated female incidence of suicide in the spring, as in the northern hemisphere. They suggested that a rapid increase of light in spring stimulates the pineal gland in such a way as to produce or increase vulnerability to certain affective disorders (see also discussion on seasonal affective disorder in Chapter 3). There was indeed a rapid increase in luminosity at the onset of spring, with a corresponding increase in the re-admission of those with depression and with the peak incidence of female suicides. Nayha (1982), studying the seasonal variation in suicides in Finland, suggested there might be two peaks: a 'natural' seasonal peak, which is probably universal, occurring in spring and summer, while there might be an autumnal peak which might characterize those living in urban, man-made environments.

Suicides can occur in secure institutions. Stengel (1975) noted how in the period between 1920 and 1947, the rates for suicide in mental hospitals in England and Wales was about 4–5 times that for the general population while Copas and Robin (1982) showed that the relationship between hospital and general population suicides had not changed for 50 years. For psychiatric hospital in-patients, suicide risks are highest in males, in the first week of admission and for depressed patients. The tendency to suicide of violent offenders is also underlined by the figures produced by Topp (1979), who found the suicide rate in male prisoners was some three times that of the general population, with the highest rates among those who had received a life sentence. Here again there was another variable. The expectation of a sentence greater than that of 18 months' duration was associated with a higher risk of suicide, and thus it is not possible to attribute the suicide solely to the violent propensity of the men. Only a small proportion of suicides had been thought to be at risk, which shows that even in an institution with a captive population, close supervision of individuals and a ready access to medical staff, it is not always possible to prevent suicide.

In a rural study, Myers and Neal (1978) noted that suicides had behaved violently in the past, experienced a broken marriage or had previously deliberately harmed themselves, often by violent means. There are few clinical pointers to suicide, and these will be considered in a later section. However, it is of interest to consider whether suicide, and other violent behaviour is a feature *per se* of depression as the outward manifestation of a neurobiological change or whether it may be related to depressed mood which, as was shown in Chapter 4, is a universal feature in psychiatry and is pervasively found in neurology. Schizophrenia is a case in point. Suicide is a not uncommon feature of schizophrenic illness. Markowe *et al.* (1967) suggested that schizophrenics were 50 times as likely to kill themselves as a member of the general public. Depression is a not uncommon feature of schizophrenia. However, depression does not appear to have been directly

190

implicated in suicides who have killed themselves (Barraclough *et al.*, 1974; Falloon and Talbot, 1981; Wilkinson, 1982). Schizophrenic suicides, on the other hand, appear to be young, single patients who have had a chronic illness, have been irritable, had previous multiple suicidal attempts, have had a relapse or persistence of hallucinations and delusions, and suicide has occurred early in the course of treatment.

Durkheim (1897, 1970), to whose work several references have been made, presented a sociological view of suicide, and distinguished between three groups of suicide on the basis of the relationship between the individual and society.

(1) *Egoistic suicide* – this occurs when a person becomes too individualistic, cuts himself off from society and its protection which lead to his 'selfish' suicide.

(2) *Altruistic suicide* – a person gives up his life for the sake of society, which might be represented symbolically as the officers with whom their men die during battle, or as in the case of Japanese officers who committed *hara kiri*, or wives who leapt into their husbands' funeral pyres, or the elderly and the sick who wish to relieve society of their burden by this 'selfless' suicide.

(3) *Anomic suicide* – if the regulatory functions of society in terms of political, religious and social codes are weakened, the ensuing permissiveness or moral anarchy could facilitate a form of 'stateless' suicide, with the power of the state (broadly interpreted) withering away.

Durkheim's views may be studied in relation to suicide among immigrants and in the medical profession. Transcultural aspects of depression are taken up in Chapter 8, but it may be stated here that, as expected, rates for suicide are also high. A high incidence of suicide among Polish immigrants was noted by Myers and Neal (1978), whereas the rates in Poland itself were considerably lower, especially for women. They have speculated upon the reasons and suggested that isolation may be a major factor. Political upheaval in Poland rather than systematic immigration has led to these migrants being in Britain with a higher ratio of men to women and also with a larger number of divorced men. There are difficulties with language (see also Chapter 8), and there is a large enough community to sustain itself but not so large that culturally normative forces can operate. There is, the authors argue, an estrangement from society that Durkheim regarded as a potent factor in suicide.

All the evidence points to an increased risk of suicide in certain professional groups, most notably doctors. There is also an increase in both alcohol-related and drug-related problems in the medical profession. The reasons commonly given are that doctors have both an awareness of disease as well as the agents (and access to them) that help kill them. This is undeniably true, but it has to be shown that doctors choose agents which are different to that by which the ordinary public kills itself, more particularly by using chemicals that are toxic. More recently, the explanations have also taken into account the stresses doctors face in their occupation, though why this should be greater than the stresses faced by, say, police officers and social workers in modern society is not clear. The fact is that doctors, by nature of their training and practice, are often socially isolated. The work is demanding, often exhausting, in the earliest years of practice when work habits are first laid down. Advancement in a career depends on dedication on the part of the doctor; the more dedicated he is, the more isolated he will find himself from the real world. This is also connected to the problems of high rates of marital breakdown. There must be considerable truth in the view that the life style of doctors plays an important part in their eventual suicides, which are of the egoistic type in Durkheim's terminology, or a result of personal 'anomie'.

Even among doctors it is alleged there is a hierarchy of risk. Psychiatrists come out on top, at least when the older data or anecdotes are taken into account. As has been argued, it may not be the nature of the calling but some factor in the make-up of those doctors who answered the call. These may not necessarily apply now when doctors often make psychiatry their first choice of speciality. The number of failed physicians and surgeons turning to psychiatry has dwindled. Those who choose to make it their career have experienced life in a variety of training schemes that are on offer. Better training, as opposed to the gathering of experience by default, can be said to have improved knowledge and given more relevant experience. It cannot be said that the life of a psychiatrist is any longer more stressful than that of a doctor in any other speciality. Indeed, when one considers the poor prospects for promotion in some specialities, one might argue that more stress was being experienced elsewhere. Furthermore, a more 'normal' doctor, given access to some aspects of the world which exist outside medicine, which is the case with psychiatric training has, at least in theory, a better understanding of those aspects of his life which are necessary for fulfilment in life. The hypothesis would be that suicides among psychiatrists, if they really were increased in the past, must become no higher than in any other branch of medicine, and if the incidence has fallen, some of these explanations may serve.

Deliberate self-harm

Not every patient who attempts to kill or harm himself is depressed, and not every depressed patient thinks or acts in a manner likely to harm himself.

The epidemic of deliberate self-harm that began in the West in the 1960s will be briefly referred to as a culturally-influenced mental disorder in Chapter 8. Every year over 100 000 cases of self-harm are admitted to hospital in the United Kingdom.

The nomenclature on the subject is somewhat confusing. 'Attempted suicide' would imply that there was intention to take life which was thwarted for accidental reasons. This is clearly not the case in a large number of cases of self-harm, which also differ in clinical, social and epidemiological respects from successfully completed suicide. The terms 'parasuicide' or 'deliberate self-harm' are largely descriptive terms, which include both self-poisoning and self-injury, and, therefore, are preferred for this reason.

Women have always outnumbered men in this behaviour, although the proportion of men has increased more recently. Women outnumber men by a factor of 2:1. It is thus a behaviour different in sex ratio to suicide. It is the middle-aged and the elderly who successfully kill themselves; whereas self-harm is a problem of the adolescent and the young adult. As a further contrast to successful suicide, deliberate self-harm is found in socially deprived inner cities among the poorer classes, though the single, the separated and the divorced are still more prone to deliberate self-harm. A considerable number among those who harm themselves in this way are in the process of informal or legal separation from their partners, and it is the process of being made single that features in this group of patients. Suicides, on the other hand, have been single in most instances. As might be expected with a younger age group, there are more immediate difficulties and disruptions in the family background. Financial problems and the cessation of employment, or the imminence of it, are given as reasons for the act. This is, as one might expect, more common in inner city areas. Alcohol appears to be a major factor in either preceding the act or being used in combination with the agent employed in the act of self-harm. Surprisingly, for a young age group, there is a considerable incidence of concurrent physical illness, some of it of a serious nature, which themselves are the subject of current medical attendance.

An important clinical distinction between deliberate self-harm and suicide is that in only a minority of cases of the former is formal mental disorder found. The vast majority of acts take place in relation, or as a reaction, to the kind of social difficulties which have been noted before. Even when there is mental disorder, alcohol- and drug-related problems with an underlying personality disorder are considerably more commonly found than more formal psychiatric illness, though it is moot as to whether a diagnosis of personality disorder should be made in someone whose immature personality may well be due to incomplete development. A persistent depression preceding the act cannot be said to account for more than 5% of cases.

Being a reaction to chronic social difficulties and as an impulsive act, even when the problems giving rise to it might have been chronic, the decision to harm oneself deliberately appears to be a sudden one. Indeed the question of premeditation does not arise, and this is the reason why drugs or agents at hand are used in the attempt. Premeditation would have led to the purchase or accumulation of more lethal agents. The fact that coal gas is now detoxified, and is generally known to be non-lethal, may account for the fact that it is so rarely used in self-harm attempts. A high proportion of attempts are made under the influence of alcohol and/or other drugs, circumstances in which the judgement is clouded and any remaining inhibitions removed. On questioning, a substantial proportion of cases admit they had wished to die, and although this is a retrospective response, there is usually no reason to disbelieve the claim. The fact that some common household drugs, with various serious consequences in overdose

193

e.g. aspirin, paracetamol are common agents of known lethality must make one suspect that spur of the moment though the decision might have been, the result could easily have been fatal. In this behaviour, the correlation between premeditation, agent employed and death is a very small one, and only chance seems to have stood in the way of another suicide statistic.

As the numbers of those doing deliberate harm to themselves are great, the yield of formal mental disorder being small, and resources limited, the patients are not usually subjected to extensive psychiatric follow-up. This raises some anxiety in relatives, in GPs, in other services, and not least in the psychiatrist. There is foundation for this anxiety as, previous behaviour being the best predictor of future behaviour, a proportion of patients can be expected to repeat the act. It has been estimated that 20% will repeat the attempt within a year; the risk being greatest in the first 3 months after the act; 1% will die by suicide by the end of 1 year and 3% would have killed themselves within 3 years. The risk of suicide in someone who has attempted it before is calculated as being 100 times greater than that of the general population, and 50% of suicides, when their records are studied, give a history of a previous attempt. It is thus important to be able to make a reasoned prediction as to who might be most at risk from graduating from deliberate self-harm to successful suicide.

Buglass and Horton (1974) have suggested features that are predictive of further attempts which need not necessarily be suicidal. Previous behaviour is the single most important factor. Others include alcohol- or drug-related problems, personality disorder, previous history of psychiatric treatment, living by oneself, a criminal record, unemployment and lower social class. It is readily seen that it is personality and its consequences added to a variety of indices of deprivation that might have led to the reasons for the initial attempt persisting thereby preparing the ground for another attempt.

As has been already observed, there are important clinical, social, demographic and epidemiological differences between deliberate self-harm and suicide. It may be reasonable to expect those cases of deliberate self harm who correspond most closely to those who successfully complete suicide to be most at risk. Pallis *et al.* (1982, 1984) tested this hypothesis by using risk scales of clinical and socio–demographic factors, and found that they could predict suicides on follow-up with these indices. Their findings demonstrated that the closer a suicide attempter resembles a suicide in personal and clinical characteristics as well as in the manner of carrying out his suicidal act, the higher the risk for a further and fatal suicide attempt. Beck *et al.* (1974) have noted that leaving a suicide note, admitting to suicidal intent, secretive preparations such as collecting and hoarding tablets, making a will or organizing insurance, concealing intent from potential helpers, extensive premeditation and the circumstances in which the act was carried out, i.e. in isolation, with steps taken to avoid discovery and intervention, all point to seriousness of intent and lead one to suspect the patient survived by chance, and not design. The other factors that make one anxious about a patient are atypical features in a case of deliberate self-harm. If the patient is male, middle-aged and has made a previous attempt by violent means, one is justifiably anxious. A single (separated, widowed, divorced) state, unemployment, physical illness or mental disorder (depression as well as personality disorder with alcohol- and drug-related problems) raise the index of suspicion. Briefly, the more like a suicide a case of self-harm is, the greater the likelihood of successful suicide in the future. The numbers of deliberate self-harm patients who fit this description are relatively small, and psychiatric resources could be profitably deployed in their active follow-up.

Deliberate self-harm patients are available for questioning, which makes them different in that respect, too, to patients who have killed themselves. James and Hawton (1985) found there were marked differences between the reasons chosen to explain overdoses by the relatives and friends of patients who had poisoned themselves, and the reasons chosen by the patients themselves. Vastly more of the patients claimed they wished to die than those who believed them. Relatives and friends were wont to believe there was manipulation involved in acts of self-harm which was directed against others, but both patients and informants agreed that the act alleviated distress, and it was felt that sympathy as well as guilt and anger had been evoked in significant others.

At least a third of patients claim they had wished to die. Others claim a need to escape, or gain relief, from a difficult situation. However, they deny they have been communicating in any way or manipulating others. James and Hawton suggest there are at least three clinical implications from these findings. The first is to bear in mind that different interpretations may be obtained from the patients and the informants at assessment. While there is sympathy shown to patients by relatives and friends, there is also guilt and anger, and the clinician may make more headway in eliciting the former by letting individuals ventilate the latter. Thirdly, the clinician could focus on the need for communication as being the reason for the act and thereby focus on any faulty communication that might have been present. Any improvement in communication may well reduce the likelihood of a repetition of the behaviour.

To be considered in the same context as adolescent self-harm is the question of childhood suicide and self-harm which are further taken up in Chapter 8. Before the age of 16, suicidal behaviour is uncommon, and below the age of 12, rare. However, some 7–10% of referrals in childhood and early adolescence are for threatened or attempted suicide (Shaffer, 1974). In young suicides, 70% are male and the male to female ratio is 2:1 (Anderson, 1981; McClure, 1984). On the other hand, 80–90% of young parasuicides are female (Anderson, 1981). Suicide is involved with 'getting into trouble' (see Chapter 8), but deliberate self-harm is associated with getting back at others, trying to get others to change their behaviour, gaining relief from stress, but is rarely to get help (Hawton, 1982). Hawton also found that only a minority of young patients who had deliberately harmed themselves had formal psychiatric illness. The figure has been put at 20% (Lumsden Walker, 1980). Depression is more likely to be found in male youngsters. Self-injury has been associated with depressive disorder in children (Taylor and Stansfeld, 1984). Hawton (1982) found greater evidence of disturbed

195

behaviour in those who repeated the act, and Shaffer (1974) put a figure of 50% of childhood suicides who had had emotional or behavioural problems.

Assessment of suicidal risk

Factors that put a patient at risk of suicide have been referred to at several points in the foregoing discusssion. For completeness, the following points made by Stengel (1975) with regard to the assessment of suicidal risk in a depressed patient may be noted. The features include:

(1) Depression with guilt feelings, self-depreciation and self-accusation associated with tension and agitation;
(2) Severe hypochondriasis;
(3) Insomnia with pre-occupation with sleeplessness;
(4) Fear of loss of control, or of hurting self and others;
(5) Previous suicidal attempts;
(6) Suicidal pre-occupations including communication of this to others;
(7) Social isolation, which can be the result of lack of sympathy in others;
(8) History of suicides in the family;
(9) History of a broken home before the age of 15;
(10) Serious physical illness, especially if it is incurable and associated with severe pain;
(11) Alcohol and drug-related problems;
(12) The recovery phase of depressive illness when psychomotor retardation or agitation may be ameliorated so that the patient is provided with the physical means of killing himself;
(13) Dreams of catastrophes, falls and self-destruction – dreams might have been suppressed by hypnotics and tricyclic antidepressants only to re-emerge when treatment is discontinued; and
(14) Unemployment and financial difficulties.

Stengel lists the following as being positively correlated with suicide rates: male sex, increasing age, widowhood, single and divorced state, childlessness, high density of population, residence in big towns, a high standard of living, economic crisis, alcohol and drug consumption, a broken home in childhood, mental disorder and physical illness. Among factors he lists as being inversely related to suicide rates are female sex, youth, a moderate density of population, rural occupation, religious devoutness, the married state, a large number of children, membership of the lower socio-economic classes and war.

In assessing suicide potential one must, of course, bear in mind the individual nature of the patient's problems. The long lists given of 'risk factors' is a general guide derived from statistical studies. They may be of little use in assessing the suicidal risks in an 'atypical' patient. Ordinary clinical judgment taking into account all available information is the only practical device. The doctor is best served here by putting his head together with other professionals from a variety of services. Not only will he obtain more information but, as will follow in the next section, he would have shared his patient's problems with those who might be able to assist him.

A criticism of much of the sociological theory of suicide is that little or no attention is paid to the individual. While certain broad classes may exist, e.g. depression, socio–demographic details etc, every individual act is unique. Experienced psychiatrists never cease to teach their juniors that every suicide can teach the doctor something, and that is because the details of the circumstances of every act point to some unique set of circumstances. It is for this that a clinical or administrative 'post-mortem', as opposed to the forensic pathological kind, is advised where a multidisciplinary team can review the facts relating to the patient or subject. The details that emerge are different in each case, and point to some clinical management or administrative point that might have been overlooked or dealt with better.

Management of violence

In the management of the suicidal and/or homicidal patient, the problem, for purposes of the present discussion, is simplified by the assumption that the patient is depressed. Other considerations obviously arise when another diagnosis, or no diagnosis, is made. A way of preventing a person whose balance of mind, to use the old phrase, is disturbed taking his own life is by recruiting any friends or relatives who might have accompanied the patient or are in contact with the patient. There is everything to be gained by revealing one's findings and one's fears to relatives. It goes without saying that the patient's agreement has been sought to speak to relatives and it is only rarely that one comes across a situation where this permission is refused. The practice of speaking only to the patient alone and friends and relatives separately is to be deprecated. On the contrary, the practice of speaking at some stage to the patient and those who accompany him together has much to commend it. The possibility of misunderstandings and misinterpretations is minimized, one's concerns regarding suicidal risk are publicly aired and any directions for medication and the safe holding of drugs may be stated in front of the patient and, also, in this litigious age, witnesses are present to good practices.

The problem arises if the patient is single or has arrived at the doctor's by himself. Here the doctor must make an effort to seek any existing relatives or friends there might be and, failing in that, find allies among professional colleagues. General practitioners and social workers are two who come to mind, though they may not be readily accessible. Community nurses and district nurses, both, like GPs and social workers, capable of visiting the homes of depressed patients are also valuable professional allies. It is a counsel of perfection, of course, but the doctor will do well to visit the patient at home as soon as possible after the consultation if he is thought to be at risk. Not only will the doctor assure the patient that his complaints, problems and symptoms are being taken seriously, which may be all that is necessary to shift the balance in the equation of ambivalence towards preservation of life, but the doctor may find neighbours who by their concern and helpfulness may convince both the doctor and the patient that no man is truly an island. There is a question of confidentiality involved in apprising all and sundry of the suicidal intent of a patient, but one cannot imagine the powers that be, at least in this country, taking to task a doctor who has behaved reasonably and in good faith. When he visits the patient's home, the doctor may also discover a cache of drugs or other items collected by the patient in order to take his life.

The question of hospitalization for the suicidal patient is a vexed one. In general the practice is to be avoided, if only to forestall a trend that may result in large numbers of ill-affordable hospital beds being filled by anxious doctors who have been informed by the questionable practice of defensive medicine. Also, admission to hospital engenders a false sense of security in staff and relatives. A patient who is determined to kill himself can do so as well, probably better, in a busy hospital, as anywhere else. One is aware of the number of tragedies that have occurred in even the best regulated hospitals. Crammer (1984) has reviewed the subject. The findings of Topp (1979) make a similar point as regards prison. However, making rigid rules is as dangerous in this business as in any walk of life. The genuinely uncertain doctor must have access to hospitalization, and here the practice in some hospitals of admitting patients overnight in an informal, largely document-free fashion is a sensible one. The practice involves frequent re-assessment and review and the whole basis of the practice is crisis containment. There is no expectation of prolonged admission on either side and the time bought by knowledge of the patient being in temporarily secure care for a few hours, may be utilized to set in motion the practices described in the previous paragraph. Apart from that, the doctor is enabled to seek the advice of senior colleagues. It is one of those instances in medicine where a second opinion may be sought as much for one's peace of mind as for the diagnosis and management of a patient's condition.

Physical treatment may be considered for the suicidal patient. The details of drug therapy have been considered in Chapter 5, but drug treatment takes time to act and ECT is often the agent of choice. The absurd requirements of the Mental Health Act of 1983, which requires a second opinion in cases under compulsory order, appears simply to be a device to invoke second thoughts. Whatever might not be known about its modes of action, ECT is an effective treatment and it is remarkably safe. The only serious objections to its use are based on ideology and doctrine. One would have thought that 50 years of use was sufficient for the authorities to make up their minds if the treatment is to be permitted or banned, instead of which a situation is created in which the treatment is grudgingly sanctioned and obstacles put in the way of its smooth use.

In the management of depressive violence, whether potential suicide, homicide or other violent behaviour, the diagnosis is obviously important, but the overall management depends on other factors as well. As has been discussed before, the actual diagnosis of depression, its severity and the symptoms present may have little to do with the actual act of violence which is being prevented or contained. To this end, the circumstances in which the act might be perpetrated, and the presence of any 'trigger' or provoking factors must be noted.

The actual personal contact between doctor (or other professional) and patient is probably the single most important factor in preventing a violent act. Certainly, in the case of suicide, the fact that the patient has turned to a doctor or another person in the caring professions is sufficient proof that the patient (1) has doubts about the proposed course of action to deal with his perceived difficulties, i.e. suicide and (2) thinks the person turned to is able to help him. It is an enduring source of mystery that the most deluded of patients still turn up in hospitals seeking a medical solution to problems which one might have imagined they could not perceive as being medical. It is the business of the doctor in situations such as this to use his authority. However mad a patient might be, he still seems capable of recognizing disinterested authority and agreeing to the reasonable demands the average doctor makes, but not apparently with the demands other, less beneficient figures in the family or the law might make. This authority is the doctor's chief weapon. His expression of concern, his professional interest not only in the problems of the patient but in the evolution of his illness (the medical air that emanates from taking down symptoms and eliciting signs may be most helpful in dealing with suicidal patients; if the doctor looks for an illness, perhaps there may be treatment for it, which helps to introduce more doubt in the patient's mind and shift the balance between living and killing oneself), and his formulation of the difficulties of the patient may be the first occasion when anyone has tried to make sense of what to the patient might have seemed an insoluble problem. It would appear that a large section of the population have no access to disinterested help. They may have friends and family, of course, but these often have a variety of emotional axes to grind. The doctor can approach the problem in the way he might a gangrenous leg. Whereas the patient is attached in more ways than one to his leg, his friends and family have other interests besides reading the situation that requires detachment. Too often they exhibit a vicarious proprietorial interest in limbs which are not directly linked to pathological considerations.

Violence directed against other people often occurs in a setting of fear and suspicion, if not downright persecutory delusion. Here again the presence of those nominally closest to the patient may actually exacerbate the feelings of the patient, and the doctor's initial role is one of reassurance and support. However, as with suicidal patients, the doctor must seek to enlist the help of other professionals. With homicidal or otherwise violent patients, the potential victim needs to be warned in the clearest possible terms. Others who may need to be alerted are social workers, the police, community nurses and, not least, general practitioners.

The immediate management of violent incidents is outside the purview of this study, but a note may be made of the sedation used to control the patient. This applies to emergencies regardless of the diagnosis, and is surprisingly not widely known when a parallel emergency procedure such as resuscitation is well known to a variety of professions. Parenteral drug therapy may be indicated. Chlorpromazine 50–200 mg i.m. and haloperidol 5–30 mg i.m. are probably the drugs of choice at present. They may be repeated every 4 hours, even though their effect is cumulative. The

199

question of consent on the part of the patient is an interesting philosophical one, but an emergency remains just that. Waiting for the machinery of the Mental Health Act to move is not advised in cases of imminent psychotic violence. The only proviso is that if one is a junior doctor, the advice and support of a senior colleague is best solicited as soon as is practicable. Once again reasonableness and good faith will help keep the doctor out of trouble.

The authority of the doctor has been mentioned in connection with making contact with the patient. This authority may also have to be deployed in another connection, when it comes to the management of violent psychotic patients – the taking of decisions. Partly through taking a very legalistic view of things, partly through uncertainty born out of inexperience and a rather deplorable defensiveness, many multidisciplinary teams are rendered impotent by a crisis relating to a violent patient. The doctor needs to take an informal decision and implement it in conjunction with his nursing colleague. Crises do not await unanimity in committees.

Deliberate self-harm has been referred to in an earlier section: a few remarks must be addressed to the assessment of the patient after the act. The history is far more informative than the present mental state which often reveals only bland recognition or the after effects of the drugs used in the attempt. Almost always the patient is interviewed the day after in a general medical bed, sometimes with the monitors of vital function still in place. A curtain around the bed is often the only guarantor of privacy, and the examiner at the foot of the bed finds he is unlikely to gain much detail. This cursory examination, which is usually to help the physicians discharge the patient, must be followed-up at least to the extent of the patient being seen in out-patients' with a reliable informant. The circumstances in which the act was undertaken may be reviewed, as can a more objective appraisal be made of the problems facing the patient. The rest of the history can be filled in and some assessment can be made of the family relationships which, as has been said already, often contribute to the pressures on the patient, though they might not have been the immediate precipitating factor. It is only a minority of patients who require psychiatric supervision or treatment. The vast majority may be discharged, it being made clear to all concerned, including the general practitioner, that a more appropriate response might be preventive, involving the psychiatric services when the pressure was actually building up and not when the dam broke with some maladaptive response following in its wake. Referral to social, housing and other local authority services may be appropriately made at this time.

The lack of contact with the psychiatric services among the potentially suicidal has been remarked upon in various studies. The fact that a high proportion of suicides have previously had contact with their doctors has been confirmed in many studies (Jacobson and Jacobson, 1972; Barraclough et al., 1974; Myers and Neal, 1978). Even when there has been contact, the inadequacy of the treatment needs to be explained. Difficulties in diagnosis can only be part of the explanation as a precise diagnosis of depressive illness, as opposed to depressed mood in the context of other symptoms, is not of great moment, provided an antidepressant agent is exhibited in appropriate dose. The fact that anxiety is commonly associated with

200

depression might have meant the prescription of an anxiolytic agent such as, in an earlier age, barbiturates or, later, benzodiazepines which themselves are able to exacerbate the depression, in both cases are potentially able to release aggression and, in the case of the former, be the instrument of suicide itself. The fact that antidepressant drugs have also been known to be toxic in overdose might also have led to undue caution being shown in their prescription, a state of affairs which may change with the relatively safer drugs now on offer.

This inability of the services to reach potential suicides appears to extend to homicides. Some years ago an opportunity arose to study (with Dr Pamela Taylor of the Institute of Psychiatry, London) depressed patients who had committed homicide and were remanded whilst awaiting trial at Brixton Prison in London. In keeping with the picture of depressive homicidal offending, these were men of largely unexceptionable previous histories and each of the victims was a woman (one a wife) with whom the offender had had a turbulent relationship eventually ending in tragedy. There were five such men, and each of them had been in contact with their own general practitioner. Not one had been referred to the specialist psychiatric services, although there had been significant depressive symptomatology (even though noted in retrospect). In no case was the diagnosis of depression missed, but the treatment, seen admittedly from the perspective and resources of a specialist service, was, in all cases, inadequate or incomplete. One had the impression that contrary to what one expects from the ordinary run of offenders, the general practitioners had become emotionally entangled in the care of these patients. Perhaps the specialist psychiatric service referral was at variance with the perceived need for empathy on the part of the patients. These offenders were largely of stable and successful background before their illnesses and the sympathies of the GPs might have been engaged rather forcefully. Having detected pathology, a sense of detachment might have prevented the attitude of over-protection that seemed to have prevailed. It is not unfair to repeat that the very human qualities of understanding and sympathy may stand in the way of proper professional care of the patient.

8
Depressed minds, diverse souls: transcultural aspects of depression

The incidence and variety of depression across nations and cultures have been matters of quite considerable interest for some centuries, and attention was drawn to a few points of interest in Chapter 1. Paralleling the interest in the rise of the mentally handicapped in the period immediately after the French Revolution (Mahendra, 1985c) was an interest in the increase in mental illness generally and, as it then appeared, the racial variation in rates of disorder. In 1820, Burrows paid attention to this in a climate in which considerable interest had been generated by George III's madness. There did not appear to be an absolute increase in the numbers of the insane when Burrows studied case registers and hospital superintendents' reports, but the subjects in the constituent countries in the kingdom apparently displayed different rates. The relatively lower incidence among the Scots was put down to their moral fervour and intellectual character, and the relatively high prevalence in the hapless Irish was put down to the widespread use of alcohol, and the deprivation their country suffered from.

Halliday in 1828 produced a curious forerunner of an argument that would then run for over a century. He attributed both the frequency and the seriousness of mental illness in the civilized nations of Western Europe to the excessive use of mental and bodily powers which led consequently to the 'derangement of the vital functions that react upon the brain and damage its operations'. In contrast the rarity of mental illness in the savage tribes of Africa or the slaves in the Caribbean or the peasantry of the Welsh mountains, the Western Hebrides and the more remote parts of Ireland were attributable to their simple existence and contentment. This view that mental illness is a by-product of civilization is of ancient lineage, and Democritus in the fifth century BC and Lucretius in the first century BC expressed a similar view.

Daniel Hack Tuke (1878) reviewed the prehistoric incidence of madness in Jews, Egyptians, Greeks and Romans and laid to rest the notion that they might have been spared the inroads of mental illness. However, he concluded that mental illness was probably much rarer in primitive society than in societies which had become more developed. But he was aware of the danger of looking at absolute figures of incidence at a time when life expectancy was necessarily restricted. As for the contemporary period, Tuke attributed the rise in mental illness to different causes in the upper and lower classes. Those at the top of the social tree became insane because of loose morals, the use of stimulants and as a result of the complexities of modern life; the lower classes became mentally disordered because they led a deprived life, suffered, among other privations, malnutrition and were predisposed to abuse alcohol. To Tuke mental illness was an inevitable by-product of progress, and the only way out was to seek methods of prevention. He believed mental illness was the penalty superior man had to pay for his greater sensitivity. 'Civilisation involves risks because it entails a higher form of mental life, and our highest wisdom consists in thankfully accepting this boon and escaping one of these risks by the prevention of insanity'.

This view of mental illness in different 'cultures' did not undergo substantial revision until well into the second half of the twentieth century. Indeed it might be argued that there was a regression in later years, as while these older writers were describing differential incidence in a particular country, those who succeeded them, especially in the early years of this century, followed the conquerors into lands that were opened up and compared people of one country with another on a different continent, in a different hemisphere, with different ways of life and, indeed, different patterns of disease. It was also common to find descriptions of the people of one continent, e.g. Africa, in terms suggesting that they might belong to one homogeneous, monolithic tribe. As we know to our cost, the tribes of Africa differ in every conceivable way and on virtually any index one chooses to apply. (To give an example from personal experience (Mahendra, 1981), an interest in catatonia was kindled not only by the low incidence among patients at the Maudsley Hospital but by talking there to a psychiatrist from East Africa who was very familiar with the condition, and another from West Africa who had but a nodding acquaintance with it. It was quite clear that the conventional social explanations provided for the decline in incidence of catatonia were not applicable in this instance – the East African represented a country with relatively well developed psychiatric services with reasonable access to modern physical treatments and he himself was one of a growing number of trained psychiatrists; the West African represented a poor country, with no medical school, where native treatments predominated and he was training to be their first qualified psychiatrist). Furthermore, western psychiatrists who made the study of psychiatry among the 'savage races' were not comparing like with like. Comparison was being made between native patients who had had a chance encounter with the 'Western' medical system in some undeveloped country and, usually, a middle or upper class patient in Britain or Western Europe. As we shall see shortly, the differences between the 'savage' and the 'civilized' mind diminish when the 'savage' is compared with members of the lower classes, children or the mentally handicapped, i.e. patients who take a simpler, less sophisticated view of the world.

EXOTIC DEPRESSIVE SYNDROMES

However, the pre-occupation with the exotic brought forth a number of exotic psychoses which have traditionally adorned the pages of textbooks and taxed generations of examination candidates. Those which are depressive in nature are described briefly, for what they are worth, but already their cultural specificity is being questioned as more and more case reports emerge from cultures other than in which they were thought to exist exclusively. For instance, Berrios and Morley (1984) and Ang and Weller (1984) described cases of *Koro* in non-Chinese patients. These are in addition to cases which have now been reported from the North American and European continents. The latter authors presented the case of a 20-year-old Greek Cypriot immigrant youth in Britain with a family history of depression who presented with depressed mood, panic, elective mutism, abdominal pain and the conviction that his penis was shrinking into his abdomen. He improved on a neuroleptic drug given with an antidepressant but later experienced a hypomanic episode. Four years later he had a major hypomanic bout requiring treatment with chlorpromazine and lithium. Following this was a depressive episode requiring amitriptyline. In this case the koro-like symptomatology was in the midst of clear, recurring manic depressive illness. These authors believe koro is not specific to a particular diagnostic category, but that it may occur as a symptom of anxiety with delusional colouring in affective or schizophrenic illness. Berrios and Morley (1984) concluded that koro-like symptoms may be considered as behavioural phenotypes, being over-valued ideas, sometimes amounting to delusions, found in a variety of psychiatric conditions. The symptom improves when the underlying clinical condition improves. It is seen that not only has koro ceased to be 'culture bound', it is no longer considered to be a disease entity. The only value in having a cultural conception of koro, these authors reasonably conclude, is that when it occurs in the original culture, appropriate and socially meaningful psychotherapeutic interventions might be applied. Outside that culture its 'exotic' nature may, in fact, only distract the clinician from making what, that symptom apart, might be a straightforward diagnosis, which would be amenable to standard treatments which are now available in any culture.

Amok was originally described in parts of South East Asia. It is almost always seen in men and the clinical presentation is one of withdrawal followed by violent aggression directed towards people, animals and objects. The attack subsides when the patient becomes exhausted, or when he kills himself, or is killed by the onlookers in the process of restraint. It seems to have some similarities to the reactive depressive psychosis described in Chapter 2. Its incidence is, however, showing decline. Murphy (1973) has discussed features of this condition. He contends that it was only after the onset of civilization *viz.* the middle of the 19th century that amok was considered a pathological syndrome. Before that it was recognized as a valid, if excessive, means of letting off steam if a socially underprivileged member of that society felt hard done by in dealing with his superiors. It was sanctioned protest against unfairness and, perhaps, fraud.

A not dissimilar condition found in Eskimo women was *Piblokto*, where, once again following a period of depressive withdrawal, sudden activity would occur in which the patient would run into the snow or plunge into freezing waters. The violence was excessive, and both homicide and suicide could occur. Kiev (1972) notes the *Windigo* psychosis occurring among certain North American Indian tribes. He considers it to be a depressive condition reflecting the mythologies of the tribe. The myth at the heart of this condition is the Windigo, a cannibalistic monster. In winter, when food is scarce and starvation imminent, a member of the tribe becomes depressed, claims he has been possessed by, or transformed into, the Windigo and attacks his fellow tribesmen with a view to eating them. Once again, shorn of the detail, this appears to be a reactive depressive psychosis. The form in these three exotic syndromes is the same; the content, influenced by culture, is different.

Too much may be made of the exotic nature of these depressive disorders. Cultures are obviously different, but the forms the illnesses take have many features in common. Added to this is the device of protest, or a 'cry for help', a phrase more familiar to Western psychiatry. It could be submitted that the epidemic of parasuicide, or deliberate self-harm (see Chapter 7) might have appeared culture-bound to observers from those exotic cultures that gave us Koro, Amok, Piblokto and Windigo. In parts of Western Europe, amidst material plenty, one finds young women of the lower social classes, faced with difficulties at work or with parents or partners, slash their wrists or swallow a variety of chemicals. If they die, it is usually an unintended consequence of their actions. There are, for every suicide, some ten of these acts. The explanation for these gestures, apart from a 'cry for help' is lacking; they seem to be impulsive and have been attributed to immaturity in the personality in the individual concerned and his lack of adjustment to the society he lives in. To the 'native' in exotic lands, doing injury or using poison other than to kill, or be killed, might have seemed no less 'exotic'.

TRANSCULTURAL DEPRESSION IN TRANSITION

The evolving nature of depression in so-called undeveloped societies may be illustrated with reference to the situation in certain parts of East Africa, where the growth in psychiatric services has also led to a corresponding increase in the number of scientific papers documenting the nature of the change. Changes in the perception of depression have implications for the provision of services, and this consequently has repercussions in a part of the world not known for a prodigality of natural resource.

There have been three phases in the study of depression in Africa. In the first, the widespread view that 'savages' were not subject to depression was upheld. In the second, depression was conceded to exist, but the presentation was thought to be predominantly in physical guise, as opposed to the pattern in European countries. In the third, and current, phase, depression is said to exist for all practical purposes in the European or 'advanced' mode, and the aetiological factors are now alleged to be broadly similar.

Prince (1968) reviewed reports published between 1895 and 1957 discussing depression in Kenya, South Africa, Nigeria, Uganda, Tanganyika and Ghana. Virtually all the papers pointed to a difference between European and African cultures in the presentation of depression. Pfeiffer (1968), in turn, reviewed published accounts of depression in 22 non-European countries and showed that the 'core' symptoms were mood change, diurnal variation, loss of appetite, sleep, libido and some somatic complaints; those that showed cultural variation were guilt, hopelessness and suicidal tendencies.

There now seems little doubt that considerable psychiatric morbidity is to be seen in all parts of Africa, comparable to the incidence and prevalence in Western Europe and North America. In Ethiopia psychiatric illnesses were as common as communicable diseases until the situation changed with the onset of famine. In Nigeria, they appear to be as common as malaria (Mbanefo, 1971). A quarter of the adult population in some small villages in Uganda had psychiatric disorders (Orley and Wing, 1979). Other countries with a comparable incidence of psychiatric incidence include Tanzania (Holmes and Speight, 1975) and Kenya (McEvoy and McEvoy, 1976; Ndetei and Muhangi, 1979).

As Dhadphale et al. (1983) have commented, there were several features common to all these studies. Not less than 20% of all patients presenting at medical clinics had psychiatric illness, and almost all these patients had somatic pains or vague ill-defined symptoms; the treatment prescribed was for physical illness and many of the clinicians seemed unaware they were dealing with mental disorder, either limiting treatment to the symptomatic features or investigating unnecessarily. Often psychiatric patients were converted to long-term attenders at medical clinics in an attempt to have their illness treated. Dhadphale et al. (1983), in their study, found a prevalence of psychiatric morbidity of 29%, with anxiety and depression predominating. There was no significant sex difference; they found psychiatric symptoms were easily elicited and they also found that the psychiatric patients had been ill longer than non-psychiatric patients.

These findings are confirmed by the work of Majodina and Johnson (1983) on an urban population in Ghana. They reported on a common core of depressive disorder and commented on how the mode of presentation in African patients had changed over 30 years. The treatment now prescribed would appear unexceptional – tricyclic antidepressants with one or more of the following: a major tranquillizer, a minor tranquillizer, ECT and supportive psychotherapy.

It is not possible to account for this changing incidence of depressive and other psychiatric morbidity solely in terms of the instruments of advance and civilization casting a shadow over Africa. Dhadphale et al. (1983) could show no difference between psychiatric and non-psychiatric patients with respect to literacy, socio–economic class, education and tribe. The obvious rejoinder that modernization and urbanization might have been responsible would not account for the rural incidence of depression which is now held to be of the same magnitude as in urban areas, and gives similar figures to Shepherd *et al.* (1966) in Britain. The answer may lie partly in the perceptions and expectations of the practitioners. Not only are many of these workers trained psychiatrists but their training has been in situations where the ideas of Western psychiatrists are current. It is also possible that with the relative decline of major contagious disease in parts of Africa, depression and other psychiatric morbidity have become more apparent. Also the established efficacy of physical antidepressant treatment may play a role. One must also not deride the effects of cultural contagion – apeing the West may result in psychiatric complications, not merely a developing taste for transistor radios, jeans and coca-cola.

It is now a fact that psychiatric morbidity may materially inconvenience the economic workings of a developing country. It used to be held that psychiatric illness, even if acknowledged to be present, was relatively trivial in its effects in the Third World; acute psychosis of possibly 'organic' origin rather than chronic, 'functional' disabling illness. The family and social systems were such, it was suggested, that not only was the illness of good prognosis but where, exceptionally, it ran a chronic or, even, malignant course, an extended social network would take over the burden from the state – community care provided by the community and not the state. This is a myth which anyone who has worked in a Third World country can explode for himself. Mental illness in those parts is a reality much as it is anywhere else in the world; the disabilities are as real; the cost not being borne by the state means hardship to families already living at subsistence level. The cost, in those materially disadvantaged, deprived societies, can be enormous.

A recent attempt was made by Westermeyer (1984) to study the cost of mental illness in 27 villages in Laos. He found that losses in productivity as a result of mental illness were consistently high; acute losses were relatively small. He concluded that his data suggested that major psychiatric disorder comprises a significant economic loss and, for most victims, is an incapacity even in a developing society.

One is here dealing with an unmet need for standard or conventional modes of treatment, not for expensive and time-consuming procedures such as formal psychotherapy. As the East African studies show, the immediate ambition is a rather modest one. It is to elicit the existence of depression and subject it to tricyclic antidepressants, ECT and/or supportive psychotherapy, mostly in a primary care setting. This is not at variance with the view, held by a growing number of psychiatrists, that unwarranted claims by psychiatrists result in a large number of people with problems and distress calling on psychiatrists for help; numbers that grow unmanageably as psychiatry expands, correspondingly, at a spiralling cost, which starves the needy with chronic mental disorder of resources. Richman and Barry (1985) have given expression to this view, support for which will undoubtedly grow in the present socio–political climate. They argue that the vast increase in perceived needs for mental health is due, in large measure, to the broadening of traditional boundaries. The factors include psychiatrists increasingly directing attention to conditions which precede mental illness proper, i.e. the pre-psychotic or pre-breakdown stage. Secondly, behavioural disorder of the kind which has been previously excluded or dealt with only cursorily have more recently been encompassed within standard psychiatric therapy. Such conditions which formerly would have come within the remit of ministers of religion and social workers have been taken over by psychiatrists. The psychiatric profession has taken to heart the World Health Organization definition of health as being a state of complete physical, mental and social well-being, rather than the absence of disease, and has responded accordingly. These views serve as a cautionary example to those in the Third World that when services expand, they should not go beyond boundaries that can be sustained by facts, empirical research and resources. The problems of mentally ill patients, whether in the West or in the Third World, are, of course, far removed from these considerations. They have traditionally suffered neglect; there is genuine unmet psychiatric need and it is necessary to emphasize this. To argue the opposite is to support the discredited view that savages did not have depression, or that it all had a 'physical' basis.

Undoubted though the social and industrial advances have been, some findings from studies in developing countries are still not comparable to those in Western Europe. The incidence in women is one such. Whereas in virtually all Western studies, women are in the majority among depressed patients, in East Africa, Kenya in particular, there appears to be an absence of a sex bias. A similar point has been made by Giel *et al.* (1968) in Ethiopia. This cannot be explained solely in terms of differential attendance at clinics as Orley and Wing (1979) also failed to find any difference in a community survey in Uganda. A suggested explanation is that African women are more accepting and tolerant of distress and pain than are men, and that this stoicism masks a natural tendency for a higher incidence of depression in women, an explanation also put forward by Ananth (1978) for Indian women to account for the absence of a sex difference in Indian culture for depressive illness. Dhadphale *et al.* (1983) go further in seeking a sociological explanation, and invoke support from the findings of workers in the West (Brown and Harris, 1978; Briscoe, 1982). They point to the evidence that unemployed women staying at home have a higher incidence of depressive and other psychiatric morbidity, explained in terms of social isolation and the perceived lack of fulfilment and satisfaction in domestic duties. In Africa, on the other hand, despite rapid industrialization and modernization, the situation, and the perception of it, is quite different. The African woman has her hands full – bringing up children, feeding the animals, tending the crops, not to mention the role she has to play in the extended social network. There is no social isolation, even less when she is at home; there is no time or opportunity to experience boredom. She has to get on with things. However, times change, with them, no doubt, the role of the African woman, and as several authors have predicted, the natural pattern of depressive incidence, if indeed it existed, may emerge.

The extent to which social factors may influence the onset and progression of depression in the Third World has been taken further by the work of Vadher and Ndetei (1981). They compared black Kenyan patients with matched non-psychiatrically disturbed controls in the community, and found that the depressed group had significantly more life events in the 12 months preceding their depression than the controls. They found that 68% of a sample of depressed Kenyan patients had experienced at least one independent severe life event in the 12 months preceding the onset of their depression, while the figure for depressed women in London had been 67% (Brown and Harris, 1978). The 'vulnerability' factors discussed by Brown and Harris have been dealt with in Chapter 2. In the Kenyan study events involving loss were predominant and about half of them were related to separation, or perceived or threatened separation. Separation in a Kenyan context involved family members, friends or lovers or the departure of family members in pursuit of work. It was also seen in this study that there was a female preponderance. The views and fears expressed before that a female preponderance is the natural state for depression might have already come to pass.

In a further study of depressed patients in an urban area of Kenya, lack of regular income or employment, and being first born were noted to be vulnerability factors (Ndetei and Vadher, 1982). However, having an intimate, confiding relationship or active religious affiliation did not seem to protect against depression. Being first born was the most significant vulnerability factor, and it is speculated that in the Kenyan culture the first born has a special responsibility in that he may be charged with the care and provision in an extended social network that may even be in excess of the role played by his parents. The resulting stresses and the subsequent life events may lead to his depression (cf the work on social mobility and depression in Western cultures, discussed in Chapter 2). Another cultural variant was that the number of children aged 14 and below bore no relationship to depression, which may indicate the support a mother derives in child-minding from an extended family network.

It is thus seen that within a generation the perception of depression in several parts of Africa has undergone dramatic change. From the view that the African is incapable of being depressed emerged the idea that he presented, when depressed, with somatic features. Later it became apparent that somatization is a not invariable feature, and now the view is held that social factors can influence the onset of depression. The few remaining sceptics who argue for an essentially 'physical' basis to most depressions in African patients do not sound convincing. As was seen, a few studies already hint at a female preponderance, as in the West. The pattern of depression in modern Africa is likely to be as in the West, and the requirements for services, as far as one can tell, will be as those in the West.

SOMATIZATION, AND THE PERCEPTION OF DEPRESSION

The idea that depression presented partially or wholly in terms of bodily dysfunction has dominated transcultural considerations of depression. It has already been mentioned that it has been known even in industrially advanced societies for members of the lower socio–economic classes to present with somatic symptoms when depressed. But it is now necessary to consider why the somatic presentation was for so long held to be the mode of presentation of depression in traditional cultures. Reports of somatic presentation are widespread, and have come from large parts of Africa, India, Pakistan, Sri Lanka, Bangla Desh, the West Indies and Hong Kong.

Rack (1982) has described the presentation of depression in the Indian or Pakistani patient. The patient, usually a woman, complains of pain and weakness. The pain may be described as being in the back, limbs, head or as a diffuse bodyache. Discomfort in the chest or abdomen is thought to be particularly common and the weakness in the body is a generalized one. Male patients describe sexual dysfunction, and it appears that description and aetiology are often confused, patients tending to attribute the cause and the site of the lesion as the heart or bowels. It becomes clear that it is the presentation of the disorder that is somatic as the appropriate questions elicit the features of depression readily enough. It seems whereas a patient in the West expresses the psychological features of depression first and then volunteers the somatic symptoms afterwards, or only on direct questioning, the Asian patient does it the other way round. One suspects there is no overall difference in the type of symptomatology between the Asian patient and the depressed patient in the West if all the questions are explicit and put directly to the patient.

The practice of depression in a Third World country is instructive in this respect. In Sri Lanka, patients with depression often presented with a symptom of 'burning' over their chest and upper abdomen. It was quite clear that the term used covered several meanings. A free translation into English turned out to be burning (see the later discussion of the nuances of language in describing what may be culturally significant) and doctors, often middle-class and preferentially English speaking, accepted this description as if it were that of some specific entity. Experience seemed to suggest that many of the words or terms used did not arise spontaneously in the patient's mind but were the result of a native practitioner of traditional medicine suggesting the diagnosis or its causation. One explanation for 'somatization' is that the concepts of one culture, perhaps, are being transferred via free translation to another, and from one language to another. Much of the research appears to have been done with non-English speaking individuals in the same culture. A bias enters immediately – those who speak English belong to a higher class, are urban, better educated and considerably more likely to be affected by concepts of depression current in the West. Aspects of somatization of depression found in classes of patients who take a different view of life from that of the average adult – viz. children, the mentally handicapped, and the elderly – are validly compared to depressives in Third World, and this will be taken up in later sections.

Other explanations are available for the 'somatization' of depression. One which is applicable to both Asian and African cultures is part cultural and part economic. Until recently, and even now in many parts of the world, consulting a Western-trained doctor was both expensive and discouraged for cultural reasons. The obvious triumphs of Western medicine became

211

most clearly apparent in the treatment of infectious illness, in particular, and with physical illness generally. Populations in Third World countries gradually accepted alien methods of care for these conditions, but continued to show a preference for their native healers where mental disorder was concerned. Wig *et al.* (1980) sought opinions as to the appropriate treatment for physical and mental symptoms from community leaders in parts of the Sudan, the Phillipines and India. It was shown that help for physical symptoms was acceptable from Western-style doctors, while substantial numbers of respondents in all three countries believed mental symptoms were best dealt with by native or traditional healers. In a rural population of Nigeria, Harding (1973) found that 91% of those questioned preferred the traditional practitioner for mental disease, whereas only 66% chose the native healers for epilepsy. Kapur (1975) in India showed that fits were seen as more appropriately treated by the Western practitioner than some symptoms of mental illness which were believed to be the province of the traditional healer. When case vignettes of epilepsy, psychosis and tuberculosis were given by Dale and Ben-Tovim (1984) to a population in Botswana, they found that indigenous care was most favoured for epilepsy, and least for tuberculosis, psychosis taking an intermediate position. As the Western-style doctor deals with physical symptoms, the patient presents accordingly, whatever might be the parent condition giving rise to such physical symptoms. If the patient has depression which does not give rise to physical features he goes to the native healer or, if the distress is not pressing, puts up with it or has it dealt with by family or friends. This symptomatological dichotomy is reflected in the patterns of consultation, but community surveys in these parts of the world, working among unselected, representative groups of patients with a systematic inventory of symptoms elicited by direct questioning, bring out a prevalence of depression which is not dissimilar to that in any Western country. It is also important to realize that the pattern of depressive or any other illness seen in a hospital population in the Third World would have factors other than the purely cultural affecting it – the availability of hospital services, cost of transport, whether payment for the consultation was made at source, loss of wages if a day was taken off to visit hospital, arrangements to look after children, or, indeed, if there was a war going on. In these circumstances there is much greater justification for presenting at a clinic with a depression which has bodily pain or discomfort attached to it than with a depression which has merely produced chronic unhappiness. There are more important things in the minds of people in most parts of Africa and Asia than some mild dysphoria.

The other ready explanation comes from the knowledge that mental illness has been, and remains in many instances, a stigma. In Asian cultures the 'shaming' aspects of mental illness remain a potent force to discourage treatment. Indeed, in many of these cultures, such infectious illnesses as leprosy and tuberculosis, and neuropsychiatric disorders such as epilepsy are considered tragedies affecting the whole family. The indisputable hereditary basis to mental illness has not helped erase the dismay, shame and fear associated with psychiatric disorder. However, these considerations apply in the main to psychotic disorders. But, as was seen in the discussion of reactive psychosis in Chapter 2, psychotic behaviour may present with aggression, violence and destruction which, however redolent of stigma, is occasionally beyond containment in the family or even in the village. Traditional practitioners do not have recourse to antipsychotic agents; their strength lies in psychotherapy. Thus once the psychotically violent patient gets to hospital, more for restraint, only secondarily for a cure, the traditional villager cannot prevent a diagnosis of mental disorder, with all the refinements of medical diagnosis, being made by Western-trained clinicians. This is why the major psychoses, especially those causing excitement, could always be sought and found in any culture. Their incidence and prevalence, in broad terms, has been comparable to those in the West. The higher incidence of psychoses with a physical basis has an obvious explanation. The 'stigma' is to come to terms with attempts at culturally-sanctioned explanations, e.g. excessive stress in the individual, perhaps an evil spirit invoked by envious neighbours. The minor psychiatric disorders such as common depression may not have such obvious (to the villagers, at least) precipitants; the symptoms are vague and ill-defined; ill-understood by family and neighbours; lassitude may be seen simply as a disinclination to work; the symptoms are not socially disruptive and are containable within the family, and the traditional healer may have an efficacious remedy. Mere low spirits cannot conceivably be a disease within this framework. The 'stigma' may be more easily understood in these forms of mental disorder.

This is a social view of the interpretation of depression. But there is an individual factor, too. The insight that is present with milder forms of depression may enable the patient to quite consciously emphasize the physical and the somatic to justify obtaining medical treatment. Whether this desire can also be unconscious we do not know. But Rack (1982) regards the unconscious mechanism as being significant. He sees this as a hysterical manoeuvre, as with any hysteria in which some unacceptable internal conflict may be 'converted' into physical symptoms. It follows that in any such patient with a diagnosis of 'hysteria', underlying depression must be sought for with an awareness of cultural factors that may be playing a part. The fact that Western psychiatrists may see 'hysteria' and depression as antithetical conditions, the somatic features counting in favour of the former and directing attention away from depression, is a handicap when the diagnosis of depression in patients from other cultures is considered. This is certainly a plausible view in that the decline of the somatic features and their substitution by more understandable psychological symptoms of depression may parallel the socio—cultural changes which have led to the decline of gross hysterical stigmata. Certainly, any view that proposes looking deeper into alleged cases of hysteria, in whomsoever and wherever it is found, must be welcomed.

The role of language must be examined in any study involving explanations for the somatization of depression in non-European patients. There is, for instance, the question of misunderstanding, even when the language used is arguably a common one. West Indian patients in Britain take a literal, and barometric, view of the phrase 'low feelings', equating this with weakness, lassitude and a low level of activity. There is, in similar vein, the confusion that arises from the use of idiom. A use of such a phrase as 'heart broken' may result in a literal physical counterpart to psychological distress being referred to. Rack quotes work on Asian patients, especially those speaking Urdu, who complain of 'heart distress'. Various malfunctions of the heart are referred to by patients, and their traditional healers interpret them accordingly. The heart is taken as expressing emotion in Muslim culture, and traditional healers give due regard to those symptoms they believe arise from the diseased organ. This is partly done by verbal exchange, partly by the patient demonstrating physically, as by pounding the chest or squeezing the hand to demonstrate what he is feeling and partly by the practitioner examining the pulse. As Rack points out, the Western patient may also express these idioms and metaphors but has recourse to a larger fund of language and is able to refer directly to the emotional experience that he feels. The Asian and African patient may prefer the somatic metaphor. We see again that the experience of depression may be similar but the artifice of language and the chance possession of one which may be rich in its terminology of the emotions, enables one patient to be more exact in describing his feelings than another. We thus have to consider not merely the feelings that might be present in depression, but their interpretation by the individual patient, his society and his healers. It is not difficult now to understand that what we might call the phenotype of depression may vary the world over.

We have briefly touched on how one language rather than another may provide a richer fund of words and phrases to depict depressive symptomatology. It is reasonable to assume that various languages and related dialects sprang up to make sense of situations and experiences in given localities. The resulting pre-occupations of peoples may be apparently different. To take an example, the British pre-occupation with the weather has provided, or so we think, a rich seam of words which we see mined every day on radio, television and the newspapers to describe minor variations in the weather which might seem bizarre to anyone living in the tropics who has to contend merely with the dry season and the wet season. But this profligacy of the English language pales almost into inarticulacy when one considers the well-known example of the Laplander's obsessively minute description of the snow that is his pre-occupation. Leff (1973) has noted that when one's eyes are drawn to the differentiation of the snow and its practical implications, it would be perfectly possible to appreciate the finer points in the distinction of something which one had regarded before as some homogeneous and inconvenient mass.

Similarly, certain concepts hold greater cultural importance than others. Rack has given examples from the English and various African languages. English is rich in words that may be used to describe mood states. These are not synonymous but portray nuances of thought and speech as regards moods such as depression, a large number of which are in current, if not colloquial, use and are available both to the articulate patient and his doctor. In African languages, the vocabulary as regards mood states is a meagre

214

one. In Yoruba, one word stands for 'sad' and 'angry'. In Ghana, three words exist to cover all the unpleasant emotions, one of these being for their somatic manifestations. This richness of the English language for describing mood states is taken to be indicative of a pre-occupation with the inner workings of the mind, an obsessive introspection. In some other languages, the variety of the language extends to the description of relationships between people using that language; in others it is a pre-occupation with some practical matter involving nature as it affects the area where the language is spoken, e.g. the Laplanders and their pre-occupation with the minute linguistic description of snow and its properties. The lesson is clear. It is to take a latitudinous view of matters pertaining to cultures, their languages and the words that describe inner states such as depression.

It is not necessary to go 'exotic' to seek these differences in the use of language. The ubiquity of usage of English, modified by a variety of dialect and usages, brings with it the paradox that not all will use the language, its words or idioms in the same way. There may be scope for misunderstanding. An example from West Indian usage was cited above. Others follow when groups of individuals in the *same* culture but with different, often limited, grasp of language are considered. The difficulties in articulation and literacy among such groups as those of a poorer class, children, the mentally handicapped and the elderly are often alluded to, though most often in the more literate sections of the press, than in medical textbooks. These groups generally have a less sophisticated grasp of the nuances of language and the description of depressive symptoms is correspondingly simpler, more concrete, less introspective and often at variance with the models of depression textbooks and teachers of psychiatry provide. Depression in these individuals has often to be inferred; the evidence is indirect; the results of treatment are controversial. But it is a problem that needs to be acknowledged and, certainly, for the first generation, if not later, immigrants, the same principles may need to be applied. Pre-occupation with language must not hinder concerted, even ingenious, efforts from being made to find out what people are experiencing, and suffering from.

The limitations of clinical psychiatry, dependent as it is on the subjective description of mood states by way of language, is exposed. One may take a visionary view and await the arrival of biological markers and indices that circumvent language and, indeed, any active role on the part of the patient whatever language he speaks, but a more immediate practical solution is to train psychiatrists not merely in the nuts and bolts of his speciality, but to be aware of the complexity and diversity of the world, its occupants and their problems. The plea must go out again for the widest possible education (not merely training) for psychiatrists. A liberal education now seems to have a more immediate and practical application quite apart from the merits traditionally attributed to it.

As has been noted already, Pfeiffer (1968) made a distinction between 'core' symptoms which, in a sense, are culture-free and those features such as guilt, hopelessness and suicidal tendencies which are more likely to be determined by culture. Guilt needs to be considered as a separate culturally

215

determined variable. The view has been expressed that Christian teaching of original sin and the possibility and means of redeeming onself brings with it an element of free-will. In the presence of diminished mood, an individual may feel guilt at his moral incompetence in not having lived or acted appropriately in his pre-morbid existence. In non-Christian cultures, the element of free-will may be reduced or abandoned altogether. The patient's life and fortunes are determined by fate and other forces quite beyond his control. Even in the depths of depression, even when it has been attributed to physical or natural causes, the patient in these cultures is less likely to be afflicted by a sense of guilt; his whole life has been determined for him by some authoritarian force over which he has no control. He cannot blame himself for any act of omission or commission. This plausible explanation for the differential incidence of guilt and self-blameworthiness in different cultures has been given in the context of Christian teaching and in terms of the Hindu concept of Karma by Rao (1973). Another explanation for the differential incidence is given by Rack (1982). He draws a distinction between societies which may be 'guilt-based' and those which are 'shame-based'. The discussion is allied to that surrounding the introspective nature of Western culture and the views on stigma which have already been taken up. In Western, Christian culture, the patient who is given to introspection is concerned not only with his current, pathological mental state but also with his previous thoughts and actions. These views are not dependent on the views, attitudes, opinions or judgements of those who live around him in his culture. Guilt arises, therefore, as a personal symptom. In non-Western, non-Christian cultures, shame may be felt by the patient for his past and present thoughts and actions, but, more importantly, it is the family and sometimes other people who express and feel shame for the symptoms or the behaviour of the patient. As opposed to individualistic guilt, one has the communal shame. These symptoms of depression are culturally determined and are not, therefore, part of the core symptomatology of depression.

The recent shift in the subject matter of transcultural psychiatry has been made from the study of peoples living in industrially undeveloped cultures to the study of quite heterogeneous groups of people emigrating to countries of the West. There has been no uniform pattern to this immigration. In the past 50 years there has been an influx from the Jewish populations of advanced industrial countries in the face of persecution; large numbers of East Europeans have arrived from industrially advanced countries following political ferment and the expression of dissent; West Indians have emigrated from culturally disparate parts of the Caribbean for largely economic reasons; Asians came not only for these reasons from parts of the Indian sub-continent but other Asians came via East Africa, where they had lived for many years, following political turmoil. The fact that these immigrants are not only from a variety of cultures but have emigrated for differing reasons is important, as the suggested causes of increased mental disorder in emigrants differ in those whose emigration was voluntary as opposed to being involuntary (Odegaard, 1932; Mezey, 1960). Briefly, the former are believed to emigrate partly as a result of some factor that may predispose to mental disease – restlessness as a result of dissatisfaction with the *status quo*, perhaps paranoia (prophets not without honour save in their own lands are often classic examples of paranoid personality). The latter are essentially refugees and their predisposition to a higher incidence of mental illness is, perhaps, due to stress.

Once they have emigrated, their acclimatization and adjustment may be far from complete, and it is revealing to note that children of original immigrants may still have to be considered in the same light as their parents. Hitch and Rack (1980) studied patients in Bradford who were members of ethnic groups and who had been refugees during World War II. They confirmed that foreign-born subjects had more illness than the native born, and that morbidity was greater among Poles than in Ukranians. They could also show that this was not due to 'culture shock', as the onset of illness was often many years after migration. Their explanation is given in terms of social cohesion in migrant groups. The Ukranian community is said to be wellknown as affording mutual support and having an identity of its own even in a foreign land. They seem to be self-sufficient and are not fully integrated. The Polish community, on the other hand, appears to be less self-contained, and its members do not engage in the same degree of social support as do the Ukranians. But the Poles do not appear to have integrated fully into British society. The authors comment on the striking extent to which a large number of Polish patients, especially women, had problems with language to the extent that effective doctor–patient communication was affected. The differences, not merely in the incidence of disease, but the social factors that could account for the differences in morbidity are revealing in that to the casual observer – a term that takes in most doctors and members of health and social care teams – the difference between Poles and Ukranians would have been thought to be minimal. Such is the complexity of the subject that a comparative study of various factors in the diversity of immigrant life and living conditions is not easily made. Yet, it is clear that a sweeping generalization regarding depression or mental illness in immigrants – who in Britian may include Jews from several countries, East Europeans, Asians, negroes from Africa as well as the Caribbean, among others – cannot be made as though they were one homogeneous group.

There is no reason to suppose that the neurobiological basis of depression differs in various parts of the world. The causation of depression may vary. Until recently, a high proportion of depression and other mental disorders in non-European cultures was in all probability due to, or influenced by, physical illness consequent upon infectious and other physical causes. Industrialization and advances in public health measures have caused these factors to decline in importance. Now the proximate cause of depression in these countries is closer to that of the West *viz.* social and personal. The manifestation of depression was presumably different because the peoples of these populations took a different, perhaps less complex, view of their world, and their relationship to one another and to their healers. Evidence suggests that as societies evolve into a state of greater industrialization, they become more open to influences from outside their cultures and have

217

consequently a more 'Western' outlook on the world. The presentation of depression then takes the form we are familiar with in the West. The influence of Western-trained and Western-influenced doctors in the changing presentation of depression is likely to have been crucial.

It is now necessary to consider depression in three groups who occupy a position different to the mainstream in any society – the mentally handicapped, children and the elderly – in order to test the hypothesis that was put forward before, *viz.* modification of the features of depression seen in other cultures may be understood by reference to the characteristics of depression seen in those groups of any culture who take a simpler, less sophisticated view of the world.

Depression in mental handicap

Neurobiological and social factors compel the mentally handicapped to take a simpler and different view of the world, materially different from the view taken by more 'normal' members of society. It has been known for some considerable time that while depression exists among the mentally handicapped, the presentation of the condition may differ in that mood change may not necessarily be a primary feature but may have to be inferred from such motor features as agitation and increased activity, and from social withdrawal. This is especially so in those patients whose severity of handicap may include deprivation of verbal ability. In place of responses to questions, one relies on relatives' and experienced nurses' reports of suspected mood change, and then confirms it with observations in the spheres of level of activity, social responsiveness, feeding and sleeping habits, and from a knowledge of family history of mental illness (Reid, 1982).

Even if speech is available, it may be too simple in form and meagre in content to describe the complexities of depressed mood and its associations. It is quite common to find actions replacing speech in the form of aggressive and assaultive behaviour, though irritability and unco-operativeness may not always find a physical outlet. Somatic features such as headache or abdominal pain are commonly encountered, as is hypochondriasis: symptoms for which a physical basis cannot be found, and therefore labelled 'hysterical' include fits, odd gaits or the inability to walk. Interestingly, as with childhood, where the older the child is, the more 'adult' its depressive features, less handicapped individuals may present with the commoner symptoms of depression, although their manifestation may be modified by intellectual and social handicap. A more obvious depressed mood, feelings of guilt, depressive delusions and mood-appropriate hallucinations, attempted suicide and even successfully completed suicide may be seen in the mildly impaired patients (Wright 1982).

Depression in childhood

The received wisdom has been that depression in childhood, in terms that are applicable to adults, is rare, and exceptionally rare before puberty (e.g. Anthony and Scott, 1960). This is in contrast to anxiety states which come

218

under the heading of 'emotional disorders'. Whether the view that a strict distinction may not be validly made between anxiety states and depression in adults (see Chapter 4) will be followed in child psychiatric practice is not clear. However, the emotional disorders produce symptoms which may be seen in adult depression. These include, apart from anxiety, disorders of sleep and appetite, phobic features, motility symptoms such as fidgetiness and restlessness, withdrawal, somatic features such as vomiting and headaches and poor attention and concentration.

One of the difficulties in assessing childhood mood disorders is that, even within normal variation, mood in children is labile. Persistence of depressed mood is, therefore, not seen. However, reported symptoms of depression have included change of mood, an unaccustomed look of sadness and misery, disinclination for play and social activity, physical complaints, irritability and impaired concentration (Wolff, 1978). Frommer (1968), after studying 190 depressed children, noted that the illness in childhood presented most commonly as a non-specific somatic malaise, often with abdominal pain as the reason for referral. She also claimed that these children benefited from antidepressant medication. The issue is complicated by the fact that phobic children, too, respond to antidepressants, as do children with conduct and emotional disorders coupled with mood change. Frommer *et al.* (1972), comparing depressed, anxious and aggressive children, found the depressed group showed the highest incidence of sleep problems, abdominal pain, enuresis and anorexia.

Frommer (1967) and Cytryn and McKnew (1972) described childhood mood disorders, and proposed their sub-classification. Frommer (1967) divided childhood depression into three groups: enuretic depressives, phobic depressives and pure depressives. The enuretic depressives were described as moody, immature, weepy, hostile and aggressive; the phobic depressives as irritable, weepy and tense. Frommer states, 'they rarely showed a frank depressive picture or its typical mood disorder, and sometimes even denied any feeling of depression'. As for the 'mood disorder' group, they are described as weepy, irritable, with temper outbursts and sleep disturbances, some with quite serious antisocial behaviour. It is clear from this study that Frommer was not attempting to diagnose children to fit the adult depressive syndrome. Rather, she seems to have discerned from clinical experience that certain children appeared to benefit from antidepressant drugs, and therefore reasoned on this basis that they might have been depressed.

Cytryn and McKnew (1972) isolated three categories of possible childhood depression. In masked depression – again an analogy from adult life – hyperactivity, aggression, somatic features, hypochondriasis and delinquency are seen in the midst of severe temperamental and family problems. Another of their groups presented a more conventional picture of depressive illnesss – there was a persistent sad affect, social withdrawal, hopelessness, helplessness, psychomotor retardation, anxiety, social difficulties, school failure, sleep and appetite problems and suicidal thoughts or attempts.

Persistent depressed mood by itself is rare, and it is more common to have indirect behavioural evidence of depression such as aggression, pain or other somatic complaints, sleep, appetite or bladder control problems. Typically, adult features such as guilt, self-reproach and futility are not seen. Sleep problems may be associated with early insomnia or early morning awakening, and there is a high incidence of primary nocturnal enuresis and EEG abnormalities have been noted.

Puig-Antich et al. (1978) also suggested that there were children in whom an adult pattern of depression could be observed. Severe forms of depression could be seen in this group in whom hallucinations, retardation, suicidal thoughts and anhedonia were seen, in addition to a depressed mood. Given the apparent clinical similarity between child and adult depression with regard to clinical symptomatology, family history and response to imipramine, they suggested some children and adults experienced a similar illness. This view has been put in formal terms in the DSM-III of the American Psychiatric Association (1980) where no distinction is made in the diagnostic criteria for pre-pubertal, adolescent and adult depression. In addition, Puig-Antich et al. (1979) have also reported cortisol hypersecretion as occurring in some depressed pre-pubertal children. The pattern of cortisol hypersecretion is said to be indistinguishable from that seen in the adult (see Chapter 3).

The traditional practice with childhood depression has been to infer psychopathology in the child through observation and through reports from parents and teachers. This, while being a necessary process, does not reveal symptoms such as depression, guilt, obsessions, lowered self-esteem, suicidal pre-occupations, and anxiety which may not necessarily lead to a change in behaviour that forms the basis for observation. These are likely to be experienced by the older child, who may also exercise a growing capacity for privacy by concealing these experiences. Thus, as with patients in the Third World, direct inquiry reveals the experiences of some depressed children to be not unlike depressed adults.

Rutter et al. (1970) found that the occurrence of depressive symptoms within the three groups of emotional disorder, conduct disorder and mixed emotional and conduct disorders was broadly similar. A rough distinction between early and middle childhood and later adolescence could also be discerned. The point is also made that there was little agreement between parents and teachers as to whether a child was miserable, more an illustration of the transient nature of the mood disturbance in children rather than a reflection of the different methods of inquiry of parents and teachers. The diagnostic problem eases slightly when middle childhood is reached, as children can then present with apathy, social withdrawal, pain, loss of appetite, psychomotor retardation and express wishes such as a desire to run away which may reflect unhappiness. As puberty and adolescence are entered, a cognitively more mature child can indicate hopelessness and guilt, and the picture gradually evolves into an illness that is seen in adults. We are then led to making the diagnosis of depression in children in ways which are broadly similar to that for adults – the presence of a sad mood which persists beyond the precipitating cause, the term 'persistence' being used in a relative sense.

Hyperactivity and school refusal have been considered by some workers to be depressive equivalents in children (see Chapter 2, for a note on adult depressive equivalents). However, when hyperactive children grow up, there is no evidence that they are more prone to depression than normal children are. In school refusal (Hersov, 1961) one occasionally notes a history of depression in the mother. The child itself, often timid, well-behaved and bright, has feelings of panic which prevents it from attending school; this is accompanied by such somatic features as vomiting and abdominal pain. Antidepressant medication may produce good results. Thus, there are a number of factors which point indirectly to school refusal being a species of depression.

As was discussed in Chapter 7, suicide is rare before puberty; the incidence increases slightly during adolescence. Some of the more obvious reasons for the rarity of the phenomenon include the lack of ability to plan the act, the inability to secure the means of committing the act, a view of death as something reversible and, therefore, not final and also the relative scarcity of such depressive symptoms as hopelessness and futility. Shaffer (1974) made a study of childhood suicide and observed several characteristics in the child who had killed itself. It had above average intelligence and possibly a consequent conceptual maturity which might have made it take an adult view of death; a disturbed family background, e.g. divorce or non-communication; involvement in antisocial behaviour and school non-attendance; a personal experience of suicidal behaviour in a close friend or relative; a depressed mental state in which guilt was a feature, i.e. a picture corresponding to the mental state in the adult suicide; the prospect of imminent disciplinary action, e.g. a court appearance, or parents being about to be informed of some misdemeanour; a feeling of abandonment either socially or within the family. Actual suicide in children and adolescents, when it occurs, seems to be rarely impulsive but bears all the hallmarks of successful planning and execution.

As for a psychological explanation as to the roots of later depression being found in childhood behaviour, it is instructive to quote the work of MacFarlane et al. (1954). Aggressive behaviour found in very young boys and girls disappears in girls earlier than in boys; girls thus lead boys in social learning and in the exercise of social control. The authors believe the later incidence of timidity, anxiety and depression in girls is a result of internalizing aggressive feelings which boys are free to express more openly. The authors emphasize that this is not a biological phenomenon, but that different social roles allotted to boys and girls in Western society are sufficient to account for this.

This presentation of some of the features of childhood depression in a section in a chapter on transcultural depression is no mere idiosyncrasy but an attempt to show how the features of a condition may vary when the patients take a different view of the world, a consideration that applies to the study of depression in non-European cultures. In children, obvious biological immaturity is an important element; in non-European cultures, until recently, physical illness co-existing with, or actually causing depression, was an important factor. The somatization of depression is a feature common to both groups. The question of masked depression or depressive equivalents has also to be addressed in both traditional populations and children. The fact that depression had to be inferred from the behaviour of non-European adults finds an echo in child psychiatric practice where considerable discrepancies may exist between the assessments of teachers, parents and clinicians. It is said that 'adult' features of depression such as guilt, self-reproach and hopelessness are not found among children; the reasons for their absence in non-European cultures have been discussed in an earlier section. Moreover, one must remember childhood is not some unvarying and homogeneous age group. As the Rutter *et al.* (1970) study showed, as early childhood gives way to middle childhood and, then, adolescence, the pattern of depression may undergo a change. Non-specific features of depression give way to more recognizable features such as apathy, retardation and loss of appetite; then, to guilt and hopelessness and the increasing possibility of suicide. Here, intriguingly, the differences between childhood suicide and non-European suicide become more marked. The suicide of adolescents in European cultures becomes possible because the child more nearly approximates to the adult who kills himself – has a higher intelligence, a more mature conceptual framework, alienation from family or conflict with society, the possession of features of depression, e.g. guilt, which are associated in adults with suicidal ideas. In non-European suicidal acts, suicidal behaviour is impulsive and has much more to do with personal adversity, e.g. disappointments, betrayal, humiliations than with any feature of illness. It is interesting that the behaviour which is seen later in childhood bears the least similarity to non-European traditional culture.

This comparison between non-European depression and childhood depression is not meant to demean the former in any way. The comparison is used merely as a vehicle to discuss how those who take, in Western terms, a less complex and less sophisticated view of the world may present with an apparently different version of an illness which may eventually be seen to have common biological roots. The child makes up for his lack of neurobiological maturity with active fantasy; a person in a non-European culture compensates for lack of 'industrialized society' sophistication with a rich traditional source of myth and legend. The sophisticated approaches to child psychiatric disorder deserve to be extended to the study of depression in non-European cultures.

Depression in the elderly

Some aspects of the cognitive impairment associated with depression in the elderly were considered in Chapters 3 and 4. In this section attention will be paid to the course and symptomatology of depression in old age insofar as it differs from the general presentation of depression. Much of the work in this area was pioneered by Dr Felix Post, Emeritus Physician to the Bethlem Royal and Maudsley Hospitals, and as this discussion will show, his findings are still relevant to present-day considerations.

Dysphoric mood states in the elderly include minor mood disorders which are not associated with significant changes in behaviour, mild to moderate depressions which have a high incidence of neurotic symptoms, more severe depressions of a non-psychotic kind and severe, psychotic depressions. It is, of course, to be expected that depressions which have had an onset in earlier life may continue beyond the age of 65. Thus, milder but chronic depressions marked by neurotic features have an onset between 35 and 45 years, whereas the more severe depressions with a cyclical, self-limiting course have their onset between 55 and 65 years. Thus most depressions have had their onset before the senium, and the prevalence of depression diminishes after the age of 75. As was shown in the discussion in Chapter 1, all the features seen in younger patients may be seen with, perhaps, an increased incidence of hypochondriacal and somatic symptoms.

In a sample of in-patients, Post (1972) found that 37% had severe depression characterized by both retardation and agitation. There were problems with regard to food intake, loss of weight and insomnia. Delusions of worthlessness, poverty and personal hygiene were present. Ideas regarding bodily function were related to alimentary and urinary functions, the shrinking of organs, the emptiness of cavities and delusions of enormity. In a minority of patients there was severe retardation and mutism. 24% of patients were in an intermediate category with paranoid ideas and some delusional ideas, with the same content as described above. The rest (39%) were classed as 'neurotic' depressives. Here hypochondriacal ideas were common, though not of delusional intensity. Similarly, ideas of low self-esteem and self-reproach were present. These patients tended to blame others and showed histrionic behaviour. There was also importuning behaviour, restlessness and nocturnal disturbance. As the discussion in Chapter 7 showed, suicidal behaviour assumes greater importance in later life. Conversely, deliberate self-harm is reduced in incidence. 30% of all suicides are shown to occur after the age of 65, and only 5% of all cases of deliberate self-harm.

The follow-up of elderly depressive patients provides a less encouraging picture of prognosis than in the younger patient. Post found that over a 3-year follow-up, only 26% remained completely well. In 37% there were further bouts of depression characterized by good recovery, 25% had not recovered fully and carried with them such sequelae as insomnia, poor appetite, anxiety, hypochondriacal symptoms, and had made a poor social adjustment. 12% remained continuously ill. 4% had commited suicide and another 5% had made an attempt. Of serious adverse prognostic import was age over 70 years, the onset of dementia and serious non-cerebral physical disease.

Those elderly patients with depression do not appear to be more prone to any of the common neurological forms of dementia. This includes those patients whose cognitive dysfunction may amount to dementia, with reversal following treatment of the depression. A possible ameliorating effect of depression in dementia was the subject of speculation in Chapter 4.

The cognitive dysfunctions associated with depression have been discussed in Chapters 3 and 4. Although there are exceptions, the general features of depressives with cognitive deficits include greater age, later onset of depression, lower recovery from the illness, lower discharge rates and poor social adjustment (Cole and Hickie, 1976). A correlation between CAT scan changes and increased mortality on follow-up has been discussed in Chapter 3. It seems likely that remission in cognitive dysfunction in depressives over 60 years of age with a late onset of depression is limited, and some psychophysiological indices such as barbiturate sedation threshold, do not revert to normal in these patients (Cawley *et al.*, 1973).

In old age, the scope for adverse life events increases. The social, occupational and physical status of patients undergo an impairment. Bereavement, and geographical isolation from family and friends are other factors. Thus the interactionist hypothesis of the onset of depression (see Chapter 2) may be studied with profit. The stronger the genetic loading, the earlier depression occurs in general (Mendlewicz, 1976). Also, workers have noted a reduced morbidity risk in older patients. Thus the genetic contribution in the interactionist model is restricted, and a correspondingly more important role is played by environmental factors. Thus, up to 80% of patients may show evidence of exposure to life events. These include bereavements, physical illness (which may also have more specific effects other than being a life event), especially diseases of the heart and malignancy, financial loss including retirement, and such seemingly mundane events as moving house.

Murphy (1983) described a prospective study of elderly depressed patients and showed that in only a third of cases was there a good outcome. Poor outcome was associated with severity of initial illness, those with depressive delusions having a particularly poor outcome. Outcome was also influenced by physical health problems and severe life events in the follow-up year. There were also social class differences in the experience of severe life events. There was no evidence that an intimate relationship protected against relapse in the face of continuing life stress.

Over half of depressed patients were re-admitted within a year of their previous episode, considerable resources from the psychogeriatric services having to be devoted to caring for the relapsing group. Patients in Murphy's series had the full range of treatment in hospital, day hospital and out-patient settings, but the prognosis was as bad as Post had reported. She speculated that the less severe cases were now being successfully treated by general practitioners and only the more persistent or severe cases were referred to psychiatrists.

With the thrust of psychogeriatric care being in the community, there may be a change not merely in the emphasis of the service but in the prognosis. A cohort of patients is being established in Salford for the purposes of a follow-up study of depression in old age. The patients are seen first in their homes and referral is by the general practitioner. It appears that only a small minority of patients need to be admitted for in-patient care, a number that is expected to fall even further when a projected day hospital for the 'functionally' ill opens in the near future. The early impressions are that the prognosis of depression is by no means as bad as the figures of Post and Murphy lead one to fear. It may be true that the resolution of symptoms is not as complete as in the depression of younger patients, but social adjustment is better preserved if in-patient admission is avoided. It may well turn out that the crucial issue is in not breaking-up the social network of the patient by admitting him; restoring it is difficult. The later involvement of the GPs, community nurses and others is more difficult when this hiatus is present. With a 'functional' illness day hospital, out-patient ECT, attendance at day centres and a vigorous policy of rational pharmacotherapy, one suspects the picture may change substantially for the better.

An important point to note in most studies on the prognosis of depression of old age is the relationship between poor outcome and indifferent physical health. It is essential, therefore, to be aware of the possibility of existing physical illness, not something that comes naturally to many psychiatrists, either as a result of temperament or training. Murphy (1983) noted that the severity of the initial illness and the patient's continuing physical health took precedence as the two most important factors in determining the outcome of depression in old age.

9
Depressed mind, distinguished art: a pathography of depression

The belief that creative ability and insanity may be related in some way has been present for centuries. The romantic Aristotleian view of melancholia and the prowess for creating which left others in wonderment has been noted in Chapter 1, and mention was also made of the influence of that view at least into Elizabethan times. However, earlier pre-occupation was with the work and abilities of those with florid insanity, the demon of the demonstrably mad. Certainly in more recent times considerable evidence has been brought to bear in support of the view that schizophrenia in its florid form is *not* conducive to creative production. Schizophrenic artists, it is said, create in spite of, not because of, their illness, and this view, with one or two dissenting voices, is now the established one.

A more recent attempt has been to promote the notion that these strictures may apply to schizophrenia but that, on the contrary, depression and manic-depressive illness may have a facilitating role on creativity. A recent (*The Guardian*, 24 September 1984) such attempt was a report of a study by an American psychologist, Dr Kay Jamison, who surveyed British painters, sculptors, playwrights, poets and novelists. She found that half the poets had received some form of treatment for depression or mania, and that 38% of all her subjects had been on medication for such conditions. She was led to conclude that, overall, artists and writers are 35 times more likely to receive treatment for mood disorders than the general population.

Noll and Davis (1984) while commenting on the influence of depressive illness on the life and work of William James, the Huxleys, Virginia Woolf, Ernest Hemingway and Albert Einstein, quote from a recent review of the lives of 400 eminent people of the 20th century that 'there are many references to periods of acute depression in the biographies and autobiographies of eminent men and women'. They also remark that in the follow-up to the Stanford University study of gifted children, by the average age of 50, 22 of the original 1500 had died by suicide.

In a more recent report (*The Guardian*, 25 November 1985) of a survey undertaken by the National Centre for Orchestral Studies, half of British orchestra players surveyed in a study of anxiety in European orchestras said they had bouts of unexplained sadness.

However, this implied relationship between creativity and depression has been questioned by others. Indeed, in the last study quoted, a significant proportion of the players admitting to unexplained sadness said the mood change had an adverse effect on their performance. Levels of stress were considerably higher among British performers than Continental European ones, and the reasons given were not artistic but mundane. They blamed their heavier workload, the British players having twice as many engagements, inadequate rehearsal time and, frequently, bad conductors. 'The most important cause of stress is the conductor, most of whom are vastly overpaid and are in the main incompetent, and in quite a few cases downright vindictive.' There was no mention of this stress and the mood change it produced actually aiding virtuosity, so the attractive idea of precipitating dysphoria through a harsh environment in order to enhance creative ability finds no support. (It is not a very original idea; the public schools have been at it for years in order to strengthen character, and fluency in the classics and Euclid.)

An example of manic-depressive illness which did not assist creativity at all but stifled a career of established achievement was that of Vivien Leigh (1914–1967), who was married to Laurence Olivier, and whose life and work has been reviewed by Lasky and Silver (1978). Her first depressive episode was at the age of 30 following a miscarriage. The features of the depression were not unusual but Leigh, chain-smoking, drinking heavily, trying to keep pace with Olivier's energy, and refusing medical help, neglected herself. Soon, the early signs of tuberculosis appeared. Recovery from the chest complaint was followed by depression which, very soon, gave rise to rapidly alternating moods. She was about 38 when she became afflicted with frequently occurring manic illness. Her judgment and understanding were seriously impaired. And even though her tuberculosis was well established she continued with heavy smoking and drinking. Some drinking bouts precipitated mania. Pregnancy, miscarriage, a broken marriage and divorce followed in the next few years. The career was over; so was the marriage. Life was to end in 1967. She was 53. No reading of her biography could conceivably attribute any creative advantage in having a manic depressive illness.

More generally, Sir William Trethowan (1979) in his *Art of Madness* quotes the Wittkowers' investigation of the character and conduct of artists up to the time of the French Revolution. The Wittkowers (1963) were able to identify only a few who could be considered to be mentally ill, and these, for the most part, suffered from melancholia. They were able to discover only 14 suicides (four of them doubtful) among European artists between the years 1350 and 1800, and most of these occurred towards the end of the period and none before the year 1500. Eliot Slater (1979) in a study of 27 German musicians – as a preliminary to the wider study of German creative genius – found only one, Robert Schumann, who seemed to have had recurrent depressive illness.

228

Lewis (1961), in a characteristically sceptical contribution, pointed to mental illness being a common affliction and said unless it could be shown to exist significantly more frequently in men of genius than in the general population matched for age, sex and nationality, its occasional appearance in the former could not be taken as indicating a common root for genius and illness. He referred to the work of Catherine Cox and Professor Terman who collected full biographical data in some 300 of the most eminent people who had lived since 1450, eminence being reflected in the space allocated to such individuals in encyclopaedias and reference books. They concluded the majority of persons were above average in terms of both character and social attributes, and did not differ significantly from the average in their emotional make-up and control. He also referred to the work of Dr Adele Juda (also cited by Eliot Slater) who collected the most eminent scientists and artists of the German-speaking countries since 1650. This was a cosmopolitan group including artists, sculptors, architects, musicians, poets, scientists, theologians, philosophers, historians, jurists, Field Marshals, statesmen and inventors. Taking the artists, she found more than two-thirds of them were free from psychological abnormality. An eighth had a history of psychotic disorder, but in virtually all cases this was due to organic brain disease of late-onset. Neurotic and psychopathic disease had been present in less than a third. Psychiatric disorder in parents, sibs, children and in second degree relationships did not appear to be significantly increased. All in all, the data indicated, to a remarkable extent, that artists and their families were free from mental disorder.

The mental make-up of scientists was even more impressive. Three-quarters of them were free from any mental abnormality, and only 4% showed manic-depressive illness. Neurotic disorders and personality disorders occurred chiefly among the philosophers. Furthermore, there was a diminution, or suspension, of creative activity during spells of manic and depressive illness with full restoration on recovery. Studies of parents and children of scientists showed an even smaller incidence of mental disease and psychopathic disorder than amongst the relatives of artists. An intermediate group of professional men showed much the same incidence of mental illness and psychopathic disorders. The conclusion reached by Juda (quoted by Lewis, 1961) is that 'there is no definite relationship between the highest mental capacity and mental health or illness and no evidence to support the assumption that the genesis of the highest intellectual ability depends on psychological abnormalities....'

A pervasive problem in studies such as these is that the term depression is used in so many different senses and, certainly in non-technical studies and texts which provide much of the data for diagnosis, is not necessarily to be equated with the strict diagnostic term. Furthermore, diagnostic differences between countries, cultures and across centuries would appear to mount formidable obstacles in the way of accurate diagnoses. Even if it is alleged that so many poets had been on psychotropic medication, this is less than conclusive evidence, given the widespread use – and abuse – of such drugs, not least in the ability of those with creative gifts to obtain and abuse prescribed and unprescribed drugs. Suicide is a behaviour so enormously

229

influenced by socio-cultural factors that its relationship to depression – often established by retrospective inference – must always be moot. In any historical survey, the near impossibility of a re-creation of the state of society and its cultural values must be taken into account. Did suicides occur more commonly in the harsh market place in which artists competed unsheltered by social welfare, Arts Council grants and creative writing fellowships? Or was society so strictly constrained by a myriad taboos that suicide was a rare event even in the midst of unimaginable deprivation and poverty? Or are geniuses never simply bound by any such considerations applicable to the common man?

The point about the essential sanity of genius is made by Charles Lamb in his essay on the *Sanity of True Genius* (1833):

> So far from the position holding true that great wit has a necessary alliance with insanity, the greatest wits, on the contrary, will ever be found to be the sanest writers .... The greatness of wit, by which the poetic talent is here chiefly to be understood, manifests itself in the admirable balance of all faculties. Madness is the disproportionate straining or excess of any of them ... the ground of the mistake is that men, finding in the raptures of the higher poetry a condition of exaltation, to which they have no parallel in their own experience, besides the spurious resemblance in dreams and fevers, impute a state of dreaminess and fever to the poet. But the true poet dreams being awake. He is not possessed by his subject but has dominion over it.

The essence of Lamb's thesis is the incomprehensibility of creative genius and its products to lesser mortals. It finds an echo in a feature which bedevils the whole of psychiatric practice, the necessary distinction that needs to be drawn between abnormality, in a statistical sense, and pathology. It implies the existence of attitudes to non-conformism which finds parallels from history to the present day, and one manifestation of recent public concern has followed the ascribing of political and religious dissent in parts of Eastern Europe to the presence in the dissenter of mental disorder. If, as with the creative process, the final product of a state of mind is an abnormal production, i.e. something that is not generally to be produced by the preponderant majority of members of a society, then comprehension is sought in deeming that mind to be pathological. Political and religious dissent are obvious subjects from the pages of history, but two other examples of some interest to psychiatrists come from the attitudes of society to witchcraft and homosexuality. Both sets of attitudes had political, religious, social, cultural and legal overtones. In both the legal and medical world viewpoints overlapped. In both, a harsh legalistic interpretation of the abnormality was opposed by an apparently enlightened, medical point of view – 'They need treatment'. Abnormality in behaviour, even when it involves the production of aesthetic or creative merit, is readily understood, therefore, in terms of the pathology of the mind. The other, and by no means invalid interpretation is in terms of envy. If mental illness used to be a social stigma, not merely those who dissent, are awkward or wicked, such as dissenters, rebels, subversives, witches and homosexuals, but those who create beyond our imagination or understanding may be seen to be mad, and we may thus find solace in our inability to match or compete with them. The extraordinary deference to royalty and others with inherited wealth and privilege may be compared to the envy and hostility that is directed against the prosperity and material success of neighbours and colleagues. The former cannot help it; we, for our part, were not born lucky, so there is nothing we can do, and there is no point in complaining. The exalted state of our neighbours is, on the other hand, a constant reminder of what we might have been, or had; it kindles a feeling of guilt as well. To see the gifted in terms of madness is to see them in constitutional terms, to use a pun, and that restores our wellbeing.

Be that as it may, some associations of depression – the mood, the personality, the drive to work to avoid depression and so on – may have a facilitatory influence on creativity unconnected with depression as an illness. It is these factors which we must examine to seek why depression continues to be held as being helpful to the creative process. In order to do this, we must first consider some psychological aspects of the creative process.

SOME PSYCHOLOGICAL ASPECTS OF THE CREATIVE PROCESS

One may note the psychological factors which are relevant to the role the symptomatology and associated factors of depression may play in the creative process.

There is a speculative link between the slowing of conscious processes in sleep and the psychomotor retardation of depressive illness. The synthetic function of sleep and dreams is attested to in the work especially on REM sleep. There are also well documented – and wellknown – examples of creative discovery during pre-sleep, sleep and dreaming. These are described by Koestler (1964), and it is instructive to compare the state in which these discoveries arise with the mental state in depression. Henri Poincare, the French mathematician, has described how he came by his discovery of the theory of Fuchsian functions. For 15 days he had striven to disprove this theory. Then one evening he took an unaccustomed late night drink of black coffee and could not sleep. Ideas crowded his mind and, very much as in a hypnagogic state, collided with each other to combine in a whole. By the next morning he had established a class of Fuchsian functions. The creative process, which had started off in the period between sleeping and waking, did not end there. Over the next few weeks sudden insights – resembling, in effect, primary delusional experiences – helped Poincare make further connections. In the first, he went on a journey and at the moment he placed his foot on a bus the idea came to him, without any prior notice, that the transformations he had used to define the Fuchsian functions were identical to those of non-Euclidean geometry. He then turned his attention to other matters but, frustrated by the lack of success, took himself off to the seaside and attempted to forget his work. One morning, while walking, the idea occurred to him with 'just the same characteristics of brevity, suddenness and immediate certainty' that the

231

arithmetic transformations of indeterminate ternary quadratic forms were identical to those of non-Euclidean geometry. Poincare notes, 'most striking at first is this appearance of sudden illumination, a manifest sign of long, unconscious prior work. The role of this unconscious work in mathematical invention appears to me incontestable . . .'.

Three separate ideas were connected by an idea which sprang in a state of pre-sleep. A more direct relationship to dreams in a state of sleep is illustrated by the example of Friedrich August Von Kekulé, Professor of Chemistry in Ghent, who in 1865 fell asleep and dreamt what became acknowledged as a major advance in organic chemistry. He dreamt atoms were dancing before him. These atoms became larger and of various configurations, long rows of them, some far apart and others closely fitted together. They became entwined and twisted in snake-like fashion. Then, suddenly, one of the snakes had seized hold of its own tail and the form danced. At this point Kekulé awoke. The image of the snake swallowing its tail had given him the idea that the benzene molecule was not an 'open' structure but 'closed'.

Neuroscience has its own example in Otto Loewe's discovery in 1920 of the chemical basis to neural transmission. This involves not pre-sleep or dreams but the process of sleep itself. One night he awoke, turned on the light and jotted down his thoughts on a piece of paper. Then he fell back into sleep and awoke again at 6am. The feeling crept on him that he might have written down something during the night but, to his chagrin, he could not decipher his scrawl. However, the next night, actually at 3am., the idea returned and, fortunately, Loewe awakened fully. It was the experimental design to fit the hypothesis of chemical transmission he had enunciated some 17 years before. He went to his laboratory straight away and put the design to the test on a frog's heart – showing essentially that the nerve endings when stimulated produced acetyl choline which when collected in the solution in which the heart lay slowed another heart without further neural stimulation. There is an addendum to this anecdote. 35 years later, Loewe, while preparing a bibliography of all the work involving his laboratory, found that the 'nocturnal design' did not spring *ab ovo* from the dark, but the process of sleep had actually synthesized these early experiments with the hypothesis of 1903 to produce the idea that made him wake-up and run to the laboratory. He commented that, 'most so-called 'intuitive' discoveries are such associations suddenly made in the unconscious mind'.

Lewis (1961), while disputing that the psychiatrically disturbed can be capable of creative scientific thought which requires preparation, incubation, illumination and verification, has pointed to how a transient toxic disturbance may produce illumination in an otherwise 'normal' mind which has carried on with the business of preparation and incubation. He gives the example of Alfred Russel Wallace, the co-begetter with Charles Darwin of the theory of evolution by natural selection, who found the solution to his questions during a bout of malarial fever. A more literary example is the process by which Coleridge's remarkable poem *Kubla Khan* was composed. In the summer of 1797 Coleridge took two grains of opium

232

to check an attack of dysentery. He then either fell asleep or drifted into a state of disturbed consciousness – 'a reverie', in his own words. At the moment he was drifting into one or other states, he was reading an account of how the Kubla Khan had commanded a stately palace with a garden to be built. During the state of changed consciousness, images of places and monuments and general grandeur floated through his mind. On awakening, or recovering, he recollected the whole and wrote the entire account of the *Kubla Khan*. He did not actually finish his composition for he was interrupted, by what appears to have been a commercial traveller from Porlock in Somerset, and held up by this person for an hour. When Coleridge returned to his composition after the visitor had left, he found the inspiration had vanished except for a handful of lines and images.

It thus appears, in anecdotal terms at least, that processes of disturbed consciousness, pre-sleep, dreams, toxic confusion or other may aid the creative process. There is in all these states a distinct change in the mental state. However, in depression, a cardinal feature is the preservation of consciousness, but the point that is being argued is that even if a patient and his mental processes are inaccessible, it does not necessarily follow that the mind is fallow – creation and synthesis might be going on. It is readily conceded that in relation to depression this hypothesis appears, at present, excessively speculative, but the analogy is at least capable of helping us understand. Moreover, the actual execution of creative ideas takes place only on recovery from states of disturbed consciousness, and this appears to hold true for depression also. In trying to examine a possible relationship between depression and creativity, we may not actually suggest execution of ideas – by which creativity is judged – in the phase of depressed mood. As Kretschmer noted, creative production tends to emerge from a 'psychic twilight', a state of lowered consciousness and diminished attention to external stimuli. The example of Virginia Woolf in a later section may convince us that a latent process of creative activity goes on while mental functions are apparently in abeyance.

THE ABNORMAL PERSONALITY: THE PROPENSITY TO DEPRESSION

Creative expression and the production of what is deemed to be exalted is abnormal in the statistical sense. It is logical to assume that some, if not most, of those engaged in such creative activity will have personalities which must be at some variance with the general population's, whose members are not destined for such creative distinction. This is indeed the case, as the incidence of abnormal personality is considerably greater than the incidence of psychosis, including manic-depressive illness. It is a common observation that depression, even if not of illness proportions, is commonly to be found in such individuals. Obviously, these individuals can become depressed like anyone else. However, the more usual picture is a somewhat more equivocal one – the mood change is less permanent, the response to the environment much more marked, the response to treatment less definite. Much ink has been consumed in arguing whether such a picture amounted to a form of depression. Nevertheless, there is little doubt that creative persons with an abnormal outlook are prone to such dysthymia.

One reason for this is that they are constantly at odds with the rest of society. The non-conformity of genius is generally acknowledged. Samuel Butler noted that the characteristic of genius was not, as Carlyle had remarked, a transcendent capacity for taking trouble but a transcendent capacity for getting its possessor *into* trouble and keeping him there. Lewis (1961) quotes Butler:

> Genius points to change, and change is a hankering after another world, so the old world suspects it. It disturbs order; it unsettles mores and hence it is immoral ... the uncommon sense of genius and the common sense of the rest of the world are thus as husband and wife to one another; they are always quarrelling and common sense, who must be taken as the husband, always fancies himself the master.

Being at odds with the world is a consequence of being a law unto oneself. The refusal to accept the established rules leads to exceptional creation; it also leads to exceptional characters not always so acceptable to their compatriots who might be as underwhelmed by the man as they are overwhelmed by the work. Slater (1979), in his descriptions of the personality disorders in composers, has given a graphic account of character and behaviour which may lead to unhappiness and isolation. Beethoven lived in unnecessary squalor; he was quarrelsome, miserly, sadistic, pinched and bit his pupils, was paranoid all his life, was totally self-centred, ruthless, inconsiderate, impulsive, lacking self-control, was prudish and unscrupulous in his financial dealings. The remarkable thing, of course, is the controlled, scrupulous genius one sees in his music. However, it must seem obvious that such a person will find isolation and occasional misery, though it may not amount to definable illness. Other composers who are described in a similar vein are Schubert and Wilhelm Friedemann Bach, and an impressive list of great musical psychopaths would include these three plus Brückner, Liszt, Mahler, Pfitzner, Johann Strauss the younger, Wagner and Wolf.

There are more modern examples of abnormal personality associated with exceptional creative gifts. In the biography of Peter Sellers by his children (Sellers *et al.*, 1981), a clear account of a grossly abnormal personality but no discernible formally diagnosable depressive illness emerges. Sellers was often miserable; he was also superstitious, jealous, possessive, hypochondriacal, violent and vindictive. The penalty incurred for his genius, according to his children, had to be paid for by the family which absorbed like a buffer 'whims and insanities of his incredibly complex character which would change faster than the colours of the chameleon'. The undisputed genius could give way to 'horrific black depressive moods (which) descended abruptly upon him and turned him into a snarling, malevolent beast, convinced the family and the world were against him'. He was a man totally absorbed in his work. Not only did he immerse himself in the total identity of the character he was playing, mannerisms, voice,

234

personality and all, he lived the character, unable to switch off when he came home from the studios. When he played a screen villain, the realistic portrayal of the character at home terrified the family. They did not think it was the extension of the acting. When not working, he became restless and easily bored. The desperately insecure and unhappy man had to be taken with the undisputed genius. A recent, and living, example has made this self-confession (Omar Sharif, *Sunday Times Magazine*, 13 October 1985): 'I'm very moody, in fact this probably is my greatest defect and probably the reason why I'm unable to live with someone in the same house under the same roof. I have no idea what causes my moodiness but I can be happy and cheerful and then turn sombre and not want to see anyone.

Kretschmer summarized the personality of genius:

> Men of genius show in their psychological (make-up) an unusual instability and hypersensitiveness, together with a very considerable liability to psychoses, neuroses and psychopathic complaints ... the loosening of mental structure, the hypersensitiveness to fine distinctions and remote relations, the frequent bizarre play of contrasts in the inmost parts of the personality – all these things are conditioned by the passionate quality of genius, its restlessness, internal production and its immense intellectual range, are part of the daemonic element which is identical with the psychopathic structures in the personality ... for some types of genius, this inner dissolution of the mental structure is an indispensable prelude.

Kretschmer was led to the conclusion,

> ... were we to remove the psychopathic inheritance, the daemonic unrest and mental tension from the constitution of the man of genius, nothing but an ordinary talented person would remain. The more one studies of biographies, the more one is driven to the viewpoint that the psychopathic component is not merely a regrettable, non-essential accident of biological structure but an intrinsic and necessary part, an indispensable catalyst, perhaps, for every form of genius in the strict sense of the term.

DEPRESSED MOOD AND CREATION

It is interesting to ask if the depressed mood itself can give rise to creativity. An up-to-date example is Karlheinz Stockhausen (Profile, *The Observer*, 22 September 1985), the avant garde musical composer. Despite a family history – his mother had severe, recurrent depression, dying of a mental illness – he has no definite history of depressive illness. However, he is described as solitary, self-righteous, overbearing, intolerant of criticism or opposition and falling out with his friends. In 1968, he had a 'personal crisis' which brought him near to suicide, 'but', the profile notes, 'as usual, he turned the experiences to positive creative use, recreating his 'dark night of the soul' in *Aus den sieben Tagen*, a wholly improvizational collaboration'.

Beethoven was grief-stricken when he had to relinquish guardianship of his nephew, Karl. The slow movement of his last quartet *opus 135 – 'lento assai cantante e tranquillo'* – was described by Stravinsky as 'grief-music', the second variation as a 'dirge' and the fourth variation as portraying impending death.

It would appear that individual incidents provoking or associated with sorrow or grief may lead to portrayal in creative works. It is possible that the known presence of these mood states – or following the discovery of the incidents leading to the creative act – have led to suggestions that creative artists have been suffering from depressive illness.

It is also commonplace to make the distinction between schizophrenia and manic-depressive illness partly on the full recovery that is allegedly invariably seen in the latter. Schizophrenia leaves its mark on the personality; depressive illness, however severe, leaves the character preserved in its previous essentials. Literary comparisons are made with the darkness – *'the dark night of the soul'* – with the implication that when daylight resumed, there would be no trace of the previous night. This may or may not be true as regards ordinary individuals' affliction, but there is reason to suspect the persistent influence of depression in some creative individuals. At the age of 50 Tolstoy suffered a significant depressive illness which appears to have produced a considerable change in his attitudes (Plokker, 1964). He began to advocate non-violence, voluntary poverty and asceticism. His marriage suffered as he inflicted his views on his wife, and his view of marriage in his creative work underwent a transformation. The portrayal of marital love and happiness in *War and Peace* gave way to a highly critical account of marriage and sexuality in the *The Kreutzer Sonata*, it is alleged, as a result of the change wrought by depression. Lewis (1961) referred to the effects of a 3-year depressive illness in Fechner, the philosopher. In literature, the analogy seems to be not between night and day but between death and rebirth, where there is a necessary, and sometimes essential connection, between the two states. Koestler (1964) notes that works including Coleridge's *The Ancient Mariner*, Morgan's *The Fountain*, T.S. Eliot's *The Waste Land*, D.H. Lawrence's *The Plumed Serpent* and *The Man who Died*, all of E.M. Forster's major novels, the great Russian and German literature, the works of Kierkegaard and Sartre have considered the idea of conversion, or where a hero or heroine goes through some kind of emotional fire and emerges as a changed character.

We may also note at this point the relationship between creativity and self-destruction. Lockspeiser (1973) quotes T.S. Eliot on Baudelaire: 'He had the pride of a man who feels in himself great weakness and great strength. Having great genius ... he had neither the patience nor the inclination, had he had the power, to overcome his weakness; on the contrary he exploited it for theoretical purposes'. Lockspeiser believes this explanation serves for the self-destructive impulses in such creative individuals as Debussy, Schoenberg, Berg, Stravinsky, Monet and Van Gogh.

CREATIVITY AS AN ANTIDEPRESSANT

It is a common observation that those who are creatively gifted also seem to be endowed with superior reserves of energy. The sentiment that genius is 1% inspiration and 99% perspiration, however, appears to be necessary not merely for the production of creative works of unique quality but to provide the practitioner's mental state with a stability that may not be possible in a state of idleness or non-work. This drive to exertion or creation has been discussed by Storr (1972, 1983). Storr's essential thesis is that persons of high creative ability may seek satisfaction or solace in work, whereas most ordinary people seek a parallel satisfaction in relationships with other people. Failing to find meaning and value in personal relationships, the personality disordered artist may turn to creation. The ensuing creative work, and the talents that go to make it, is valued by society and the individual finds satisfaction in this curious multi-pronged relationship. Depressives, failing to find satisfaction in ordinary human relationships, compensate by attempts to earn acclaim and vicarious love through their work, and the more distinguished the work, the more clamorous the public recognition. Whereas ordinary human beings find fulfilment in the bosoms of their families, and their self-esteem on the love received from these close relationships, depressives, denied this, seek it in the self-esteem that follows public recognition of their worth.

A slightly different point is to inquire whether depressives actually avoid depression through work that leads to creation. A case in point is Winston Churchill. Both Churchill and his father, Lord Randolph, were subject to depression, referred to by Churchill as his 'Black Dog'. Two particular episodes in his life led to a significant lowering of his mood – in one he was incapacitated by the Boers who had captured and imprisoned him. Lack of action neither prevented nor could relieve the depression. However, a prolonged period of disappointment came his way between the two world wars. This was preceded, in 1915, when, having been made a scapegoat for the failure of the Dardanelles campaign, he had to leave the government. When the war came to an end, the man of action was understimulated and in despair, described in a memorable phrase as a 'world of monstrous shadows, moving in convulsive combinations through vistas of fathomless catastrophe'. It was at this time he added the hobbies of painting and bricklaying to the accomplished art of authorship. At the age of 42, he learned painting while the Dardanelles commission was still considering his future. He had lost both public office and influence. He was frustrated in every direction and depression threatened.

His painting was influenced by Sir John Lavery who was painting his portrait at the time. Churchill found that when he painted his concentration was directed on his art; he could not think of anything else. He could not dwell on his problems; there was an escape from arguments and justifications he would face and have to resort to if he went in search of company, and he found the relief in painting almost beyond belief. His paintings, vigorous and colourful landscapes, developed to the extent that he won the praise of professionals and he sold four pictures at a show in Paris in 1921. They were seascapes with impressions of sunshine falling in water from a stormy sky. Churchill also turned to bricklaying and, learning it well, joined the Amalgamated Union of Building Trade Workers. These activities were in addition to the reading and writing he did at a phenomenal rate all during his life.

Adversity of a different kind was the constant pressure for the 5 years of the second world war that involved him at the very top. There is no evidence of depression in that period. To counter Lord Moran's allegation that impending senile decline might have assailed Churchill during the war, several of those who worked with him collaborated on a book (Wheeler-Bennett, 1968). These writers, who worked with him as both war and peace-time prime minister, agree on his voracious appetite for work. They saw him virtually every day, and are unanimous in the view that Moran was mistaken, seeing Churchill as he did in ill-health, not being part of the 'secret circle' and being handicapped by his own pre-conceptions. The essentials of the physical illnesses and the *later* disabilities due to strokes are also established. Changes in mood seem well in keeping within the normal range for the average human being. There is no evidence of any depression or purely psychogenic malaise. On the contrary, one of the contributors notes, 'he was quite impervious to depression, despair or indeed the sinking of the morale which assails people when the news is constantly bad and disaster looms ahead'.

The nearest one gets to a picture of dejection is after the 1945 general elections which his party lost – a rejection he took personally, although all the evidence even then pointed to an astonishing degree of personal affection for him, but which did not extend to his party which was not thought up to making the reforms the British people desired after the long struggle and the sacrifices of the war years. Moran's descriptions were made by a doctor who saw the patient when he was ill; he was also a physician, most sensitive to physical illness. Churchill's subordinates were with him when he was at his most active and vigorous. Neither might have seen him when he was depressed. In any case, there is no independent account of depression in Churchill in the war years. For a man who had no doubt of the reality of the 'Black Dog', a phenomenal capacity for work both in public and private life seems to have succeeded in staving off depression.

It has been suggested that Michelangelo might have been depressive (Storr, 1983), on the basis of his sonnets and his self-portrait which is seen upon the flayed skin held up by St Bartholomew in *The Last Judgment*. We are fortunate in have a rare *contemporary* account by Vasari (1550). This is percipient, if somewhat hagiographical. The evidence for depression or illness suggestive of an affective state is scant or non-existent. The evidence for personality abnormality – quite apart from homosexuality – is clearer. Vasari notes Michelangelo had an excellent constitution with strong nerves. However, he appears to have been a solitary individual, not at ease in the company of ordinary folk but seeking and apparently enjoying the company of the learned. Even this pursuit of solitude is deemed a virtue – he could work undisturbed – 'to produce works of merit, the artist must be free from cares and anxieties. Art does not permit wandering of the mind'. That he might have avoided depression through artistic exertion appears to be a more valid speculation. An austere man who needed little sleep, Michelangelo usually worked through the night. He hated idleness and when, in old age, he could not paint any longer, he worked on a piece of marble from which he tried to extract a larger than life Pieta. He died at the age of 89, working till about 6 days before his death.

Cynicism or clinical concern alone must not inform our inquiry. Even such a man as Haydn, disordered in personality and subject to depression, could have a higher motive than avoiding mere pathology in creating some wondrous work for our benefit.

> Often when I have struggled with obstacles of all kinds – when the forces of my spirit and body were sunken – a secret voice whispered to me: 'There are on earth so few happy and contented human beings, so many persecuted ones, in sorrow and in pain – perhaps your work will turn into a fountain from which the down hearted may, for a few moments at least, drink some recreation and find peace'.

Other people's misery and pain may also inspire composition.

Samuel Johnson and his 'circle'

Another interesting example of a creatively able individual who kept himself busy in order to avoid depression was Samuel Johnson. There was a family history of depression and Wain (1974) has noted how Johnson *père*, a bookseller, would fight off depression by riding off for orders. In Johnson's case the onset was early, at the age of 20. As Boswell (1791) records,

> He felt himself overwhelmed with a horrible hypochondria, with perpetual irritation, fretfulness and impatience; and with a dejection, gloom and despair, which made existence misery. From this dismal malady he never afterwards was perfectly relieved, and all his labour, and all his enjoyments, were but temporary interruptions of its baleful influence.

Johnson's chosen weapon to fight this mental anguish, as Boswell put it, was work, including activity of every kind and the active pursuit of society. Johnson advised his friends against idleness. He feared the 'stagnant idleness' of his mind not merely because of the misery, but also because obsessional religious thoughts might intrude. As Wain (1974) notes, by the time Johnson was 20, two factors had entered his life and stayed there – one was the fear of a disabling depression, the other an imaginatively terrifying view of Christianity.

Work and conversation he tried, to keep his misery at bay, conversation helping by taking him away from solitude.

The depressions he had were typical. His energy would fail, his spirits decline, he would be disinclined or unable to do anything, staring incessantly at the clock without being able to read it, and anxiety and distress came to occupy his mind. Boswell records the episode in 1766, the year after Johnson completed his monumental edition of Shakespeare,

> ... an illness overwhelmed him. It was something in the nature of a nervous collapse ... his will deserted him; he lay on his bed for weeks on end, and gloomy forebodings gnawed incessantly at his mind.

Associated with his depression there were ritualistic features, which remained, to some extent, even when he was relatively well.

239

Going along a street in which there were posts, he would carefully lay his hand on each one as he passed ... also he made a ritual of entering or leaving a door or passage in such a way as to take a certain number of steps to reach a certain point.

Johnson's circle of friends included William Cowper, William Collins and Christopher Smart, all of whom were depressives. William Cowper (1731–1800) a sensitive child to begin with, suffered from depression from early in his life. An extremely sensitive man, he had difficulty in coping with stress of any kind and broke down, attempting suicide, when he was about to be interviewed for a clerkship in the House of Lords. His recurrent depressions had religious themes with strong feelings of guilt and self-reproach. Later in his life he became engaged to a widow, the event itself provoking another depressive breakdown and a further suicidal attempt. The later death of this widow produced a severe depression which never lifted in the last 4 years of his life. Some have seen in his poems a pre-occupation with man's helplessness and isolation, symbolized by images of storms and shipwrecks. In *Human Frailty*, the last stanza reads,

But oars alone can ne'er prevail
To reach the distant coast;
The breath of heaven must swell the sail,
Or all the toil is lost.

Cowper has been described as 'meek and unassuming'. In 1792, '... his finances were now increased by a grant from royal munificence of 300 pounds a year; but such was the state of his mind, that he was disabled from receiving any enjoyment at the disclosure of the circumstance'. In the somewhat morbid, *The Castaway*, written in the last few years of his life, he concludes,

No voice divine the storm allayed,
No light propitious shone;
When, snatched from all effectual aids,
We perished, each alone:
But I beneath a rougher sea,
And whelmed in deeper gulfs than he.

Samuel Johnson said of William Collins (1721–59), '(he) languished some years under that depression of mind which enchains the faculties without destroying them, and leaves reason the knowledge of right without the power of pursuing it'. A somewhat slothful and feckless man all his life – he was pronounced too indolent even for the army – the work by which he is remembered was done before the age of 32 when he became mentally ill. He never made a full recovery.

Christopher Smart (1722—71) first fell ill in 1756 and was admitted to an asylum. He spent 4 years in private asylums, and appears to have had marked obsessional and compulsive symptoms, which included the compulsion to pray publicly and recruit others, including Samuel Johnson, into doing so with him. In 1763, he was discharged from the asylum and published *A Song to David*. In the poem there is a mathematical and mystical ordering of stanzas grouped in threes, fives and sevens, which was compared by Robert Browning to the structure of a cathedral.

Virginia Woolf (1882–1941)

The life and work of Virginia Woolf is the subject of the outstanding literary biography by her nephew, Quentin Bell (1972). Not surprisingly, there was a significant family history of depressive behaviour, if not illness. As with Samuel Johnson's father, Virginia Woolf's father appeared to counteract a 'weakness of character' by prodigious efforts at work. The man was a grim and negative character, much given to pessimistic brooding and pre-occupations with his griefs and disappointments. 'The very strength of (his family) was rooted in weakness; the prodigious capacity for hard work, the ability to take risks, the athletic feats were but the sorties of a garrison that has no walls.' (Bell, 1972). The two volumes provide a telling description of the chequered life of even an upper middle class family with some privilege at the turn of the century. There is a long catalogue of illness, bereavement and disappointment and how anyone, let along a highly sensitive girl, could hope for a well-balanced and stable personality will remain a mystery to most readers. As soon as she makes what appears to be a Herculean effort and relates to someone, winning their trust, he or she seems to die. Her first breakdown, at the age of 13, was preceded by her mother's death, her father's prolonged mourning which showed many signs of pathological grief and her sexual molestation at the hands of a half-brother. Depression intermingled with marked anxiety, and physical symptoms were prominent. She became depressed, irritable, excitable, her pulse raced, she was terrified of meeting people in the street, was given to morbid self-criticism, and self-blame and compared herself unfavourably with her sister.

The second breakdown was at the age of 22, and followed her father's last illness, his death and a state of exhaustion. Once again depression, anxiety and physical symptoms emerged. Auditory hallucinations, imperative in character, appeared for the first time. Thinking these might be due to overeating, she decided to starve herself. To her birds sang in Greek and King Edward VII lurked in the bushes mouthing obscene imprecations. Improvement in her mental state was slow, headaches persisted, but optimism returned and with it an overenergetic phase. She seems to have been at her best, in terms of mood, whilst working and, coming to the end of a novel, she was assailed by doubt and anxiety.

In 1908, she began work on *Melymbrosia*, which eventually turned into *The Voyage Out*. In March 1912 *The Voyage Out* was completed, submitted to the publishers and accepted without delay. Whilst waiting for it to appear, she was stricken with doubt. Her whole meaning and purpose in life was heading for judgment and she was quite plainly terrified of the adverse criticism that might be directed against her work, and thereby at her. The insomnia, headache and anxiety re-appeared, as did her depression and feelings of guilt. Her family feared another suicidal attempt. The delusions were bizarre – not only was she convinced she would be punished for her

241

actions which had been proclaimed by the guilt, she believed that her body, especially her mouth and belly, had become a disgusting and monstrous entity. Misinterpretations were common. She took 100 grams of Veronal, a dose which could have been lethal, and nearly died while being resuscitated. Certification and committal to an asylum were considered but rejected in favour of private care. Those around her had no doubts as to the precipitating cause of this bout of illness – 'It is the novel which has broken her up'. The anxiety and apprehension regarding its acceptance by the world at large seemed to counteract the apparently stabilizing effect of her marriage. When a 'delicate mind' such as Virginia's came across such a stress, the family were not surprised pathology was a likely outcome.

Her recovery from this bout of illness was slow, but within 3 years a manic phase ensued. Violent screaming, incoherent garrulity and an animosity towards her husband were the chief symptoms. Recovery was very slow and the sequel was that her personality appeared changed at first, especially in regard to her husband and other men. Her circle feared that this might be permanent. Not only were her attacks of madness becoming more frequent and more severe, but her character appeared changed. However, her book received generous praise, and she responded so well to this that her (and the family's) fears were seen to be unfounded. It was widely believed the favourable notices accorded her first book played an important part in her gradual return to normality.

The effects she had experienced after the completion of her first novel made her choice of the subject matter of the second work a more modest affair. In the final chapters of her first book, *The Voyage Out*, some of the torment in her mind had been relieved by expression. That, the effort of the work, and most of all, the doubts and uncertainties as to how the work might be received had driven her into insanity. She looked for something to write that would not provoke her mind into an untoward response. It is said this alternation between the ambitious and, hence, dangerous with the modest and, even, pedestrian was to be a feature for the rest of her life. Thus the lightweight would follow the profound; *Orlando* follows *To the Lighthouse*, *Flush* follows *The Waves* and *Three Guineas* follow *The Years*. *Night and Day* was considered a recuperative work.

Her recovery and subsequent stability did not prevent her apprehension when *Night and Day* was published. The signs of impending breakdown were there but they did not progress to the same extent as after her first novel. By 1923 she is thought to have completely regained her previous self. Between June 1925 and December 1928, Virginia Woolf, in what was for her a normal state, conceived her two most outstanding works, *To the Lighthouse* and *The Waves*.

Bell makes this point as regards the influence of depression on Virginia Woolf's creativity.

> The evidence suggests (it does no more) that Virginia ... could profit by her illnesses. She needed to 'float with the sticks on the stream; helter-skelter with the dead leaves on the lawn, irresponsible and disinterested and able; perhaps for the first time in years, to look around, to look up – to look, for example, at the sky.

But she also needed, if she were to cope with the exacting task of describing that which she had seen in the heavens, to be well. In 1913 she had not been strong enough to cope with her vision, but in the years between 1925 and 1932 she was just healthy enough to cope with her own maladies. Nevertheless, the effort was considerable.

In 1929, following a trip to Germany, she fell unwell again. For 6 weeks she could not work. But she considered this fallow period almost a necessary preparation for the creative endeavour that would follow.

> If I could stay in bed another fortnight ... I believe I could see the whole of *The Waves* ... I believe these illnesses are in my case – how shall I express it? – partly mystical. Something happens in my mind. It refuses to go on registering impressions. It shuts itself up. It becomes a chrysalis. I lie quite torpid, often with acute physical pain – as last year; only discomfort this. Then suddenly something springs.

Robert Schumann

Robert Schumann's medical history holds much fascination, not least because of the changing diagnoses that were made in regard to it. For nearly a century the diagnosis of schizophrenia was considered until Slater and Meyer (1959) more or less established that a recurrent depressive illness with general paresis had been the probable diagnosis.

Schumann's depressive illness had its onset before the age of 30. A more severe episode came on about the age of 34. Both were characterized by severe depressions and anxiety with marked somatic features. The latter included such features as fainting, fear of heights, fear of being poisoned and fear of insanity and other illness including cholera. He also hallucinated the muscial note A and, during the first episode of illness, tried to jump from the fourth floor of his lodgings, but was restrained.

The effects of Schumann's illness on his creativity are particularly noteworthy. During the second episode of depression he lost interest in music and could not even remember musical ideas as he forced himself to compose. Schumann's reputation lies on what he created between the ages of 23 and 33. Thereafter, paralleling the change in his personality was a decline in creative productivity. Elevated mood was associated with increase in output. The inhibiting effect of depression and the excitatory effect of what one presumes was mania is made clear by any consideration of the chronology of Schumann's output. 1840 and 1849 are generally adjudged his most productive years, and in both he was in what might be claimed an exalted mood. In 1844 there was a depressive phase that lasted a year; it is reflected in the paucity of his output. Despite the onset of 'organic' features he was, in general, free from depressive symptoms between 1850 and 1853, years which produced a considerable volume of work. The happy year of his marriage was a year of productivity, including the set of songs for which he is chiefly remembered.

It is not inappropriate here to consider the changes in Schumann's work following the onset of what was later considered to be 'organic' change. This has been discussed by Bowman (1970). He refers to the strangeness

243

and remoteness of Schumann's music that follows this change. One peculiarity of this last phase of Schumann's career was the striving for greater formal perfection in his music. There was greater concern for form than for content; for construction than for expression. A rejection of spontaneity, or an inability to bring it to expression, produced a pre-occupation with formal structure which tended to produce remote, difficult and inaccessible works in his last years. This pre-occupation with the formal and, in some ways, stereotyped in preference to the spontaneous and the abstract is a reasonable approximation to the old idea of 'concreteness' that follows brain damage or illness. The interesting point of this discussion is that while largely quantitative and occasionally contextual differences may be seen with mania and depression, a qualitative turn in an artist's work may reflect a more profound impact on brain function.

Other composers whose productivity changed with alterations in the mood state were Handel and Rossini. Handel produced a large corpus of work when his mood was elevated. In the year 1743, when he had a significant lowering of the mood, little was produced. Rossini had several lean years when he was severely depressed and suicidal. But in 1857, his depression passed after at least 4 years of torment, he began writing songs again, and his first efforts in resuming creation were dedicated to his wife for her care and support during that 'overlong and terrible illness' (Weinstock, 1968).

EFFECTS OF ANTIDEPRESSANT TREATMENT ON CREATIVITY

As we have seen in Chapter 5, the availability of antidepressants, neuroleptics and lithium salts from the 1950s and 1960s enabled a more effective attempt to be made to treat depression. If depressive illness was indeed associated with the facilitation of creativity, there might have been, it could be argued, significant consequences of treatment. Schou (1979) noted the effects on creativity seen after treatment with lithium. Twenty-four manic-depressive artists, in whom prophylactic lithium had diminished or prevented recurrence of illness, were questioned about their creativity during treatment. Twelve artists reported increased productivity, six unaltered productivity and six lowered productivity. Schou concluded that the effect of treatment on artistic productivity depended on the severity and type of illness, on individual factors, and also on whether manic episodes of illness were taken advantage of in creative production.

Schou attributed the rise of productivity during lithium treatment to its prophylactic actions. Before lithium treatment depressive and manic episodes had interfered with the artist's life and work, leading to long, unproductive periods or to undistinguished work, sometimes even to spells of idleness in hospital. When lithium therapy brought the disease under control, the artists not only remained creative, but in fact produced more and better work than before. They felt that treatment had led to stabilization of their work habits, to better emotional control, greater maturity and stricter artistic discipline. In a second type of response to lithium therapy, artists with unaltered productivity noted a possible qualitative change in their work. Finally, a group of artists who felt their productivity decreased during lithium therapy were inclined to default from treatment. While a lithium-induced feeling of lack of well-being might have been a factor, there were also factors such as increasing age and the onset of somatic illness to be considered in these cases.

Response to lithium seemed to depend on the severity of the illness before its use, the type of illness, on previous habits of using manic periods as times of inspiration, and also on an individual response to the actions of lithium. Almost invariably artists described their depressive periods as grey, barren and unproductive of intellectual and emotional material that was of use to them in their artistic creation.

Schou provides summaries of the 24 cases, and a reading of those of relevance to this discussion is revealing. Case 1 was a 40-year-old male painter who suffered from manic and depressive illness from the age of 20. During depressions the patient's paintings were characterized by melancholy themes and dark colours, his productivity declined and at times he stopped painting altogether, because of his lack of initiative and his self-criticism. During the manic spells he was prolific, the subjects gay and the colours bright. Lithium improved both personal and artistic life, improving his depressions and hence his productivity, and preventing his manias getting out of hand. During the year of therapy, the patient felt he had been more productive and his works of better quality.

Case 4 was a 42-year-old male publisher and amateur painter who had suffered from recurrent depressions and an incapacitating anxiety since adolescence. He had taken up painting to afford himself a means of self-expression. Lithium therapy had been begun 2 years before and had led to fewer and less severe spells of depression. He felt lithium had helped his artistic productivity by reducing his states of dysphoria.

Case 5 was a 35-year-old female author who had suffered from the age of 16 from both depression and mania. On lithium treatment for 3 years, her mood had stabilized. The depressions before treatment had been masked by apathy and uninspired work. Two years after treatment begun, she felt full of inspiration, her steady mood state leading to regular habits, regularly emerging ideas and steady productivity. Her work on lithium was 'defined and informative'; previously it had been 'misty and indistinct'.

Case 6 was a 49-year-old journalist and author who had suffered for 20 years with a manic depressive illness. Lithium led to the disappearance of his manic spells which brought him initiative. He was in no doubt that treatment brought him a higher general level of productivity. The lithium prevented not only the excessive and promiscuous overproductivity of the manic spells, but prevented the lack of productivity of the depressive spells. He was also able to get back to journalism as, with lithium, he was able to keep assignments more reliably.

Case 7 was a 37-year-old male amateur painter who had both manic and depressive illness. With lithium not only did his productivity increase but his style had changed from realistic portrayal to abstract art. He put his rise in productivity down to a stability in his mood state and possibly more frequent hypomanic episodes.

245

Case 9 was a 44-year-old male painter with both mania and depression for about 20 years. With lithium the uninspired work during his depression has given way to more motivated work accomplished more quickly.

Case 11 was a 44-year-old theatre producer and author with a history of mania and depression. With lithium his mood had stabilized and his productivity had increased considerably, whereas previous depressive spells had been marked by barrenness and the manic episodes by unproductive overactivity.

Case 13 was a 46-year-old male composer who was at his creative best at the onset of depressive and manic episodes, there being a decline when the episodes developed fully.

This and other cases exhibited an unaffected and decreased productivity. It seems clear that the effect of lithium, in general, was to stabilize the mood and increase the productivity, though the individual variation was marked.

Of those who complained of lowered productivity only one could claim the previous depressive episodes were inspirational. A 42-year-old female painter complained her creative power diminished whilst on lithium, and this was attributed to a direct action of the drug. It also came to light that she had been bereaved during lithium treatment.

The overwhelming conclusion is that depression as part of manic-depressive psychosis is not useful creatively, and that a substantial proportion of patients with the condition who were subjected to lithium therapy were enabled to be more creative; if there was any loss of creative ability or productivity, it was due to the reduction or disappearance of the manic episodes.

BIOLOGICAL AND SOCIAL ADVANTAGES OF DEPRESSION

The prevalence, indeed the universality of depression, must lead one to consider whether depression may have biological and social advantages. Work and achievement have been considered already. Even if depression, by itself, does not lead to an increase in productivity and social achievement – indeed, the contrary can be shown to be the case – there is little doubt there is a large and, in the nature of things, incalculable number who avoid depression, either as illness or as a disabling mood state, through work and exertion. There may or may not be overt depressive illness in such individuals who therefore are underestimated in statistics pertaining to illness.

It is generally taken that the Judaeo-Christian work ethic has helped the advance of Western culture and ideas through large parts of the world. This has two implications for the future. If work, or officially sanctioned work, is not to be part of this ethic, will the influence of those cultures which are based on the achievement, effort and advance decline? Secondly, if the work ethic features as part of another culture, will that culture advance to envelop the declining work-based cultures of Western Europe?

The next point to be made is regarding the prevalence of depression in its biological context. Major depressive illness has an undisputed genetic element. Despite its undeniable disadvantages, the genes have remained

246

and the incidence of true depression has not shown a decline. On the contrary, if lesser forms of depression – those closer to distress – are taken into account, the incidence of dysthymia may indeed be shown to have increased. While the foregoing paragraph makes a case for the spread and persistence of depressive genes, another may be made from the biological angle. Sections of this book have hinted at the advantages to be had from the influence of depressive symptomatology on a variety of not uncommon and possibly related disorders. These include such conditions as schizophrenia and Parkinson's disease as well as primary dementing illnesses, e.g. Alzheimer's disease and Huntington's chorea. In general, these illnesses tend to run a relatively more benign course in the presence of depressive symptomatology, the patients perhaps living longer, being socially less disabled and, perhaps, are more fertile. It is interesting that it is the less malignant – and more common form of Alzheimer's disease that tends to show depression among its symptoms. What this may mean is that there is large bank of depressive genes in the population quite apart from those associated with primary depressive illness. Obviously, a benign course of illness may equally favour the spread of the genes of the primary or parent illness. Little work has been done on this aspect of the spread or persistence of disease, and it may well repay detailed consideration.

The ethological or anthropological arguments for the origins and persistence of depression have been put with varying degrees of conviction. Price (1975) seeks an explanation in terms of the adaptive phenomena seen in lower animals, viz. hibernation and behaviour following a change in dominance hierarchy. The adoption of a submissive role follows a decline in dominance and resembles depression in that there is an unwillingness to compete for food and sexual partners, the avoidance of others and a refusal to assert oneself. Price (1975) has extended the discussion. The starting point in the discussion is that depression is part of our behavioural repertory, ready to be called on in appropriate circumstances to perform some useful function. This leads one to suspect that if we knew the function depression was performing we might be enabled to replace it with something less disagreeable.

The different degrees of motility seen in depressed patients may be explained within this framework as supporting the view that being static or dispersing would be of value socially in different situations. Hibernation suggests itself as a condition akin to depression associated with retardation; activity is reduced, so is the need for food, which may be advantageous to the whole group. The retardation, avoidance of contact and loss of libido may be seen in the same terms. However, it is not possible to explain such common symptoms as insomnia, unless one wished to suggest the hibernating animal had to keep an eye open for a predator, perhaps even a cannibalistic colleague, when its lack of motility might have to be seen as a fatal disadvantage. Furthermore, hibernation is associated with the winter months, when only some forms of depression are seen (see Chapter 2).

Increased motility associated with a general restlessness and dissatisfaction with surroundings may be helpful to the individual and, by communication from one individual to the next, the group in moving from one area to another, perhaps more fertile territory. This has obvious advantage to the group in colonizing different areas of the land, but whether a highly mobile individual with depression will have sufficient authority to promote this move is debatable. This is countered by Price with the argument that the inefficiency, indecisiveness and inattentiveness which in modern man is to be equated with depression in the individual might have in an earlier period served for the welfare of his social group. An element of altruism might have crept in so that members of the group with such features would have dropped out of the herd. Why a reversible condition needed to have such a drastic solution is not explained.

As for the value of depressive behaviours in the dominance hierarchy it is suggested that the minor, chronic depressions and associated behaviour might have helped keep certain members low in the hierarchy, while the more severe, phasic depressions would have helped those members who fell in the hierarchy to make a less disruptive adjustment to their lowlier status.

The changes in sociability and increase in libido might have helped in outbreeding (before formal exogamy came into being) small groups which might have gathered periodically (perhaps at the time of the full moon).

It is interesting, even though the proviso must be entered into that conventional achievement must not be equated with genius, to look into the educational and occupational achievements of those with depression. Woodruff et al. (1968) studied 100 patients with primary affective disorder, comparing them in these respects with their siblings of same sex. The data provided no clear evidence that persons suffering from primary affective disorder demonstrated exceptionally greater occupational or educational achievement, or, on the contrary, that their achievements were impaired as a result of illness. The authors were testing the hypothesis that primary affective disorder is an affliction affecting striving individuals who manifested greater need for social success and approval as compared to those members of their family who did not have affective illness. Apart from the fact that conventional social achievement was being considered, the category of 'primary affective disorder' is at once too restrictive (it has connotations of illness as opposed to mood change) and too wide (in its considerations of affective illness as opposed to depression) for the purposes of the present argument. There is also a more fundamental objection which is discussed in Chapter 3. This is that manifest depression is but the outward and visible effects of some underlying neurobiological process. The process may well occur equally in all members of a family. However, some and not others, will show depression for reasons which are of obvious aetiological importance but still not clear. The strict criteria required for a diagnosis of 'primary affective disorder' precludes transient depressive changes which may occur in members of the family who are excluded from a pathological category.

A further study by Monnelly et al. (1974) confirmed the expected finding that socio-cultural factors influenced social achievement even in the presence of affective illness. Families of patients who have had private hospitalization showed higher achievement when the diagnosis was bipolar illness than when it was unipolar illness. The significance disappeared when the patient was in a public hospital. Their conclusion was that there was not only no evidence for significant differences in social achievement in sibs who had primary affective illness and those who had been spared it, but the hypothesis that social achievement is associated with bipolar illness cannot be sustained in unbiased samples. It would appear that a case for manic-depressive illness, as opposed to pure depressive illness, as favouring creative achievement in relation to mental pathology in its strict sense as opposed to mood change, cannot be upheld.

There is also the speculative argument that creative individuals are somehow 'balanced' by nature by being made more predisposed to depression. Creativity in a competitive society – whether in the primitive jungle or modern society – gives an individual a headstart in survival. Depression, with all its disadvantages and increased mortality due to several causes, will counterbalance that advantage. The selection of the most creative by the evolutionary process could, then, account for the apparent increase in depression which has occurred in parallel with social and technological advance. Its increase may also account for the diminished virulence of conditions such as schizophrenia, which was discussed in Chapter 4.

References

Abou-Saleh, M. T. and Coppen, A. (1983). Classification of depression and response to antidepressive therapies. *Br. J. Psychiatry*, **143**, 601–3

Abraham, K. (1924). A short study of the development of the libido, viewed in the light of mental disorders. In *Selected Papers in Psycho-Analysis*. (London: Hogarth Press)

Abse, D. W., Wilkins, M. M., Brown, R. S. *et al.* (1974). Personality and behavioural characteristics of lung cancer patients. *J. Psychosom. Res.*, **18**, 101–13

Adelstein, A. and Mardon, C. (1975). Suicides 1961–1974. In *Population Trends* No 2. (London: HMSO) (quoted in McClure, 1984)

Albert, M. L. (1978). Subcortical dementia. In Katzman *et al.* (eds.) *Alzheimer's Disease: Senile Dementia and Related Disorders.* (New York: Raven Press)

Albert, M. L., Feldman, R. G. and Willis, A. L. (1974). The subcortical dementia of progressive supranuclear palsy. *J. Neurol. Neurosurg. Psychiatry*, **38**, 121–30

Alexanderson, B. and Borga, O. (1972). Individual differences in plasma binding of nortriptyline in man – a twin study. *Eur. J. Clin. Pharmacol.*, **4**, 196

Ananth, J. (1978). Psychopathology in Indian females. *Soc. Sci. Med.*, **12B**, 177–8

Anderson, L. S. (1981). Notes on linkage between the sexually abused child and the suicidal adolescent. *J. Adol.*, **4**, 157–62

Ang, P. C. and Weller, M. P. I. (1984). Koro and psychosis. *Br. J. Psychiatry*, **145**, 335

Angst, J. (1966). Zur Ätiologie und Nosolie endogener depressiver Psychosen: *Monographien aus der Neurologie und Psychiatrie* No 112. (Berlin: Springer-Verlag) (Translation: The aetiology and nosology of endogenous depressive psychoses: A genetic, sociological and clinical study).

Angst, J. (1973). Affective psychoses among the relatives of schizo-affective 'mixed' psychotics. *Foreign Psychiatry*, **2**, 35–7

Angst, J., Baastrup, P., Grof, P. *et al.* (1973). The course of monopolar depression and bipolar psychosis. *Psych. Neurol. Neurochir.*, **76**, 489–500

Annear, M. W. (1979). *Aspects of the psychopathology of witchcraft from the middle ages to the 17th century.* (Welwyn Garden City, Hertfordshire: Smith Kline and French Laboratories Ltd)

Anthony, E. J. and Scott, P. D. (1960). Manic-depressive psychosis in childhood. *J. Child. Psychol. Psychiat.*, **1**, 53–72

Appleton, W. and Davis, J. (1980). *Practical Clinical Psychopharmacology.* (Baltimore: Williams and Wilkins)

Asberg, M., Cronholm, B., Sjoqvist, F. and Tuck, D. (1971). Relationship between plasma levels and therapeutic effect of nortriptyline. *Br. Med. J.*, **3**, 331

Asberg, M., Traskman, L. and Thoren, P. (1976). 5-HIAA in the cerebrospinal fluid. A biochemical suicide predictor? *Arch. Gen. Psychiatry*, **33**, 1193–7

Avery, D. and Winokur, G. (1978). Suicide, attempted suicide and relapse rates in depression. *Arch. Gen. Psychiatry*, **35**, 749–53

251

Bagley, C. (1973). Occupational status and symptoms of depression. *Soc. Sci. Med.*, **7**, 327–39

Bahnson, C. B. (1980). Stress and cancer: The state of the art. Part 1. *Psychosomatics*, **21**, 975–81

Bahnson, C. B. (1981). Stress and cancer: The state of the art. Part 2. *Psychomatics*, **22**, 207–20

Bakker, K. (1977). *The Influence of Lithium Carbonate on the Hypothalamic–Pituitary–Thyroid Axis.* (Groningen: Wolters-Noordhoff Grafische)

Ball, J. R. B. and Kiloh, L. G. (1959). A controlled trial of imipramine in treatment of depressive states. *Br. Med. J.*, **2**, 1052–5

Ballenger, J. C., Goodwin, F. K., Major, L. F. and Brown, G. L. (1979). Alcohol and central serotonin metabolism in man. *Arch. Gen. Psychiatry*, **36**, 224–7

Barbeau, A. (1983). Advances in Parkinson's disease. McNaughton Prize Lecture. Canadian Neurological Society. Quoted in Calne, D. B. and Langston, J. W. (1983). Aetiology of Parkinson's disease. *Lancet*, **2**, 1457–9

Barraclough, B., Bunch, J., Nelson, B. and Sainsbury, P. (1974). A hundred cases of suicide: clinical aspects. *Br. J. Psychiatry*, **125**, 355–73

Bartrop, R. W., Luckhurst, E., Lazarus, L. *et al.* (1977). Depressed lymphocytic function after bereavement. *Lancet*, **1**, 834–46

Beck, A. T. (1967). *Depression: Clinical, Experimental and Theoretical Aspects.* (New York: Harper and Row)

Beck, A. T., Schuyler, D. and Herman, I. (1974). Development of suicidal intent scales. In Beck, A. T. *et al.* (eds.) *The Prediction of Suicide*. Bowie, Maryland: Charles Press.

Bell, Q. (1972). *Virginia Woolf A biography.* Vol. 1, 1882–1912; Vol. 2, 1912–1941. (London: The Hogarth Press)

Berrios, G. E. (1985). The psychopathology of affectivity: Conceptual and historical aspects. *Psychol. Med.*, **15**, 745–58

Berrios, G. E. and Morley, S. J. (1984). Koro-like symptom in a non-Chinese subject. *Br. J. Psychiatry*, **145**, 331–34.

Bieliauskas, L. A., Shekelle, R. B., Garron, D. *et al.* (1979). Prospective studies of psychological depression and cancer. Read before the *87th Annual American Psychological Association Convention,* Sept 1, 1979, New York (quoted in Bahnson, 1980).

Binnie, E. H. (1982). Mianserin hydrochloride and L-tryptophan compared in depressive illness. *Br. J. Clin. Soc. Psychiatry*, **1**, 9–10

Bioulac, B., Benezech, M., Renaud, B. *et al.* (1980). Serotoninergic dysfunction in the 47, XYY syndrome. *Biol. Psychiatry*, **15**, 917–23

Birtchnell, J. (1975). Psychiatric breakdown following recent parent death. *Br. J. Med. Psychol.*, **48**, 379–90

Blackburn, I. M., Bishop, S., Glen, A. I. M. *et al.* (1981). The efficacy of cognitive therapy in depression: A treatment trial using cognitive therapy and pharmacotherapy, each alone and in combination. *Br. J. Psychiatry*, **139**, 181–9

Bleuler, E. (1923). *Textbook of Psychiatry.* (London: Allen and Unwin)

Blumberg, E. M., West, P. M. and Ellis, F. W. (1954). A possible relationship between psychological factors and human cancer. *Psychosom. Med.*, **16**, 277–86

Bond, A. and Lader, M. (1984). The psychopharmacology of aggression. In Gaind, R. *et al.* (eds.) *Current Themes in Psychiatry* Vol 3. (London: Macmillan)

Boswell, J. (1791). *The Life of Johnson* (Hibbert, C. (ed.), 1979). (Harmondsworth: The Penguin English Library)

Bowie, P. C. W. and Beaini, A. Y. (1985). Normalisation of the dexamethasone suppression test: A correlate of clinical improvement in primary depressives. *Br. J. Psychiatry*, **147**, 30–5

Bowman, P. (1970). Robert Schumann's life. *Psychiatr. Commun.*, **13**, 19–27

Brain, R. and Henson, R. A. (1958). Neurological syndromes associated with cancer. *Lancet*, **2**, 971–5

Bridges, P. K. (1983). Point of View. *Br. J. Psychiatry*, **142**, 676–7

Bridges, P. K. and Bartlett, J. R. (1977). Psychosurgery: Yesterday and today. *Br. J. Psychiatry*, **131**, 249–60

Briscoe, M. (1982). *Sex difference in psychological well-being.* (Cambridge: Cambridge University Press)

Brown, G. L., Ballenger, J. C., Minichiello, M. D. and Goodwin, F. K. (1979). Human aggression and its relationship to cerebrospinal fluid 5-hydroxy indoleacetic acid, 3-methoxy-4-hydroxy phenyl glycol and homovanillic acid. In Sandler, M. (ed.), *Psychopharmacology of Aggression*. (New York: Raven Press)

252

REFERENCES

Brown, G. L., Ebert, M. H., Goyer, P. F. et al. (1982). Aggression, Suicide and Serotonin: relationships to CSF amine metabolites. *Am. J. Psychiatry*, **139**, 741-6

Brown, G. L., Goodwin, F. K., Ballanger, J.C. et al. (1979). Aggression in humans correlates with cerebrospinal fluid amine metabolites. *Psychiatry Res.*, **1**, 131-9

Brown, G. W., Bhrolchain, M. N. and Harris, T. (1975). Social class and psychiatric disturbance among women in an urban population. *Sociology*, **9**, 225-54

Brown, G. W. and Harris, T. O. (1978). *Social Origins of Depression*: A study of psychiatric disorder in women. (London: Tavistock Publications)

Brown, G. W., Harris, T. and Copeland, R. (1977). Depression and loss. *Br. J. Psychiatry*, **130**, 1-18

Brown, G. W., Harris, T. O. and Peto, J. (1973). Life events and psychiatric disorders. Part II. Nature of causal link. *Psychol. Med.*, **3**, 159-76

Brown, J. H. and Paraskevas, F. (1982). Cancer and depression: cancer presenting with depressive illness: an autoimmune disease? *Br. J. Psychiatry*, **141**, 227-32

Brown, R. P., Sweeney, J., Loutsch, E. et al. (1984). Involutional melancholia revisited. *Am. J. Psychiatry*, **141**, 24-8

Brown, W. A. and Qualls, C. B. (1981). Pituitary-adrenal disinhibition in depression: Marker of a subtype and characteristic clinical features and response to treatment? *Psychiatr. Res.*, **4**, 115-28

Brown, W. A. and Shuey, I. (1980). Response to dexamethasone and subtype of depression. *Arch. Gen. Psychiatry*, **37**, 747-51

Brugha, T., Conroy, R., Walsh, N. et al. (1982). Social networks, attachments and supports in minor affective disorders: a replication. *Br. J. Psychiatry*, **141**, 249-55

Bucher, K. and Elston, R. C. (1980a). The transmission of manic-depressive illness. I. Theory, description of the model and summary of results. *J. Psychiatr. Res.*, **16**, 53-63

Bucher, K., Elston, R. C., Helzer, J. and Winokur, G. (1980b). The transmission of manic-depressive illness. II. Segregation analysis of three sets of family data. *J. Psychiatr. Res.*, **16**, 65-70

Buglass, D. and Horton, J. (1974). A scale for predicting subsequent suicidal behaviour. *Br. J. Psychiatry*, **124**, 573-8.

Burnet, F. M. (1976). *Immunology, Ageing and Cancer*. (San Francisco: W. H. Freeman)

Burrows, G. D., Vohra, J., Hunt, D. et al. (1976). Cardiac effects of different tricyclic antidepressant drugs. *Br. J. Psychiatry*, **129**, 335

Burt, C. G., Gordon, W. F., Holt, N. F. and Horden, A. (1962). Amitriptyline in depressive stages: a controlled trial. *J. Ment. Sci.*, **108**, 711-30

Cade, J. F. J. (1949). Lithium salts in the treatment of psychotic excitement. *Med. J. Aust.*, **36**, 349-52

Caine, E. D. (1981). Pseudodementia. *Arch. Gen. Psychiatry.*, **38**, 1359-64

Campbell, E. A., Cope, S. J. and Teasdale, J. D. (1983). Social factors and affective disorder: An investigation of Brown and Harris's model. *Br. J. Psychiatry*, **143**, 548-53

Capstick, A. (1960). Recognition of emotional disturbance and the prevention of suicide. *Br. Med. J.*, **1**, 1179-82

Carman, J. S., Post, R. M., Buswell, R. and Goodwin, F. K. (1976). Negative effects of melatonin on depression. *Am. J. Psychiatry*, **133**, 1181-6

Carman, J. S., Post, R. M., Goodwin, F. K. and Bunney, W. E. (1977). Calcium and electroconvulsive therapy of severe depressive illness. *Biol. Psychiatry*, **12**, 5-17

Carnes, M., Smith, J. C., Kalin, N. H. and Bauwens, S. F. (1983). The dexamethasone suppression test in demented outpatients with and without depression. *Psychiatry Res.*, **9**, 337-44

Carroll, B. J. (1978). Neuroendocrine function in psychiatric disorders. In Lipton, A. et al. (eds.) *Psychopharmacology: A Generation of Progress.* pp 487-97 (New York: Raven Press)

Carroll, B. J. (1982). The dexamethasone suppression test for melancholia. *Br. J. Psychiatry*, **140**, 292-304

Carroll, B. J., Curtis, G. C. and Mendels, J. (1976). Cerebrospinal fluid and plasma free cortisol concentrations in depression. *Psychol. Med.*, **6**, 235-44

Carroll, B. J. and Mendels, J. (1976). Neuroendocrine regulation in affective disorders. In Sachar, E. J. (ed.) *Hormones, Behaviour and Psychopathology*, pp 193-224

Cawley, R. H., Post, F. and Whitehead, A. (1973). Barbiturate tolerance and psychological functioning in elderly depressed patients. *Psychol. Med.*, **1**, 39–52

Celesia, G. C. and Wanamaker, W. M. (1972). Psychiatric disturbances in Parkinson's disease. *Dis. Nerv. Syst.*, **33**, 577–83

Cerletti, U. and Bini, L. (1938). L'elettroshock. *Arch. Gen. Neurol. Psychiatr. Psychoanal.*, **19**, 266–88

Charney, D. S. and Nelson, J. C. (1981). Delusional and non-delusional unipolar depression – further evidence for distinct subtypes. *Am. J. Psychiatry*, **138**, 328–33

Checkley, S. A. (1979). Corticosteroid and growth hormone responses to methylamphetamine in depressive illness. *Psychol. Med.*, **9**, 107–16

Checkley, S. A. (1980). Neuroendocrine study of adrenoreceptor function in endogenous depression. *Acta Psychiat. Scand., Suppl.* **280**, 211–17

Checkley, S. A., Slade, A. P. and Shur, E. (1981). Growth hormone and other responses to clonidine in patients with endogenous depression. *Br. J. Psychiatry*, **138**, 51–3

Chen, Char-Nie (1979). Sleep, depression and antidepressants. *Br. J. Psychiatry*, **135**, 385–402

Clare, A. W. (1985). "The other half of medicine" and St Bartholomew's Hospital. *Br. J. Psychiatry*, **146**, 120–6

Clayton, P. J. (1982). Bereavement. In Paykel, E. S. (ed.) *Handbook of Affective Disorders* (Edinburgh: Churchill Livingstone)

Clayton, P. J. and Darvish, H. S. (1979). Course of depressive symptoms following the stress of bereavement. In Barrett, J. D. (eds.) *Stress and Mental Disorder* (New York: Raven Press)

Clayton, P. J., Rodin, L. and Winokur, G. (1968). Family history studies. III. Schizoaffective disorder, clinical and genetic factors including a one to two year follow-up. *Compr. Psychiatry*, **9**, 31–49

Cohen, M. B., Baker, G., Cohen, R. A. *et al.* (1954). An intensive study of 12 cases of manic depressive psychoses. *Psychiatry*, **17**, 103–37

Cohen, S. I. (1980). Cushing's syndrome: A psychiatric study of 29 patients. *Br. J. Psychiatry*, **136**, 120–4

Cole, M. and Hickie, R. N. (1976). Frequency and significance of minor organic signs in elderly depressives. *Can. Psychiatr. Assoc. J.*, **21**, 7–12

Conolly, J. (1849). *On Some of the Forms of Insanity*. Croonian Lectures. (London: Royal College of Physicians)

Cooper, A. J., Moir, A. J. B. and Guldberg, H. C. (1968). Effect of electroconvulsive shock on the cerebral metabolism of dopamine and 5-hydroxytryptamine *J. Pharm. Pharmacol.*, **20**, 729–30

Cooper, S. J., Kelly, J. G. and King, D. J. (1985). Adrenergic receptors in depression. *Br. J. Psychiatry*, **147**, 23–9

Copas, J. B. and Robin, A. (1982). Suicide in psychiatric in-patients. *Br. J. Psychiatry*, **141**, 503–11

Copeland, J. R. M. (1985). Depressive illness and morbid distress. Onset and development data examined against five-year outcome. *Br. J. Psychiatry*, **146**, 297–307

Coppen, A. (1967). The biochemistry of the affective disorders. *Br. J. Psychiatry*, **113**, 1237–64

Coppen, A. J. and Metcalfe, M. (1963). Cancer and extraversion. *Br. Med. J.*, **2**, 18–19

Coppen, A., Abou-Saleh, M. T., Milln, P. *et al.* (1981). Lithium continuation therapy following electroconvulsive therapy *Br. J. Psychiatry*, **139**, 284–7

Coppen, A., Abou-Saleh, M. T. Milln, P. *et al.* (1983). Dexamethasone suppression test in depression and other psychiatric illness. *Br. J. Psychiatry*, **142**, 498–504

Coppen, A., Bishop, M.E., Bailey, J. E. *et al.* (1980). Renal function in lithium and non-lithium treated patients with affective disorders. *Acta Psychiatr. Scand.*, **62**, 343–55

Coppen, A., Milln, P., Harwood, J. and Wood, K. (1985). Does the dexamethasone suppression test predict antidepressant treatment success? *Br. J. Psychiatry*, **146**, 294–6

Coppen, A., Prange, A. J. and Whybrow, P. C. (1972). Abnormalities of indoleamines in affective disorders. *Arch. Gen. Psychiatry*, **26**, 474–8

Coppen, A., Swade, C. and Wood, K. (1978). Platelet 5-hydroxytryptamine accumulation in depressive illness. *Clin. Chim. Acta*, **87**, 165–8

Coughlan, A. K. and Hollows, S. E. (1984). Use of memory tests in differentiating organic disorder from depression. *Br. J. Psychiatry*, **145**, 164–7

Crammer, J. L. (1984). The special characteristics of suicide in hospital in-patients. *Br. J. Psychiatry*, **145**, 460–76

Crisp, A. H. (1970). Some psychosomatic aspects of neoplasia. *Br. J. Med. Psychol.*, **43**, 313–31

REFERENCES

Crow, T. J. (1984). A re-evaluation of the viral hypothesis. Is psychosis the result of retroviral integration at a site close to the cerebral dominance gene? *Br. J. Psychiatry*, **145**, 243–53

Curzon, G., Kantamaneni, B. D., Van Boxel, P. *et al.* (1980). Substance related to 5-hydroxytryptamine in plasma and in lumbar and ventricular fluids of psychiatric patients. *Acta Psychiat. Scand., Suppl.* **61**, (280), 3–19

Cutting, J. C., Clare, A. W. and Mann, A. H. (1978). Cycloid psychosis: An investigation of the diagnostic concept. *Psychol. Med.*, **8**, 637–48

Cytryn, L. and McKnew, D. J. (1972). Proposed classification of childhood depression. *Am. J. Psychiatry*, **129**, 149–55

Dale, J. R. and Ben-Tovim, D. I. (1984). Modern or Traditional? A study of treatment preference for neuropsychiatric disorders in Botswana. *Br. J. Psychiatry*, **145**, 187–92

Deakin, J. F. W., Ferrier, I. N., Crow, T. J. *et al.* (1983). Effects of ECT on pituitary hormone release: relationship to seizure, clinical variables and outcome. *Br. J. Psychiatry*, **143**, 618–24

D'Elia, G. (1974). Unilateral convulsive therapy. In Fink, M. *et al.* (eds.) *Psychobiology of Convulsive Therapy*. (Washington: Winston)

D'Elia, G. and Perris, C. (1973). Cerebral dominance and depression. *Acta Psychiatr. Scand.*, **49**, 191–7

De Lisi, L. E., King, A. C. and Targum, S. (1984). Serum immunoglobulin concentrations in patients admitted to an acute psychiatric in-patient service. *Br. J. Psychiatry*, **145**, 661–6

De Montigny, C., Grunberg, F., Mayer, A. and Deschenes, J.-P. (1981). Lithium induces rapid relief of depression in tricyclic antidepressant drug non-responders. *Br. J. Psychiatry*, **138**, 252–6

De Paulo, J. R. and Folstein, M. F. (1978). Psychiatric disturbances in neurological patients: Detection, recognition and hospital course. *Ann. Neurol.*, **4**, 225–8

Dhadphale, M., Ellison, R. H. and Griffin, L. (1983). The frequency of psychiatric disorders among patients attending semi-urban and rural general out-patient clinics in Kenya. *Br. J. Psychiatry*, **142**, 379–83

Diagnostic and Statistical Manual of Mental Disorders (1980) 3rd edition. (DSM-III) (Washington, D.C.: American Psychiatric Association)

Dick, D. A. T., Dick, E. G. and Naylor, G. J. (1981). Plasma vanadium concentration in manic depressive illness. *J. Physiol.*, **310**, 24

Doering, C. H., Brodie, H. K. H., Kraemer, H. *et al.* (1974). Plasma testosterone levels and psychologic measures in men over a two month period. In Friedman, R. C. *et al.* (eds.) *Sex Differences in Behavior.* (New York: Wiley)

Dolan, R. J., Calloway, S. P., Fonagy, P. *et al.* (1985). Life events, depression and hypothalamic–pituitary–adrenal axis function. *Br. J. Psychiatry*, **147**, 429–33

Dreyfus, G. L. (1907). *Die Melancholie* (Jena: Fisher)

Durkheim, E. (1897, 1970). *Le Suicide* Paris. (Engl. Transl. *Suicide: A Study in Sociology* by J. A. Spaulding and C. Simpson [London: Routledge and Kegan Paul])

Eagles, J. M. (1983). Delusional depressive in-patients, 1892 to 1982. *Br. J. Psychiatry*, **143**, 558–63

Eagles, J. M. and Whalley, L. J. (1985). Ageing and affective disorders: The age at first onset of affective disorders in Scotland, 1969–1978. *Br. J. Psychiatry*, **147**, 180–7

Eccleston, D. (1982). The biochemistry of affective disorders. *Br. J. Hosp. Med.*, **27**, 627–30

Eccleston, D. and Nicolaou, N. (1978). The influence of L-tryptophan and monoamine oxidase inhibitors on catecholamine metabolism in rat brain. *Br. J. Pharmacol.*, **64**, 341–5

Eichelman, B. (1977). Neurochemical studies of aggression in animals. *Psychopharmacol. Bull.*, **13**, 17–19

Eichelman, B., Elliot, G. R. and Barchas, J. D. (1981). Biochemical, pharmacological and genetic aspects of aggression. In Hamburg, D. A. and Trudeau, M. B. (eds.) *Biobehavioural Aspects of Aggression* (New York: Alan R. Liss)

Elithorn, A., Bridges, P. K., Hodges, J. R. and Joen, M. T. (1969). Adrenocortical responsiveness during courses of electroconvulsive therapy. *Br. J. Psychiatry*, **115**, 575–80

Faergeman, P. M. (1963). *Psychogenic Psychoses.* (London: Butterworths)

Fahy, T. J. (1974). Pathways of specialist referral of depressed patients from general practice. *Br. J. Psychiatry.*, **124**, 231–9

Falloon, I. R. H. and Talbot, R. E. (1981). Persistent auditory hallucinations: Coping mechanisms and implications for management. *Psychol. Med.*, **11**, 329–39

255

Fava, G. A., Munari, F., Pavan, L. and Kellner, R. (1981). Life events and depression: A replication. *J. Affect. Dis.*, **3**, 159–65

Fink, M. and Ottosson, J.-O. (1980). A theory of convulsive therapy in endogenous depression: significance for hypothalamic functions. *Psychiatr. Res.*, **2**, 49–61

Flor-Henry, P. (1969). Psychosis and temporal lobe epilepsy: a controlled investigation. *Epilepsia*, **10**, 363–95

Flor-Henry, P. (1979). On certain aspects of the localization of cerebral systems regulating and determining emotions. *Biol. Psychiatry*, **14**, 677–98

Fras, I., Litin, E. M. and Pearson, J. S. (1967). Comparison of psychiatric symptoms in carcinoma of the pancreas with those in some other intra-abdominal neoplasms. *Am. J. Psychiatry*, **123**, 1553–62

Fraser, R. M. and Glass, I. B. (1978). Recovery from ECT in elderly patients. *Br. J. Psychiatry*, **133**, 524–8

Freeman, C. P. and Kendell, R. E. (1980). ECT: Patients' experiences and attitudes. *Br. J. Psychiatry*, **137**, 8–16

Freeman, H. L. (ed.) (1984). Scientific background. In *Mental Health and the Environment*. (Edinburgh: Churchill Livingstone)

Freeman, W. and Watts, J. (1942). *Psychosurgery* (Springfield: Thomas)

Freud, S. (1917). *Mourning and Melancholia*. (London: Hogarth Press, 1957)

Frizel, D., Coppen, A. and Marks, V. (1969). Plasma magnesium and calcium in depression. *Br. J. Psychiatry*, **115**, 1375–7

Frommer, E. A. (1967). Treatment of childhood depression with antidepressant drugs. *Br. Med. J.*, **1**, 729–32

Frommer, E. A. (1968). Depressive illness in childhood. In Cooper, A. and Walk, A. (eds.) *Recent Developments in Affective Disorders*. (London: Headley Bros)

Frommer, E., Mendelson, W. B. and Reid, M. A. (1972). Differential diagnosis of psychiatric disturbances in pre-school children. *Br. J. Psychiatry*, **121**, 71–4

Funkenstein, D. H., King, S. H. and Drolette, M. E. (1957). *Mastery of Stress*. (Cambridge, Mass.: Harvard University Press)

Galdi, J. (1983). The causality of depression in schizophrenia. *Br. J. Psychiatry*, **142**, 621–4

Garmany, G. (1958). Depressive states: their aetiology and treatment. *Br. Med. J.*, **2**, 341–4

Garver, D. L. and Davis, J. M. (1979). Biogenic amine hypotheses of affective disorders. *Life Sci.*, **24**, 383–94

Garvey, M. J., Schaffer, C. B. and Tuason, V. B. (1983). Relationship of headaches to depression. *Br. J. Psychiatry*, **143**, 544–7

Garvey, M. J., Schaffer, C. B. and Tuason, V. B. (1984). Comparison of pharmacological treatment response between situational and non-situational depressions. *Br. J. Psychiatry*, **145**, 363–5

Georgotas, A., Freedman, E., McCarthy, M. *et al.* (1983). Resistant geriatric depressions and therapeutic response to monoamine oxidase inhibitors. *Biol. Psychiatry*, **18**, 195–205

Gershon, E. S., Bunney, W. E. Jr., Leckman, J. F. *et al.* (1976). The inheritance of affective disorders: a review of data and hypotheses. *Behav. Genet.*, **6**, 227–61

Gershon, E., Hamovit, J., Guroff, J. *et al.* (1982). A family history of schizoaffective, bipolar I, bipolar II, unipolar and normal control probands. *Arch. Gen. Psychiatry*, **39**, 1157–67

Gerson, S. C. and Baldessarini, R. J. (1980). Motor effects of serotonin in the central nervous system. *Life Sci.*, **27**, 1435–51

Gibson, A. J. (1981). A further analysis of memory loss in dementia and depression in the elderly. *Br. J. Clin. Psychol.*, **20**, 179–185

Giel, R., Gezahegu, Y. and Van Luijk, J. N. (1968). Psychiatric morbidity in 200 Ethiopian medical outpatients. *Psychiatry Neurolog. Neurochir.*, **71**, 169–76

Gillespie, R. D. (1929). The clinical differentiation of types of depression. *Guy's Hosp. Rep.*, **79**, 306–44

Goktepe, E. O., Young, L. B. and Bridges, P. K. (1975). A further review of the results of stereotactic subcaudate tractotomy. *Br. J. Psychiatr.*, **126**, 270–80

Gold, P. W., Goodwin, F. K. and Reus, V. I. (1978). Vasopressin in affective illness. *Lancet*, **1**, 1233–5

Goldberg, D. P. (1982). Depressive reactions in adults. In Russell, G. F. M. and Hersov, L. (eds.) *Handbook of Psychiatry* Vol IV. (Cambridge: Cambridge University Press)

Goldberg, M. E. and Horovitz, Z. P. (1978). Antidepressants and aggressive behavior. *Mod. Probl. Pharmaco-Psychiatry*, **13**, 29–52

Goldfarb, C. I., Driesen, I. and Cole, D. (1967). Psychophysiologic aspects of malignancy. *Am. J. Psychiatry*, **123**, 1545–52

Goodwin, F. K. and Bunney, W. E. (1971). Depressions following reserpine: a re-evaluation. *Seminars in Psychiatry*, **3**, 435–48

Goodwin, F. K. and Post, R. M. (1983). 5-hydroxytryptamine and depression: A model for the interaction of normal variance with pathology. *Br. J. Clin. Pharmacol.*, **15**, 393S–405S

Gove, W. R. (1972). The relationship between sex roles, marital status and mental illness. *Soc. Forces*, **51**, 34–44

Graham, P. J. (1974). Depression in pre-pubertal children. *Dev. Med. Child. Neurol.*, **16**, 340–9

Grahame-Smith, D. G., Green, A. R. and Costain, D. W. (1978). Mechanism of the antidepressant action of electroconvulsive therapy, *Lancet*, **1**, 254–6

Greden, J. F., Gardner, R., King, D. *et al.* (1983). Dexamethasone suppression tests in antidepressant treatment of melancholia. The process of normalisation and test–re-test reproducibility. *Arch. Gen. Psychiatry*, **40**, 493–500

Green, R. and Youdim, M. (1976). Use of a behavioural model to study the action of monoamine oxidase inhibition *in vivo*. In *Monoamine Oxidase and its Inhibition*. Ciba Foundation Symposium–39. (Amsterdam, Elsevier: Excerpta Medica)

Greene, W. A. and Swisher, S. N. (1969). Psychological and somatic variables associated with the development and course of monozygotic twins discordant for leukemia. *Ann. NY. Acad. Sci.*, **164**, 394–408

Greer, S. (1983). Cancer and the mind. *Br. J. Psychiatry*, **143**, 535–43

Greer, S., Morris, T. and Pettingale, K. W. (1979). Psychological response to breast cancer: effect on outcome. *Lancet*, **2**, 785–7

Gregory, S., Shawcross, C. R. and Gill, D. (1985). The Nottingham ECT study. A double-blind comparison of bilateral, unilateral and simulated ECT in depressive illness. *Br. J. Psychiatry*, **146**, 520–4

Guze, S. B. (1976). *Criminality and Psychiatric Disorders* (New York: Oxford University Press)

Guze, S. B. and Robins, E. (1970). Suicide and primary affective disorders. *Br. J. Psychiatry*, **117**, 437–8

Hafner, H. and Boker, W. (1973). *Crimes of Violence by Mentally Abnormal Offenders* (Cambridge: Cambridge University Press).

Hagnell, O. (1966). The premorbid personality of persons who develop cancer in total population investigated in 1947 and 1957. *Ann. NY Acad. Sci.*, **125**, 846–55

Hallstrom, J. (1973). *Mental Disorder and Sexuality in the Climacteric* (Goteborg: Ostradius Boktryckeri)

Harding, T. W. (1973). Psychosis in a rural West African community. *Soc. Psychiatry*, **8**, 198–203

Hare, E. H. (1974). The changing content of psychiatric illness. *J. Psychosom. Res.*, **18**, 283–9

Hartigan, G. P. (1963). The use of lithium salts in affective disorders. *Br. J. Psychiatry*, **109**, 810–14

Hawkins, D. R. (1908). Sleep and circadian rhythm disturbances in depression. In Mendels, J. and Amsterdam, J. D. (eds.) *Psychobiology of Affective Disorders* (Basel: Karger)

Hawton, K. (1982). Attempted suicide in children and adolescents. *J. Child. Psychol. Psychiatry*, **23**, 497–503

Heimburger, R. F., Small, I. F., Milstein, V. and Moore, D. (1978). Stereotaxic amygdalotomy for convulsive and behavioural disorder. *Appl. Neurophysiol.*, **41**, 43–51

Henderson, S. (1981). Social relationships, adversity and neurosis: an analysis of prospective observations. *Br. J. Psychiatry*, **138**, 391–8

Henderson, S., Duncan-Jones, P., McAuley, H. and Ritchie, K. (1978). The patient's primary group. *Br. J. Psychiatry*, **132**, 74–86

Hendrickson, E., Levy, R. and Post, F. (1979). Averaged evoked responses in relation to cognitive and affective state of elderly psychiatric patients. *Br. J. Psychiatry*, **134**, 494–501

Heninger, G. R., Charney, D. S. and Sternberg, D. E. (1983). Lithium carbonate augmentation of antidepressant treatment. *Arch. Gen. Psychiatry*, **40**, 1335–42

Henry, A. F. and Short, J. F. (1964) *Suicide and Homicide* (New York: Glencoe Free Press)

Henry, G. W. (1932). Mental phenomena observed in cases of brain tumour. *Am. J. Psychiatry*, **89**, 415–73

Herrington, R. N., Bruce, A., Johnstone, E. C. and Lader, M. H. (1974). Comparative trial of L-tryptophan and ECT in severe depressive illness. *Lancet*, **2**, 731–4

Herrington, R. N., Bruce, A., Johnstone, E. C. and Lader, M. H. (1976). Comparative trial of L-tryptophan and amitriptyline in depressive illness. *Psychol. Med.*, **6**, 673–8

Hersov, L. A. (1961). Refusal to go to school. *J. Child Psychol. Psychiatry*, **1**, 137–45

Heshe, J., Roeder, E. and Theilgaard, A. (1978). Unilateral and bilateral ECT. *Acta Psychiatr. Scand.*, *(Suppl. 275)*

Hestbech, J., Hansen, H. E., Amdisen, A. and Olsen, S. (1971). Chronic renal lesions following long-term treatment with lithium *Kidney Int.*, **12**, 205–13

Hirsch, S. R., Gaind, R., Rohde, P. D. *et al.* (1973). Outpatient maintenance of chronic schizophrenic patients with long-acting fluphenazine: double-blind placebo trial. *Br. Med. J.*, **1**, 633–7

Hirschfeld, R. M. A. and Klerman, G. L. (1979). Personality attributes and affective disorders. *Am. J. Psychiatry*, **136**, 67–70

Hitch, P. J. and Rack, P. H. (1980). Mental illness among Polish and Russian refugees in Bradford. *Br. J. Psychiatry*, **137**, 206–11

Hobson, R. F. (1953). Prognostic factors in electric convulsive therapy. *J. Neurol. Neurosurg. Psychiatry*, **16**, 275–81

Hoch, A. and MacCurdy, J. T. (1922). The prognosis of involutional melancholia. *Arch. Neurol. Psychiatry*, **7**, 1–17 (quoted by Brown *et al.*, 1984).

Holmes, J. A. and Speight, A. N. P. (1975). The problem of non-organic illness in Tanzanian urban medical practice. *E. Afr. Med. J.*, **52**, 225–36

Horne, R. L. and Picard, R. S. (1979). Psychosocial risk factors for lung cancer. *Psychosom. Med.*, **41**, 503–14

Horovitz, Z. P. (1967). The amygdala and depression. In Garattini, S. and Dukes, M. N. G. (eds.) *Antidepressant Drugs*. (Amsterdam: Excerpta Medica)

Hunter, R. A. and Macalpine, I. (1963). *Three Hundred Years of Psychiatry, 1535–1860*. (London: Oxford University Press)

Huntington, G. (1872). On Chorea. *Med. Surg. Rep.*, **26**, 317–21

Jacobson, S. and Jacobson, D. M. (1972). Suicide in Brighton. *Br. J. Psychiatry*, **121**, 369–77

Jacoby, R. J. (1981). Dementia, depression and the CT Scan. *Psychol. Med.*, **11**, 673–6

Jacoby, R. J., Dolan, R. J., Levy, R. and Baldy, R. (1983). Quantitative computed tomography in elderly depressed patients. *Br. J. Psychiatr*, **143**, 124–7

Jacoby, R. J. and Levy, R. (1980). Computed tomography in the elderly. 3. Affective disorder. *Br. J. Psychiatry*, **136**, 270–5

James, D. and Hawton, K. (1985). Overdoses: explanations and attitudes in self-poisoners and significant others. *Br. J. Psychiatry*, **146**, 481–5

James, S. P., Wehr, T. A., Sack, D. A. *et al.* (1985). Treatment of seasonal affective disorder with light in the evening. *Br. J. Psychiatry*, **147**, 424–8

Janowsky, D. S. (1980). The cholinergic nervous system and depression. In Mendels, J. and Amsterdam, J. D. (eds.) *The Psychobiology of Affective Disorders*. (Basel: Karger)

Janowsky, D. S., El-Yousef, M. K., Davis, J. M. *et al.* (1972). A cholinergic–adrenergic hypothesis of mania and depression. *Lancet*, **2**, 632–5

Jaspers, K. (1913). *Allgemeine Psychopathologie*. (Berlin: Springer) (English translation: *General Psychopathology*. Manchester: Manchester University Press)

Jenner, P., Sheehy, M. and Marsden, C. D. (1983). Noradrenaline and 5-hydroxytryptamine modulation of brain dopamine function: implications for the treatment of Parkinson's disease. *Br. J. Clin. Pharmacol.*, **15**, 277S–289S

Jimerson, D. C., Post, R. M., Carman, J. J. *et al.* (1979). CSF calcium: clinical correlates in affective illness and schizophrenia. *Biol. Psychiatry*, **14**, 37–51

Johnson, A., Pflug, B. and Engelmann, W. (1979). Effect of lithium carbonate on circadian periodicity in humans. *Pharmakopsychiatry*, **12**, 423–5

Johnson, D. A. W. (1981). Studies of depressive symptoms in schizophrenia. *Br. J. Psychiatry*, **139**, 89–101

Johnstone, E. C., Crow, T. J., Frith, C. D. *et al.* (1976). Cerebral ventricular size and cognitive impairment in chronic schizophrenia. *Lancet*, **2**, 924–6

Johnstone, E. C., Owens, D. G. C., Crow, T. J. *et al.* (1986). Hypothyroidism as a correlate of lateral ventricular enlargement in manic-depressive and neurotic illness. *Br. J. Psychiatry*, **148**, 317–21

REFERENCES

Johnstone, E. C., Owens, D. G. C., Frith, C. D. and Calvert, L. M. (1985). Institutionalisation and the outcome of functional psychoses. *Br. J. Psychiatry*, **146**, 36–44

Jones, M. T., Hillhouse, E. and Burden, J. (1976). Secretion of corticotrophic releasing hormone *in vitro*. In Martini, L. and Ganong, W. (eds.) *Frontiers in Neuroendocrinology*. pp 194–226. (New York: Raven Press)

Jouvet, M. (1969). Biogenic amines and the states of sleep. *Science*, **163**, 32–41

Kaada, B. (1972). Stimulation and regional ablation of the amygdaloid complex with reference to functional representations. In Eleftheriou, B. E. (ed.) *The Neurobiology of the Amygdala. Advances in Behavioural Biology* Vol. 2. (New York: Plenum Press)

Kalinowsky, L. B. and Hippius, H. (1969). *Pharmacological, Convulsive and other Somatic treatments in Psychiatry*. (New York: Grune and Stratton)

Kallmann, F. J. (ed.) (1953). *Heredity in Health and Mental Disorder*. (New York: W. W. Norton)

Kallman, F. J. (1959). The genetics of mental illness. In Arieti, S. (ed.) *American Handbook of Psychiatry*. New York: Basic Books

Kapur, R. L. (1975). Mental health care in rural India: A study of existing patterns and their implications for future policy. *Br. J. Psychiatry*, **127**, 286–93

Kasanin, J. (1933). The acute schizo-affective psychoses *Am. J. Psychiatry*, **13**, 97–126

Katz, M. M., Robins, E., Croughan, J. *et al.* (1982). Behavioral measurement and drug response characteristics of unipolar and bipolar depression. *Psychol. Med.*, **12**, 25–36

Kelly, W. F., Checkley, S. A. and Bender, D. A. (1980). Cushing's syndrome, tryptophan and depression. *Br. J. Psychiatry*, **136**, 125–32

Kelly, W. F., Checkley, S. A., Bender, D. A. and Mashiter, K. (1983). Cushing's syndrome and depression – a prospective study of 26 patients. *Br. J. Psychiatry*, **142**, 16–19

Kendell, R. E. (1968). *The Classification of Depressive Illnesses*. Maudsley Monographs 18. (London: Oxford University Press)

Kendell, R. E., Cooper, J. E., Gourlay, A. T. *et al.* (1971). The diagnostic criteria of American and British psychiatrists. *Arch. Gen. Psychiatry*, **25**, 123–30

Kendell, R. E., Wainwright, S., Hailey, A. and Shannon, B. (1976). The influence of childbirth on psychiatric morbidity. *Psychol. Med.*, **6**, 297–302

Kendler, K. S. and Tsuang, M. T. (1982). Identical twins concordant for the progression of affective illness to schizophrenia. *Br. J. Psychiatry*, **141**, 563–6

Kerr, T. A., Roth, M., Schapira, K. and Gurney, C. (1972). The assessment and prediction of outcome in affective disorders. *Br. J. Psychiatry*, **121**, 167–74

Kerr, T. A., Schapira, K. and Roth, M. (1969). The relationship between premature death and affective disorders. *Br. J. Psychiatry*, **115**, 1277–82

Kerry, R. J., McDermott, C. M. and Orme, J. E. (1983). Affective disorders and cognitive performance. *J. Aff. Dis.*, **5**, 349–52

Keschner, M., Bender, M. V. and Strauss, I. (1936). Mental symptoms in cases of tumours of the temporal lobe. *Arch. Neurol. Psychiatry*, **35**, 572–96

Keschner, M., Bender, M. B. and Strauss, I. (1938). Mental symptom associated with brain tumour: a study of 530 verified cases. *J. Am. Med. Assoc.*, **110**, 714–18

Keshavan, M. S., Burton, S., Murphy, M. *et al.* (1985). Benzhexol withdrawal and cholinergic mechanisms in depression. *Br. J. Psychiatry*, **147**, 560–4

Kety, S. S. (1974). Biochemical and neurochemical effects of electroconvulsive shock. In Fink, M. *et al.* (eds.) *Psychobiology of Convulsive Therapy*. (Washington: Winston)

Kiev, A. (1972). *Transcultural Psychiatry*. (Harmondsworth: Penguin Books)

Kiloh, L. G., Child, J. P. and Latner, G. (1960). Endogenous depression treated with iproniazid – a follow-up study. *J. Ment. Sci.*, **106**, 1425–8

Kirby, G. H. (1909). Die Melancholie ein Zustansbild des Manisch – Depressiven Irreseins (book review). *State Hosp. Bull.*, **1**, 499–505 (quoted by Brown *et al.*, 1984)

Kishimoto, A., Ogura, C., Hazama, H. and Inoue, K. (1983). Long-term prophylactic effects of carbamazepine in affective disorder. *Br. J. Psychiatry*, **143**, 327–31

Kissen, D. M. (1963). Personality characteristics in males conducive to lung cancer. *Br. J. Med. Psychol.*, **36**, 27

Kissen, D. M. (1964). Lung cancer, inhalation and personality. In Kissen, D. M. and Le Shan, L. L. (eds.) *Psychosomatic aspects of Neoplastic Disease*, pp 3–11. (London: Pitman)

Kissen, D. M. and Rao, L. G. S. (1969). Steroid excretion patterns and personality in lung cancer patients. *Ann. NY Acad. Sci.*, **164**, 476–82

259

Klerman, G. L. and Schechter, G. (1982). Drugs and psychotherapy. In Paykel, E. S. (ed.) *Handbook of Affective Disorders*. (Edinburgh: Churchill Livingstone)

Knesevich, J. W., Martin, R. L., Berg, L. and Danziger, W. (1983). Preliminary report of affective symptoms in the early stages of senile dementia of the Alzheimer type. *Am. J. Psychiatry*, **140**, 233–5

Knight, G. (1965). Stereotactic tractotomy in the surgical treatment of mental illness. *J. Neurol. Neurosurg. Psychiatry*, **28**, 304–10

Knights, A. and Hirsch, S.R. (1981). "Revealed" depression drug treatment. *Arch. Gen. Psychiatry*, **38**, 806–11

Kocsis, J. H., Hanin, I., Bowden, C. and Brunswick, D. (1986). Imipramine and amitriptyline plasma concentrations and clinical response in major depression. *Br. J. Psychiatry*, **148**, 52–7

Koehler, K. and Sauer, H. (1983). First rank symptoms as predictors of ECT response in schizophrenia. *Br. J. Psychiatry*, **142**, 280–3

Koestler, A. (1964). *Act of Creation*. (London: Hutchinson)

Kolakowska, T., Williams, A. O., Ardern, M. *et al.* (1985). Schizophrenia with good and poor outcome. *Br. J. Psychiatry*, **146**, 229–46

Kowalski, A., Stanley, R. O., Dennerstein, L. *et al.* (1985). The sexual side-effects of antidepressant medication: A double-blind comparison of two antidepressants in a non-psychiatric populaton. *Br. J. Psychiatry*, **147**, 413–18

Kraepelin, E. (1896). *Lehrbuch der Psychiatrie* 5th edition. (Leipzig: Barth)

Kraepelin, E. (1919). *Dementia Praecox and Paraphrenia* (Transl. R. M. Barclay). (Edinburgh: Livingstone)

Kral, V. A. (1983). The relationship between senile dementia (Alzheimer type) and depression. *Can. J. Psychiatry*, **28**, 304–6

Krauthammer, C. and Klerman, G. L. (1979). The epidemiology of mania. In Shopsin, B. (ed.) *Manic Illness* (New York: Raven Press)

Krieger, D.T. (1979). Rhythms in CRF, ACTH and corticosteroids. In Krieger, D. T. (ed.) *Endocrine Rhythms*. (New York: Raven Press)

Kriss, A., Blumhardt, L. D., Halliday, A. M. and Pratt, R. T. C. (1978). Neurological asymmetries immediately after unilateral ECT. *J. Neurol. Neurosurg. Psychiatry*, **41**, 1135–1144

Kronfol, Z., Hamsher, K. de S., Digre, K. and Waziri, R. (1978). Depression and hemispheric functions: changes associated with unilateral ECT. *Br. J. Psychiatry*, **132**, 560–7

Kronfol, Z., Silva, J., Greden, J. *et al.* (1983). Impaired lymphocyte function in depressive illness. *Life Sci.*, **18**, 241–7

Kuhn, R. (1958). The treatment of depressive states with G-22355 (imipramine hydrochloride) *Am. J. Psychiatry*, **115**, 459–64

Kupfer, D.J., Foster, F.G., Reich, L. *et al.* (1976). EEG sleep changes as predictors in depression. *Am. J. Psychiatry*, **133**, 622–6

Lamb, C. (1833). Sanity of true genius. In *The Last Essays of Elia*. (London: Newnes)

Lasky, J. and Silver, P. (1978). *Love Scene*. The story of Laurence Olivier and Vivien Leigh. (Brighton: Angus and Robertson)

Leaf, R. C., Lerner, L. and Horovitz, Z. P. (1969). The role of the amygdala in the pharmacological and endocrinological manipulation of aggression. In Garrattini, S. and Sigg, E. B. (eds.) *Aggressive Behavior*. (Amsterdam: Excerpta Medica)

Leff, J. P. (1973). Culture and the differentiation of emotional states. *Br. J. Psychiatry*, **123**, 299–306

Leonard, B. E. (1981). Speculation on the biochemical basis of depression. In *New Directions in Antidepressant Therapy*. *46th Int. Congress and Symposium*. (London: Royal Society of Medicine)

Leonhard, K. (1959). *Aufteilung der endogenen Psychosen*. 2nd edition. (Berlin: Akademie-Verlag)

Leonhard, K., Korff, J. and Schulz, H. (1962). Die Temperamente in den Familien der monopolaren und bipolaren phasischen psychosen. *Psychiatr. Neurol.*, **143**, 416

Le Shan, L. L. and Worthington, R. E. (1956). Some recurrent life history patterns observed in patients with malignant disease. *J. Nerv. Ment. Dis.* **124**, 460–65

Levy, M. I. and Davis, K. L. (1983). The neuroendocrinology of depression. In Rifkin, A. (ed.) *Schizophrenia and Affective Disorders*. pp 1–17. (Bristol: John Wright)

Levy, R., Isaacs, A. and Behrman, J. (1971). Neurophysiological correlates of senile dementia. II. The somatosensory evoked response. *Psychol. Med.*, **1**, 159–65

Lewis, A. J. (1934a). Melancholia: A historical review. *J. Ment. Sci.*, **80**, 1–42

Lewis, A.J. (1934b). Melancholia: A clinical survey of depressive states. *J. Ment. Sci.*, **80**, 277–378

REFERENCES

Lewis, A. J. (1936). Melancholia: prognostic study and case material. *J. Ment. Sci.*, **82**, 488–58

Lewis, A. J. (1938). States of depression: their clinical and aetiological differentiation. *Br. Med. J.*, **2**, 875–8

Lewis, A. J. (1961). Agents of cultural advance *30th L. T. Hobhouse Memorial Trust Lecture* (London: Oxford University Press)

Lewis, N. and Piotrowski, Z. (1954). Clinical diagnosis of manic-depressive psychosis. In Hoch, P. M. and Zubin, J. (ed.) *Depression* (New York: Grune and Stratton)

Lieberman, A., Dziatolowski, M., Coopersmith, M. *et al.* (1979). Dementia in Parkinson's disease. *Ann. Neurol.*, **6**, 355–9

Lindsley, D. B. (1970). The role of nonspecific reticulo–thalamo–cortical systems in emotion. In Black, P. (ed.) *Physiological Correlates of Emotion*. (New York: Academic Press)

Linnoila, M., Karoum, F., Rosenthal, N. and Potter, W. Z. (1983). Electroconvulsive treatment and lithium-carbonate. *Arch. Gen. Psychiatry*, **40**, 677–80

Lipowski, Z. J. (1967). Quoted in Murphy and Brown, (1980)

Lishman, W. A. (1968). Brain damage in relation to psychiatric disability after head injury. *Br. J. Psychiatry*, **114**, 373–410

Lishman, W. A. (1978). *Organic Psychiatry*. (Oxford: Blackwell Scientific Publications)

Lloyd, G. G. and Lishman, W. A. (1975). The effects of depression on the speed of recall of pleasant and unpleasant experiences. *Psychol. Med.*, **5**, 173–80

Lockspeiser, E. (1973). *Music and Painting*. (London: Cassell)

Loomer, H. P., Saunders, J. C. and Kline, N. E. (1958). A clinical and pharmacodynamic evaluation of iproniazid as a psychic energizer. *Am. Psychiatr. Assoc. Res. Rep.*, **8**, 129

Loranger, A. W., Goodell, H., McDowell, F. H. *et al.* (1972). Intellectual impairment in Parkinson's syndrome *Brain*, **95**, 405–12

Low, A. A., Farmer, R. D. T., Jones, D. R. and Rohde, J. R. (1981). Suicide in England and Wales: an analysis of 100 years, 1876–1975. *Psychol. Med.*, **11**, 359–68

Luborsky, L., Singer, B. and Luborsky, L. (1975). Comparative studies of psychotherapies. *Arch. Gen. Psychiatry*, **32**, 995–1008

Lumsden Walker, W. (1980). Intentional self-injury in school age children. A study of fifty cases. *J. Adolesc.*, **3**, 335–46

Maas, J. W., Fawcett, J. A. and Dekirmenjian, H. (1972). Catecholamine metabolism, depressive illness and drug response. *Arch. Gen. Psychiatry*, **26**, 252–62

McAllister, T. W. (1983). Pseudodementia. *Am. J. Psychiatry*, **140**, 528–33

McAllister, T. W., Ferrell, R. B., Price, T. R. P. and Neville, M. B. (1982). The dexamethasone suppression test in two patients with severe depressive pseudodementia. *Am. J. Psychiatry*, **139**, 479–81

McAllister, T.W. and Price, T.R.P. (1982). Severe depressive pseudodementia with and without dementia. *Am. J. Psychiatry*, **139**, 626–9

McClure, G. M. G. (1984). Trends in suicide rate for England and Wales 1975–80. *Br. J. Psychiatry*, **144**, 119–26

McCreadie, R. G. and Morrison, D. P. (1985). The impact of lithium in South-West Scotland I. Demographic and clinical findings. *Br. J. Psychiatry*, **146**, 70–80

McCreadie, R. G., McCormick, M. and Morrison, D. P. (1985). The impact of lithium in South-West Scotland. III. The discontinuation of lithium. *Br. J. Psychiatry*, **146**, 77–80

McEvoy, P. J. and McEvoy, H. F. (1976). Management of psychiatric problems in a Kenyan mission hospital. *Br. Med. J.*, **1**, 1454–6

McEwen, B. S. (1980). The brain as a target organ of endocrine hormones. In Krieger, D. T. and Hughes, J. C. (eds.) *Neuroendocrinology*. pp 33–42. (Sunderland, Mass: Schauer)

MacFarlane, J. W., Allen, L. and Honzig, P. (1954). *A Development Study of Behaviour problems of normal children between 21 months and 14 years*. (Berkeley: University of California Press)

McGilchrist, J. M. (1975). Interactions with monoamine oxidase inhibitors. *Br. Med. J.*, **3**, 591–2

MacLean, P. D. (1949). Psychosomatic disease and the "visceral brain": recent developments bearing on the Papez theory of emotion. *Psychosom. Med.*, **11**, 338–53

Maddison, D. and Viola, A. (1968). The health of widows in the year following bereavement. *J. Psychosom. Res.*, **12**, 297–306

Maguire, P. (1981). Psychiatric aspects of malignant disease. *S K and F Publications*, **4**, No 2

Mahendra, B. (1977a). Stress and the major psychiatric illnesses. *Acta Psychiatr. Scand.*, **56**, 161–7

Mahendra, B. (1977b). Personality factors in neoplastic disease. *Proc. Sri Lanka Assoc. Adv. Sci.*, **33**, 3

261

Mahendra, B. (1977c). Neoplastic disease: Attitudes of patients and controls. *Proc. Sri Lanka Assoc. Adv. Sci.*, **33**, 8

Mahendra, B. (1981). Where have all the catatonics gone? *Psychol. Med.*, **11**, 669–71

Mahendra, B. (1984a). *Dementia: A Survey of the Syndrome*. (Lancaster: MTP Press)

Mahendra, B. (1984b). Some ethical issues in dementia research. *J. Med. Ethics*, **10**, 29–31

Mahendra, B. (1984d). Dementia and the abnormal dexamethasone suppression test. *Br. J. Psychiatry*, **144**, 98–9

Mahendra, B. (1985a). Dementia and Depression: The multi-faceted relationship. *Psychol. Med.* **15**, 227–36

Mahendra, B. (1985b). A malignant corpus callosum tumour in an 85-year-old demented woman. *Br. J. Psychiatry*, **147**, 94

Mahendra, B. (1985c). Subnormality revisited in Early 19th century France. *J. Ment. Def. Res.*, **29**, 391–401

Maj, P. (1981). Serotonergic mechanisms of antidepressant drugs. *Pharmakopsychiatrica*, **14**, 35–9

Majodina, M. Z. and Johnson, F. Y. A. (1983). Standardized assessment of depressive disorders (SADD) in Ghana. *Br. J. Psychiatry*, **143**, 442–6

Malick, J. B. and Barnett, A. (1976). The role of serotonergic pathways in isolation-induced aggression in mice. *Pharmacol. Biochem. Behav.*, **5**, 55–61

Mapother, E. (1926). Discussion on manic-depressive psychosis *Br. Med. J.*, **2**, 872–9

Markowe, M., Steinert, J. and Heyworth-Davies, F. (1967). Insulin and chlorpromazine in schizophrenia: a ten year comparative study. *Br. J. Psychiatry*, **113**, 1101–6

Marks, I. M., Stern, R. S., Mawson, D. *et al.* (1980). Clomipramine and exposure for obsessive–compulsive rituals: I. *Br. J. Psychiatry*, **136**, 1–25

Marmorston, J., Geller, P. J. and Welner, J. M. (1969). Pretreatment urinary hormone patterns and survival in patients with breast cancer, prostate cancer, or lung cancer. *Ann. NY Acad. Sci.*, **164**, 489–93

Marsden, C. D. and Harrison, M. J. G. (1972). Outcome of investigation of patients with presenile dementia. *Br. Med. J.*, **2**, 249–52

Mason, J. W. (1972). Organization of psychoendocrine mechanisms: A review and reconsideration of research. In Greenfield, N. S. and Sternbach, R. A. (eds.) *Handbook of Psychophysiology*. (New York: Holt, Rhinehart and Winston Inc)

Mason, J. W. (1975). Psychologic stress and endocrine function. In Sachar, E. J. (ed.) *Topics in Psychoendocrinology*. (New York: Grune and Stratton)

Mastrovito, R. C., Deguire, K. S., Clarkin, J. *et al.* (1979). Personality characteristics of women with gynaecological cancer. *Cancer Det. Prev.*, **2**, 281–7

Maudsley, H. (1868). *The Physiology and Pathology of Mind*. (London)

Mayeux, R., Stern, Y., Rosen, J. and Leventhal, J. (1981). Depression, intellectual impairment and Parkinson's disease. *Neurology*, **31**, 645–50

Mbanefo, S. E. (1971). The general practitioner and psychiatry. In *Psychiatry and Mental Health Care in General Practice*. (University of Ibadan) (quoted by Dhadphale *et al.*, 1983)

Medical Research Council (1965). Clinical trial of the treatment of depressive illness. *Br. Med. J.*, **1**, 881–6

Meltzer, H. Y., Arora, R. C., Baber, R. and Tricou, B. J. (1981). Serotonin uptake in blood platelets of psychiatric patients. *Arch. Gen. Psychiatry*, **38**, 1322–6

Meltzer, H. Y., Lowy, M., Robertson, A. *et al.* (1984). Effect of 5-hydroxytryptophan on serum cortisol levels in major affective disorders. *Arch. Gen. Psychiatry*, **41**, 366–74

Mendlewicz, J. (1976). The age factor in depressive illness. Some genetic considerations. *J. Gerontol.*, **31**, 300–3

Mendlewicz, J., Kerkhofs, M., Hoffmann, G. and Linkowski, P. (1984). Dexamethasone suppression test and REM sleep in patients with major depressive disorder. *Br. J. Psychiatry*, **145**, 383–8

Mendlewicz, J., Linkowski, P. and Wilmotte, J. (1980). Linkage between glucose-6-phosphate dehydrogenase deficiency and manic-depressive psychosis. *Br. J. Psychiatry*, **137**, 337–42

Meyer, A. (1960). Emergent patterns of the pathology of mental disease. The thirty-fourth. Maudsley Lecture. *J. Ment. Sci.*, **106**, 785–802

Mezey, A. G. (1960). Personal background, emigration and mental disorder in Hungarian refugees. *J. Ment. Sci.*, **106**, 618–37

Mindham, R. H. S., Howland, C. and Shepherd, M. (1973). An evaluation of continuation therapy with tricyclic antidepressants in depressive illness. *Psychol. Med.,* **3**, 5–17

Mindham, R. H. S., Marsden, C. D. and Parkes, J. D. (1976). Psychiatric symptoms during L-dopa therapy for Parkinson's disease and their relationship to physical disability. *Psychol. Med.,* **6**, 23–33

Moller, H. J. and Von Zerssen, D. (1981). Depressive symptomatik in statioharen Behandlungsuerlauf von 280 schizophrenen patienten. *Pharmacopsychologie,* **14**, 172–9 (quoted by Hirsch, S. R., 1982. Depression 'revealed' in schizophrenia. *Br. J. Psychiatry,* **140**, 421–4)

Monnelly, E. P., Woodruff, R. A. and Robins, L. N. (1974). Manic-depressive illness and social achievement in a public hospital sample. *Acta Psychiatr. Scand.,* **50**, 318–25.

Moradi, S. R., Mumiz, C. E. and Belar, C. D. (1979). Male delusional depressed patients: Response to treatment. *Br. J. Psychiatry,* **135**, 136–8

Morrison, D. P. and McCreadie, R. G. (1985). The impact of lithium in South-West Scotland II. A longitudinal study. *Br. J. Psychiatry,* **146**, 74–7

Mullen, P. E. (1983). Sleep and its interaction with endocrine rhythms. *Br. J. Psychiatry,* **142**, 215–20

Mullen, P. E. and Silman, R. E. (1977). The pineal and psychiatry: a review. *Psychol. Med.,* **7**, 407–17

Murphy, D. L., Lipper, S., Pickar, D. *et al.* (1981). Selective inhibition of monoamine oxidase type A: clinical antidepressant effects and metabolic changes in man. In Youdim, M. B. H. and Paykel, E. S. (eds.) *Monoamine Oxidase Inhibitors – The State of the Art.* (Chichester: John Wiley)

Murphy, E. (1983). The prognosis of depression in old age. *Br. J. Psychiatry,* **142**, 111–19

Murphy, E. and Brown, G. W. (1980). Life events, psychiatric disturbance and physical illness. *Br. J. Psychiatry,* **136**, 326–38

Murphy, H. B. M. (1973). History and the evolution of syndromes: the striking case of Latah and Amok. In Hammer, M. *et al.* (eds.) *Psychopathology: Contributions from the Social, Behavioural and Biological Sciences.* (New York: Wiley)

Murphy, J. E., Donald, J. F. and Molla, A. L. (1976). Mianserin in the treatment of depression in general practice. *Practitioner,* **217**, 135–8

Myers, D. H. and Neal, C. D. (1978). Suicide in psychiatric patients. *Br.J. Psychiatry,* **133**, 38–44

Naeser, M. A., Gebhardt, C. and Levine, H. L. (1980). Decreased computerized tomography numbers in patients with presenile dementia. *Arch. Neurol.,* **37**, 401–9

Nauta, W. J. H. (1971). The problem of the frontal lobe: A re-interpretation. *J. Psychiatr. Res.,* **8**, 167

Nayha, S. (1982). Autumn incidence of suicides re-examined: Data from Finland by sex, age and occupation. *Br. J. Psychiatry,* **141**, 512–17

Naylor, G. J., Dick, D. A. T., Dick, E. G. *et al.* (1973). Erythrocyte membrane cation carrier in depressive illness. *Psychol. Med.,* **3**, 502–8

Naylor, G. J. and Smith, A. H. W. (1981). Vanadium, a possible aetiological factor in manic depressive illness. *Psychol. Med.,* **11**, 249–56

Ndetei, D. M. and Muhangi, J. (1979). The prevalence and clinical presentation of psychiatric illness in a rural setting in Kenya. *Br. J. Psychiatry,* **135**, 269–72

Ndetei, D. M. and Vadher, A. (1982). Types of life events associated with depression in a Kenyan setting. *Acta Psychiatr. Scand.,* **66**, 163–8

Nelson, J. C. and Charney, D. S. (1981). The symptoms of major depressive illness. *Am. J. Psychiatry,* **138**, 1–13

Nelson, W. H., Orr, W. W., Stevenson, J. M. and Shane, S. R. (1982). Hypothalamic—pituitary—adrenal axis activity and tricycle response in major depression. *Arch. Gen. Psychiatry,* **39**, 1033–6

Nelson, W. H., Khan, A. and Orr, W. W., Jr. (1984). Delusional depression. *J. Affect. Dis.,* **6**, 297–306

Neumann, C. (1959). Psychische Besonderheiten bei Krebspatienten Z. *Psychosom. Med.,* **5**, 91–101 (quoted in Bahnson, 1980).

Noll, K. and Davis, J. M. (1984). Depression. In Duncan, R. and Weston-Smith, M. (eds.) *The Encyclopaedia of Medical Ignorance.* pp. 27–42. (Oxford: Pergamon Press)

Noreik, K. (1970). *Follow-up and classification of functional psychoses with special reference to Reactive Psychoses.* (Oslo: Universitetsforlaget)

Nott, P. N. and Fleminger, J. J. (1975). Presenile dementia: the difficulties of early diagnosis. *Acta Psychiatr. Scand.,* **51**, 210–17

O'Connell, R. A., Mayo, J. A., Eng, L. K. *et al.* (1985). Social support and long-term lithium outcome. *Br. J. Psychiatry*, **147**, 272–5

O'Flanagan, R. M. (1973). Clomipramine infusion and lithium carbonate: a synergistic effect? *Lancet*, **2**, 974

Odegaard, O. (1932). Emigration and insanity: A study of mental disease among the Norwegian-born population of Minnesota. *Acta Psychiatr. et Neurol. Scand.*, Suppl. 4

Odegaard, O. (1946). A statistical investigation of the incidence of mental disorder in Norway. *Psychiat. Q.*, **20**, 381–400

Oltman, J. E. and Friedman, S. (1961). Comments on Huntington's chorea. *Dis. Nerv. Sys.*, **22**, 1–7

Orley, J. and Wing, J. K. (1979). Psychiatric disorders in two African villages. *Arch. Gen. Psychiatry*, **36**, 513–20

Orvaschel, H., Weissman, M. M. and Kidd, K. K. (1980). Children and depression: the children of depressed parents; depression in children. *J. Affect. Dis.*, **2**, 1–16

Pallis, D. J., Barraclough, B. M., Levey, A. B. *et al.* (1982). Estimating suicide risk among attempted suicides. *Br. J. Psychiatry*, **141**, 37–44

Pallis, D. J., Gibbons, J. S. and Pierce, D. W. (1984). Estimating suicide risk among attempted suicides. II. Efficiency of predictive scales after the attempt. *Br. J. Psychiatry*, **144**, 139–48

Pare, C. M. B. (1985). The present status of monoamine oxidase inhibitors. *Br. J. Psychiatry*, **146**, 576–84

Parker, G. and Walter, S. (1982). Seasonal variation in depressive disorders and suicidal deaths in New South Wales. *Br. J. Psychiatry*, **140**, 626–32

Parkes, C. M. (1985). Bereavement. *Br. J. Psychiatry*, **146**, 11–17

Patrick, H. T. and Levy, D. M. (1922). Parkinson's disease: a clinical study of 146 cases. *Arch. Neurol. Psychiatry*, **7**, 711–20

Paul, S. M., Rehavi, M., Rice, K. C. *et al.* (1981). Does high affinity 3H-imipramine binding label serotonin re-uptake sites in brain and platelets? *Life Sci.*, **28**, 2253–60

Paykel, E. S. (1972). Depressive typologies and response to amitriptyline. *Br. J. Psychiatry*, **120**, 147–56

Paykel, E. S. (1978). Contribution of life events to causation of psychiatric illness. *Psychol. Med.*, **8**, 245–53

Paykel, E. S. and Coppen, A. (1979). (eds.) *Psychopharmacology of Affective Disorders*. (Oxford: Oxford University Press)

Paykel, E. S., Myers, J. K., Dienelt, M.N. *et al.* (1969). Life events and depression: a controlled study. *Arch. Gen. Psychiatry*, **21**, 753–60

Paykel, E. S. and Norton, K. R. W. (1982). Masked depression. *Br. J. Hosp. Med.*, **Aug., 1982**, 151–7

Paykel, E. S., Parker, R. R., Penrose, R. J. J. and Rassaby, E. R. (1979). Depressive classification and prediction of response to phenelzine. *Br. J. Psychiatry*, **134**, 572–81

Peet, M. and Coppen, A. (1979). The pharmacokinetics of antidepressant drugs: relevance to their therapeutic effect. In Paykel, E. S. and Coppen, A. (eds.) *Psychopharmacology of Affective Disorders*. (Oxford: Oxford University Press)

Perris, C. (1966). A study of bipolar (manic-depressive) and unipolar recurrent affective psychoses. *Actc Psychiatr. Scand.*, **42**, Suppl. 194

Perris, C. (1974). A study of cycloid psychoses. *Acta Psychiatr. Scand.*, Suppl. 253

Perris, C. (1980). Central measures of depression. In Van Praag, H. M. (ed.) *Handbook of Biological Psychiatry*. (New York: Marcel Dekker)

Perry, E. K., Marshall, E. F., Blessed, G. *et al.* (1983). Decreased imipramine binding in the brains of patients with depressive illness. *Br. J. Psychiatry*, **142**, 188–192

Perry, G. F., Shapiro, L., Fitzsimmons, B. and Irwin, P. (1978). Clinical studies of mianserin, imipramine and placebo in depression: blood level and MHPG correlations. *Proceedings of Symposium on Mianserin. Br. J. Clin. Pharmacol.*, **5**, (Suppl.) 35S–41S

Perry, T. L., Hansen, S. and Kloster, M. (1973). Huntington's chorea: deficiency of gamma-aminobutyric acid in brain. *N. Engl. J. Med.*, **258**, 337–42

Petersen, P. (1968). Psychiatric disorders in primary hyperparathyroidism. *J. Clin. Endocrinol. Metabol.*, **28**, 1491–5

Petterson, V. (1977). Manic depressive illness. *Acta Psychiatr. Scand.*, **56**, Suppl. 269

Pfeiffer, W. M. (1968). The symptomatology of depression viewed transculturally. *Transcult.*

Psychiatry Res. Rev., **V,** 121–4

Pincus, J. H. and Tucker, G. J. (1978). *Behavioral Neurology.* 2nd Edn. (New York: Oxford University Press)

Plokker, J. H. (1964). *Artistic self-expression in Mental Disease.* (London: Charles Skilton)

Pokorny, A. D. (1965). Human violence: a comparison of homicide, aggravated assault, suicide and attempted suicide. *J. Crim. Law, Crim., Police Sci.,* **56,** 488 (quoted in Stengel, 1975)

Pollitt, J. (1972). The relationship between genetic and precipitating factors in depressive illness. *Br. J. Psychiatry,* **121,** 67–70

Post, F. (1962). *The significance of affective symptoms.* (London: Oxford University Press)

Post, F. (1972). The management and nature of depressive illnesses in late life: a follow-through study. *Br. J. Psychiatry,* **121,** 393–404

van Praag, H. M. (1980). Central monoamine metabolism in depression. *Comp. Psychiatr.,* **21,** 30–43

van Praag, H. M. and Korf, J. (1971). Endogenous depressions with and without disturbances in the 5-hydroxytryptamine metabolism: biochemical classification? *Psychopharmacology,* **19,** 148–52

van Praag, H. M. (1982). Depression. *Lancet,* **ii,** 1259–64

Prange, A. J., Wilson, I. C., Lynn, C. W. et al. (1974). L-tryptophan in mania. *Arch. Gen. Psychiatry.* **30,** 56–62

Price, J. S. (1975). Genetics of the affective illnesses. In Silverstone, T. and Barraclough, B. (eds.) *Contemporary Psychiatry,* pp. 67–75. (London: Royal College of Psychiatrists)

Prince, R. H. (1968). The changing picture of depressive syndromes in Africa: Is it fact or diagnostic fashion? *Can. J. Afr. Stud.,* **1,** 177–92

Puig-Antich, J., Blau, S., Marx, N. et al. (1978). Prepubertal major depressive disorder: Pilot study. *J. Am. Acad. Child. Psychiatry,* **17,** 695–707

Puig-Antich, J., Chambers, W., Halpern et al. (1979). Cortisol hypersecretion in prepubertal depressive illness. *Psychoneuroendocrinology,* **4,** 191–7

van Putten, T. and May, P. R. A. (1981). 'Akinetic depression' in schizophrenia. *Arch. Gen. Psychiatry,* **35,** 1101–7

Quitkin, F. M. (1985). The importance of dosage in prescribing antidepressants. *Br. J. Psychiatry.* **147,** 593–7

Rack, P. (1982). *Race, Culture and Mental Disorder.* (London: Tavistock Publications)

Rampling, D. (1978). Aggression: A paradoxical response to tricyclic antidepressants. *Am. J. Psychiatry,* **135,** 117–18

Rao, A. V. (1973). Depressive illness and guilt in Indian culture. *Indian J. Psychiatry,* **15,** 231–6

Rasmussen, A. F. (1969). Emotions and immunity. *Ann. NY Acad. Sci,* **164,** 458–62

Ravaris, C. L., Nies, A., Robinson, D. et al. (1976). A multiple dose controlled study of phenelzine in depression-anxiety states. *Arch. Gen. Psychiatry,* **33,** 347–50

Reed, T. E. and Chandler, J. R. (1958). Huntington's chorea in Michigan I. Demography and genetics. *Am. J. Hum. Genet.,* **10,** 201–25

Rees, W. D. and Lutkins, S. G. (1967). Mortality of bereavement. *Br. Med. J.,* **4,** 13–16

Reid, A. H. (1982). *The Psychiatry of Mental Handicap.* (London: Blackwell Scientific Publications)

Report of the NINCDS - ADRDA Work Group (1984). Clinical diagnosis of Alzheimer's disease. *Neurology,* **34,** 939–44

Richelson, E. (1979). Tricyclic antidepressants and neurotransmitter receptors. *Psychiatr. Ann.,* **9**

Richman, A. and Barry, A. (1985). More and more is less and less. *Br. J. Psychiatry,* **146,** 164–8

Roberts, J. K. A. and Lishman, W. A. (1984). The use of the CAT Head Scanner in clinical psychiatry. *Br. J. Psychiatry,* **145,** 152–8

Robins, A. H. (1976). Depression in patients with Parkinsonism. *Br. J. Psychiatry,* **128,** 141–5

Robinson, R. G. and Benson, D. F. (1981). Depression in aphasic patients: frequency, severity and clinico-pathological correlations *Brain and Language,* **14,** 282–91

Robinson, R. G., Starr, L. B. and Price, T. R. (1984). A two year longitudinal study of mood disorders following stroke. *Br. J. Psychiatry,* **144,** 256–62

Robinson, R. G. and Szetela, B. (1981). Mood change following left hemispheric brain injury. *Ann. Neurol.,* **9,** 447–53

Rogers, S. C. and Clay, P. M. (1975). A statistical review of controlled trials of imipramine and placebo in the treatment of depressive illness. *Br. J. Psychiatry,* **127,** 599–603

Ron, M. A., Toone, B. K., Garralda, M. E. and Lishman, W. A. (1979). Diagnostic accuracy in presenile dementia. *Br. J. Psychiatry*, **134**, 161–8

Rosen, G. (1964). The mentally ill and the community in Western and Central Europe during the late middle ages and the Renaissance. *J. Hist. Med.*, **19**, 377–88

Rosenthal, D. (1970). *Genetic theory and abnormal behaviour*. (New York: McGraw-Hill)

Rosenthal, N. E., Sack, D. A., Gillin, J. C. *et al.* (1984). Seasonal affective disorder: A description of the syndrome and preliminary findings with light therapy. *Arch. Gen. Psychiatry*, **41**, 72–80

Rosenthal, S. H. and Klerman, G. L. (1966). Content and consistency in the endogenous depressive pattern. *Br. J. Psychiatry*, **112**, 471–84

Roth, M. (1963). Neurosis, psychosis and the concept of disease in psychiatry. *Acta Psychiatr. Scand.*, **39**, 128–45

Roth, M., Gurney, C., Garside, R. F. and Kerr, T. A. (1972). Studies in the classification of affective disorder. The relationship between anxiety states and depressive illnesses – I. *Br. J. Psychiatry*, **121**, 147–61

Roth, M. and Mountjoy, C. Q. (1982). The distinction between anxiety states and depressive disorders. In Paykel, E. S. (ed.) *Handbook of Affective Disorders*. (Edinburgh: Churchill Livingstone)

Rowan, P. R., Paykel, E. S. and Parker, R. R. (1982). Phenelzine and amitriptyline: effects on symptoms of neurotic depression. *Br. J. Psychiatry*, **140**, 475–83

Roy, A. (1981). Vulnerability factors and depression in men. *Br. J. Psychiatry*, **138**, 75–7

Roy, A., Thompson, R. and Kennedy, S. (1983). Depression in chronic schizophrenia. *Br. J. Psychiatry*, **142**, 465–70

Roy-Byrne, P., Post, R. M., Rubinow, D. R. *et al.* (1984). CSF 5-HIAA and personal and family history of suicide in affectively ill patients: a negative study. *Psychiatr. Res.*, **10**, 263–74

Rubinow, D. R., Gold, P. W., Post, R. M. *et al.* (1983). Cerebrospinal fluid somatostatin in primary affective disorder. *Psychopharmacol. Bull.*, **19**, 422–5

Rudorfer, M. V. and Clayton, P. J. (1981). Depression, dementia and dexamethasone suppression. *Am. J. Psychiatr.*, **138**, 701

Rush, A. J., Weissenburger, J., Vinson, D. B. and Giles, D. E. (1983). Neuropsychological dysfunctions in unipolar nonpsychotic major depressions. *J. Affect. Dis.*, **5**, 281–7

Russell, G. F. M. and de Silva, P. (1983). Observations on the relationship between anxiety and depressive symptoms during the course of depressive illnesses. *Br. J. Clin. Pharmacol.*, **15**, 147S–153S

Rutter, M. L., Tizard, J. and Whitmore, K. (eds.) (1970). *Education, Health and Behaviour*. (London: Longman)

Sachar, E. J. (1982). Endocrine abnormalities in depression. In Paykel, E. S. (ed.) *Handbook of Affective Disorders*. pp. 191–201. (Edinburgh: Churchill Livingstone)

Sachar, E. J., Hellman, L., Roffwarg, H. *et al.* (1973). Disrupted 24 hour patterns of cortisol secretion in psychotic depression. *Arch. Gen. Psychiatry*, **28**, 19–24

Sainsbury, P. (1955). *Suicide in London*. (London: Chapman and Hall)

Sainsbury, P. (1975). Suicide and attempted suicide. In Kisker, K. P. *et al. Psychiatrie der Gegenwart*. pp. 557–606. (Berlin: Springer-Verlag) (quoted by Shepherd and Barraclough, 1980)

Sargant, W. and Slater, E. (1969). *Introduction to Physical Methods of Treatment in Psychiatry*. (Edinburgh: E. & S. Livingstone)

Sassin, J. F., Frantax, A. G., Weltzman, E. D. and Kapen, S. (1972). Human prolactin 24 hour pattern with increased release during sleep. *Science*, **177**, 1205–7

Schildkraut, J. J. (1965). The catecholamine hypothesis of affective disorders – a review of the supporting evidence. *Am. J. Psychiatry*, **122**, 509–22

Schmale, A. H. and Iker, H. P. (1966). The psychological setting of uterine cervical cancer. *Ann. NY Acad. Sci.*, **125**, 807–13

Schou, M. (1979). Artistic productivity and lithium prophylaxis in manic-depressive illness. *Br. J. Psychiatry*, **135**, 97–103

Schrader, G. D. and Levien, H. E. M. (1985). Response to sequential administration of clomipramine and lithium carbonate on treatment-resistant depression. *Br. J. Psychiatry*, **147**, 573–8

Schulsinger, F., Kety, S. S., Rosenthal, D. *et al.* (1979). A family study of suicide. In Schou, M. and Stromgren, E. (eds.) *Origins, Prevention and Treatment of Affective Disorders*. (London: Academic Press)

Seager, C. P. and Bird, R. L. (1962). Imipramine with electrical treatment in depression. Controlled trial. *Br. J. Psychiatry*, **108**, 704–7

REFERENCES

Sedvall, G., Fyro, B., Gullberg, B. *et al.* (1980). Relationship in healthy volunteers between concentrations of monoamine metabolites in cerebrospinal fluid and family history of psychiatric morbidity. *Br. J. Psychiatry*, **136**, 366–74

Sellers, M. with Sellers, S. and Sellers, V. (1981). "P.S. I love you." Peter Sellers 1925–1980 (London: Collins)

Shaffer, D. (1974). Suicide in childhood and early adolescence. *J. Child Psychol. Psychiatry*, **15**, 275–91

Shaw, D. M., Tidmarsh, S. F. and Karajgi, B. M. (1980). Tryptophan, affective disorder and stress. *J. Affect. Dis.*, **2**, 321–5

Sheard, M. H. (1975). Lithium in the treatment of aggression. *J. Nerv. Ment. Dis.*, **160**, 108–18

Sheard, M. H., Marini, J. L., Bridges, K. I. and Wagner, E. (1976). The effect of lithium on impulsive aggressive behaviour on man. *Am. J. Psychiatry*, **133**, 1409–13

Shekelle, R. B., Raynor, W. J., Jr., Ostfeld, A. M. *et al.* (1981). Psychological depression and 17-year risk of death from cancer. *Psychosom. Med.*, **43**, 117–25

Sheldrick, C. (1984). The implications of a changing diagnosis in psychiatry: schizophrenia succeeded by affective disorder. In Gaind, R. N. *et al.* (eds.) *Current Themes in Psychiatry*, Vol. 3., pp. 39–50. (New York: Spectrum Publications)

Shepherd, D. and Barraclough, B. M. (1974). The aftermath of suicide. *Br. Med. J.*, **2**, 600–3

Shepherd, D. M. and Barraclough, B. M. (1980). Work and suicide: an empirical investigation. *Br. J. Psychiatry*, **136**, 469–478

Shepherd, M., Cooper, B., Brown, A. G. and Kalton, G. W. (1966). *Psychiatric illness in General Practice.* (London: Oxford University Press)

Sireling, L. I., Freeling, P., Paykel, E. S. and Rao, B. M. (1985). Depression in general practice: clinical features and comparison with out-patients. *Br. J. Psychiatry*, **147**, 119–26

Sitaram, N., Nurnberger, J. I., Gershon, E. *et al.* (1980). Faster REM sleep induction in euthymic patients with preliminary affective illness. *Science*, **208**, 200–2

Skultans, V. (1979). *English Madness. Ideas on Insanity.* (London: Routledge and Kegan Paul)

Slater, E. (1947). Genetical causes of schizophrenic symptoms. *Monatsschrift fur psychiatrie und neurologie*, **113**, 50–8

Slater, E. (1953). *Psychotic and Neurotic Illnesses in Twins.* (London: HMSO)

Slater, E. (1979). The Creative Personality. In Roth, M. and Cowie, V. (eds.) *Psychiatry, Genetics and Pathography.* pp. 89–103. (London: Gaskell Press)

Slater, E., Maxwell, J. and Price, J. S. (1971). Distribution of ancestral secondary cases in bipolar affective disorders. *Br. J. Psychiatry*, **118**, 215

Slater, E. and Meyer, A. (1959). Contributions to a pathography: Robert Schumann. *Confinia Psychiatrica*, **2**, 65–94

Smith, J. S. and Kiloh, L. G. (1981). The investigation of dementia: results in 200 consecutive admissions. *Lancet*, **1**, 824–7

Snaith, R. P. and Taylor, C. M. (1985). Irritability: Definition, assessment and associated factors. *Br. J. Psychiatry*, **147**, 127–36

Spar, J. E. and Gerner, R. (1982). Does the dexamethasone suppression test distinguish dementia from depression? *Am. J. Psychiatry*, **139**, 238–40

Spitzer, R. L., Endicott, J. and Robins, E. (1978). Research diagnostic criteria: rationale and reliability *Arch. Gen. Psychiatry*, **35**, 773–82

Squire, L. R. (1977). ECT and memory loss. *Am. J. Psychiatry*, **134**, 997–1001

Squire, L. R., Chace, P. M. and Slater, P. C. (1976). Retrograde amnesia following electroconvulsive therapy. *Nature*, **160**, 775–7

Squire, L. R. and Slater, P. C. (1983). Electroconvulsive therapy and complaints of memory dysfunction: A prospective 3-year follow-up study. *Br. J. Psychiatry*, **142**, 1–8

Srinivasan, D. P. and Hullin, R. P. (1980). Current concepts of lithium therapy. *Br. J. Hosp. Med.*, **24**, 466–75

Standish-Barry, H. M. A. S., Bouras, N., Bridges, P. K. and Bartlett, J. R. (1982). Pneumoencephalographic and computerized axial tomography scan changes in affective disorder. *Br. J. Psychiatry*, **141**, 614–17

Stanley, M., Virgilio, J. and Gershon, S. (1982). Tritiated imipramine binding sites are decreased in the frontal cortex of suicides. *Science*, **216**, 1337–9

Stavraky, K. M. *et al.* (1968). Psychological factors in the outcome of human cancer. *J. Psychosom. Res.*, **12**, 251–9

Stein, Z. and Susser, M. (1969). Widowhood and mental illness. *Br. J. Prev. Soc. Med.*, **23**, 106–10

Stengel, E. (1975). *Suicide and Attempted Suicide*. (Harmondsworth: Penguin Books)

Stenstedt, A. (1959). Involutional melancholia: an etiologic, clinical and social study of endogenous depression in later life, with special reference to genetic factors. *Acta Psychiatr. Neurol. Scand.*, **34**, (Suppl. 127) 1–71

Stones, M. J. (1973). Electroconvulsive treatment and short term memory. *Br. J. Psychiatry*, **122**, 591–4

Storey, P. B. (1970). Brain damage and personality change after subarachnoid haemorrhage. *Br. J. Psychiatry*, **117**, 129–42

Storr, A. (1972). *The Dynamics of Creation*. (London: Secker and Warburg)

Storr, A. (1983). A psychotherapist looks at depression. *Br. J. Psychiatry*, **143**, 431–5

Stromgren, E. (1961). *Psykiatri*, 7th Edn. (Copenhagen: Munksgaard)

Stromgren, E. (1969). Uses and abuses of concepts in psychiatry. *Am. J. Psychiatry*, **126**, 6

Stromgren, L. S. (1973). Unilateral versus bilateral electroconvulsive therapy. Investigation into the therapeutic effect in endogenous depression. *Acta Psychiatr. Scand.*, **52**, Suppl. 240, 8–65

Strom-Olsen, R. and Carlisle, S. (1971). Bifrontal stereotactic tractotomy. *Br. J. Psychiatry*, **118**, 141–54

Summers, M. (1926). *The History of Witchcraft and Demonology.*, (London: Routledge and Kegan Paul)

Surridge, D. (1969). An investigation into some psychiatric aspects of multiple sclerosis. *Br. J. Psychiatry*, **115**, 749–64

Sweeney, D., Nelson, C., Bower, M. *et al.* (1978). Delusional versus non-delusional depression – neurochemical differences. *Lancet*, **2**, 100–1

Swinscow, D. (1951). Some suicide statistics. *Br. Med. J.*, **1**, 1417–25

Sykes, M. K. and Tredgold, R. F. (1964). Restricted orbital undercutting. *Br. J. Psychiatry*, **110**, 609–40

Tait, A. C., Harper, J. and McClatchey, W. T. (1957). Initial psychiatric illness in involutional women: clinical aspects. *J. Ment. Sci.*, **103**, 132–45

Taylor, E. A. and Stansfeld, S. A. (1984). Children who poison themselves I. A clinical comparison with psychiatric controls. II. Prediction of attendance for treatment. *Br. J. Psychiatry*, **145**, 127–35

Taylor, J. R., Kuhlengel, B. G. and Dean, R. S. (1985). ECT, blood pressure changes and neuropsychological deficit. *Br. J. Psychiatry*, **147**, 36–8

Taylor, M. A. and Abrams, R. (1985). Short-term cognitive effects of unilateral and bilateral ECT. *Br. J. Psychiatry*, **146**, 308–11

Taylor, M. A., Redfield, J. and Abrams, R. (1981). Neuropsychological dysfunction in schizophrenia and affective disorder. *Biol. Psychiatry*, **16**, 467–78

Taylor, P. J. and Gunn, J. (1984). Violence and psychosis. I. Risk of violence among psychotic men. *Br. Med. J.*, **288**, 1945–9

Terzian, H. (1964). Behavioural and EEG effects of intracarotid sodium amytal injection. *Acta Neurochir.*, **12**, 230–9

Thalbitzer, S. (1905). Melancholie und Depression. *Allg. Z. Psychiatrie*, **775**, (quoted by Lewis, 1934a)

Thomson, K. C. and Hendrie, H. C. (1972). Environmental stress in primary depressive illness. *Arch. Gen. Psychiatry*, **26**, 130–2

Thompson, C. (1984). Circadian rhythms and psychiatry. *Br. J. Psychiatry*, **145**, 204–6

Thompson, C., Mezey, G., Corn, T. *et al.* (1985). The effect of desipramine upon melatonin and cortisol secretion in depressed and normal subjects. *Br. J. Psychiatry*, **147**, 389–93

Titley, W. B. (1936). Prepsychotic personality of patients with involutional melancholia. *Arch. Neurol. Psychiatry*, **36**, 19–33

Tomlinson, B. E., Blessed, G. and Roth, M. (1968). Observations on the brains of non-demented old people. *J. Neurol. Sci.*, **7**, 331–56

Toone, B. K., Garralda, M. E. and Ron, M. A. (1982). The psychoses of epilepsy and the functional psychoses. *Br. J. Psychiatry*, **141**, 256–61.

Tooth, G. C. and Newton, M. P. (1961). Leucotomy in England and Wales 1942–54. *Reports on Public Health and Medical Subjects* No 104. (Ministry of Health, London: HMSO)

Topp, D. O. (1979). Suicide in prison. *Br. J. Psychiatry*, **134**, 24–7

REFERENCES

Torgerson, S. (1985). Hereditary differentiation of anxiety and affective neuroses. *Br. J. Psychiatry*, **146**, 530–4

Traskman, L., Asberg, M., Bertilsson, L. and Sjostrand, L. (1981). Monoamine metabolites in CSF and suicidal behavior. *Arch. Gen. Psychiatry*, **38**, 631–6

Trethowan, W. H. (1979). *The Art of Madness*. Smith Kline and French Laboratories Ltd

Trimble, M. R. and Cummings, J. L. (1981). Neuropsychiatric disturbances following brainstem lesions. *Br. J. Psychiatry*, **138**, 56–59

Tsuang, M. T. (1965). A study of pairs of sibs both hospitalized for mental disorder. Ph.D. thesis, University of London, (quoted in Kendler and Tsuang, 1982)

Tsuang, M. T. (1979). Schizoaffective disorder. *Arch. Gen. Psych.*, **35**, 633–4

Tuke, D. H. (1878). *Insanity in Ancient and Modern Life*. London: Macmillan

Tyrer, P., Gardner, M., Lambourn, J. and Whitford, M. (1980). Clinical and pharmacokinetic factors affecting response to phenelzine. *Br. J. Psychiatry*, **136**, 359–365

Uytdenhoef, P., Portelange, P., Jacquy, J. *et al.* (1983). Regional cerebral blood flow and lateralized hemispheric dysfunction in depression. *Br. J. Psychiatry*, **143**, 128–132

Vadher, A. and Ndetei, D. M. (1981). Life events and depression in a Kenyan setting. *Br. J. Psychiatry*

Vaillant, G. (1963). The natural history of the remitting schizophrenias. *Am. J. Psychiatry*, **120**, 367–375

Varsamis, J., Zuckhowski, T. and Maini, K. K. (1972). Survival rates of death in geriatric psychiatric patients: a six year follow-up. *Can. Psychiatr. Assoc. J.*, **7**, 17–22

Vasari, Giorgio (1550). Michelangelo Buonnaroti. In Burroughs, B. (ed.) *The Essential Vasari* (1962). pp. 178–216 (London: Unwin Books)

Wain, J. (1974). *Samuel Johnson*. (London: Macmillan)

Walton, J. N. (1977). (ed.) *Brain's Diseases of the Nervous System* 8th Edn. (Oxford: Oxford University Press)

Weeks, D., Freeman, C. P. L. and Kendell, R. E. (1980). ECT III: Enduring cognitive deficits? *Br. J. Psychiatry*, **137**, 26–37

Wehr, T. A. and Goodwin, F. K. (1979). Rapid cycling in manic-depressives induced by tricyclic antidepressants. *Arch. Gen. Psychiatry*, **36**, 555–9

Wehr, T. A., Wirz-Justice, A., Goodwin, F. K. *et al.* (1979). Phase advance of the circadian sleep–wake cycle as an antidepressant. *Science, (NY)*, **206**, 710–13

Weingartner, H., Cohen, R. M., Bunney, W. E. *et al.* (1982). Memory-learning impairments in progressive dementia and depression. *Am. J. Psychiatry*, **139**, 135–6

Weinstock, H. (1968). *Rossini*. (London: Oxford University Press)

Weissman, M. M. (1979). The psychological treatment of depression: Research evidence for the efficacy of psychotherapy alone, in comparison and in combination with pharmacotherapy. *Arch. Gen. Psychiatry*, **36**, 1261–9

Weissman, M. M. and Klerman, G. L. (1977). Sex differences in the epidemiology of depression. *Arch. Gen. Psychiatry*, **34**, 98–111

Weissman, M. M. and Myers, J. K. (1978a). Affective disorders in a U.S. urban community. *Arch. Gen. Psychiatry*, **35**, 1304–11

Weissman, M. M. and Myers, J. K. (1978b). Rates and risks of depressive symptoms in a United States urban community. *Acta Psychiatr. Scand.*, **57**, 219–31

Weizman, A., Eldar, M. Shoenfeld, Y. *et al.* (1979). Hypercalcaemia-induced psychopathology in malignant disease. *Br. J. Psychiatry*, **135**, 363–6

Wells, C. E. (1979). Pseudodementia. *Am. J. Psychiatry*, **136**, 895–900

Welner, A., Welner, Z. and Fishman, R. (1979). The group of schizoaffective and related psychoses. IV. A family study. *Compar. Psychiatry*, **20**, 21–6

Welner, J. and Stromgren, E. (1958). Clinical and genetic studies on benign schizophreniform psychoses based on a follow-up. *Acta Psychiatr. Neurol. Scand.*, **33**, 377–99

West, D. J. (1965). *Murder followed by suicide*. (London: Heinemann)

West, E. D. and Dally, P. J. (1959). Effects of iproniazid in depressive syndromes. *Br. Med. J.*, **1**, 1491–9

Westermeyer, J. (1984). Economic losses associated with chronic mental disorder in a developing country. *Br. J. Psychiatry*, **144**, 475–81

Wheeler-Bennett, J. (ed.) (1968). *Action this Day*. Working with Churchill. (London: Macmillan)

Whitlock, F. A. (1978). Suicide, cancer and depression. *Br. J. Psychiatry*, **132**, 269–74

Whitlock, F. A. and Siskind, M. (1979). Depression and cancer: a follow-up study. *Psychol. Med.*, **9**, 747–52

Wig, N. N., Suleiman, M. A., Routledge, R. *et al.* (1980). Community reactions to mental disorders. A key informant study in three developing countries. *Acta Psychiatr. Scand.*, **61**, 111–26

Wilkinson, D. G. (1982). The suicide rate in schizophrenia. *Br. J. Psychiatry*, **140**, 138–41

Wing, J. K., Cooper, J. F. and Sartorius, N. (1974). *The Description and Classification of Psychiatric Symptoms* (London: Cambridge University Press)

Winokur, G. (1979). Unipolar depression: is it divisible into autonomous subtypes? *Arch. Gen. Psychiatry*, **36**, 47–52

Winokur, G. (1984). Psychosis in bipolar and unipolar affective illness with special reference to schizo-affective disorder. *Br. J. Psychiatry*, **145**, 236–42

Winokur, G., Cadoret, R., Dorzab, J. and Baker, M. (1971). Depressive disease: a genetic study. *Arch. Gen. Psychiatry*, **24**, 135–44

Wistedt, B. (1981). A depot neuroleptic withdrawal study. *Acta Psychiatr. Scand.*, **64**, 65–84

Wittkower, R. and Wittkower, M. (1963). *Born under Saturn.* (London: Weidenfeld and Nicolson). (quoted by Trethowan, 1979)

Wolff, S. (1978). Psychiatric disorders in childhood. In Forrest, A. D. *et al.* (eds.) *Companion to Psychiatric Studies* 2nd Edn. pp. 325–49. (Edinburgh: Churchill Livingstone)

Wolfgang, M. E. (1968). Suicide by means of victim-precipitated homicide. In Resnick, H. L. P. (eds.) *Suicidal behaviours. Diagnosis and Management.* pp. 90–104 (London: Churchill)

Woodruff, R. A., Robins, L. N., Winokur, G. and Walbrau, B. (1968). Educational and occupational achievement in primary affective disorder. *Am. J. Psychiatry*, **124**, (Suppl.) 57–64

Wright, E. C. (1982). The presentation of mental illness in mentally retarded adults. *Br. J. Psychiatry*, **141**, 496–502

Yap, P. M. (1962). Words and things in comparative psychiatry with special reference to the exotic psychoses. *Acta Psychiatr. Scand.*, **38**, 163–9

Yozawitz, A., Bender, G., Sutton, S. *et al.* (1979). Dichotic perception: Evidence for right hemisphere dysfunction in affective psychosis. *Br. J. Psychiatry*, **135**, 224–37

Zeiss, A. M., Lewinsohn, D. M. and Munoz, R. F. (1979). Non-specific improvement effects in depression using interpersonal skills training, pleasant activity schedules or cognitive training. *J. Consult. Clin. Psychol.*, **45**, 427–39

Zeller, E. A., Barsky, J. and Fouts, J. R. (1952). Influence of isonicotinic acid hydrazide (INH) and 1–isonicotinyl-2-isopropyl hydrazid (IIH) on bacterial and mammalian enzymes. *Experientia*, **8**, 349–50

Index

Abraham, Karl 20
adreno-corticotrophic hormone (ACHT) 87, 89–90, 93
affective psychoses 95
 see also schizo-affective psychoses
Africa, studies of depression 206–8, 209
aggression
 attack and defence behaviours 180
 control in childhood 221
 hypothalamus 178, 179
 in mania 100–1
 role of sex hormones 182
 see also violence
agitation 56–7
alcohol
 link with violence 183
 with antidepressants 126
alcoholism 46, 51
 related to malignancy 162
 serotonin activity 85
aldosterone secretion 82
Alzheimer's disease 67, 106–7, 247
 cholinergic activity 81, 111
 clinical diagnosis 106
 distinguished from dementia in parkinsonism 104
 genetic factors 18
amine action 83–5
amitriptyline 86, 120, 127
 administration 124
 anti-aggression properties 182
 clinical evaluation 130
 noradrenaline response 77
amok 205–6
amygdala, effects on violence 179
aneurysms 118

anhedonia 55
anticholinergic drugs 103
antidepressant drugs 54, 120–8
 administration 126–8
 anti-aggression properties 182–3
 anticholinergic effects 124
 antihistamine properties 124–5
 combined with psychotherapy 155–7
 dosage 127
 effect on circadian rhythms 92
 effects on creativity 244–6
 length of treatment 131
 MAO inhibitors 100
 metabolism 122–3
 mode of action 85–6, 124
 non-MAOI, non-trycyclic 128–32
 REM-suppressant 93
 side- and adverse effects 124–6
 use in general practice 28
 see also lithium salts; monoamine oxidase inhibitors (MAOI)
anxiety 56, 101–2
 distinguished from depression 101
 in bereavement 30
 in melancholia 6
 manifestations 102
aphasia, following stroke 70
appetite disturbance 57, 126
 following bereavement 31
Aretaeus of Cappadocia 3
Aristotle 3, 4
Arnold, Thomas 10
artists, mental illness 228

Bacon, Francis 5
barbiturates 183

Bartholomew Anglicus 4
Beethoven, Ludwig van 234, 235–6
benzodiazepines 183, 188–9
bereavement
    associated complaints 29
    'at risk' individuals 33
    counselling 34
    effect on immune system 163
    factors influencing behaviour 31
    management 33–4
    morbidity and mortality among bereaved
        31
    mortality rate 29
    stages 29–30
    see also grief
beta-blocking agents 101
Bible, references to psychotherapy 2–3
biological symptoms 25
blood dyscrasias 125, 126
bowel function 58
brain
    blood flow 72–3
    disorders 9–10
        and associated depression 112–17
    injury, compare with stroke 117
    neuroradiology 73–4
    psychological testing 71–2
    tumours 113–14, 160
    see also cerebral hemispheres
Bright, Thomas 6
Burton, Richard 8

calcium levels 82
    related to depression 160–1
    related to psychopathology 115–16
cancer
    depression secondary to 159, 160–1
    see also malignancy
CAT (computerised axial tomography) head
        scans 73–4
cerebral hemispheres
    dominant/non-dominant involvement 70,
        72
    head injury prognosis 114
    temporal lobe abnormalities 74
cerebrovascular disease 117–18
Cheyne, George 9
chldbirth, depression related to 37
    see also puerperal psychosis
children, depression in 219–22
chlorpromazine 199
cholinergic mechanisms 81
    dexamethasone suppression 89, 111
Churchill, Sir Winston 237–8
circadian rhythms 87, 89, 91
clomipramine 86, 120, 121–2, 127
clonidine 90
cognitive disorder 58

in the elderly 60, 223–4
    specific functions spared 66
cognitive therapy 155–7
Coleridge, Samuel Taylor 232–3
Collins, William 240
composers, abnormal personalities 234
concentration impairment 25
Conolly, John 12
convulsions 125
coping ability 27
cortisol 87
    depression in Cushing's syndrome 115
    secretion in children 220
    urinary, related to stress 35
counselling, in bereavement 34
Cowper, William 240
creative ability
    as an antidepressant 236–44
    distinction between abnormality and
        pathology 230–1
    effect of antidepressant therapy 244–6
    psychological aspects 231–3
    related to mental illness 227
    released by depresion 235–6
    self-destructive impulses 236
Cullen, William 10–11
Cushing's syndrome 115
cycles, in depression 53
cycloid psychosis 62–3, 65, 100
delusional depression 60–1
delusions 10, 20, 25, 93–4
    cortisol concentrations 88
    drug treatment 131
    in depression with Cushing's syndrome
        115
    in schizo-affective psychoses 96
    of guilt/worthlessness 56
    role of stress 35
    vulnerablity factors 94
dementia 66
    associated with depression 107–12
        age range 109
    generalized cerebral disorders 112
    in Huntington's chorea 105
    in Parkinson's disease 103–4
    praecox 14
    'pseudodementias' 108–9
    senile 73, 223
    subcortical 66–7, 108
    variable prognosis 108
    see also Alzheimer' disease
depression
    abnormal personality 233–5
    African studies 206–8, 209
    akinetic 97
    associated with Parkinson's disease 102–4
    atypical 58–60
    biological and social advantages 246–9

cognitive changes 108
common base with aggression 183
creative ability 227, 235–6
distinguished from schizo-affective
    psychosis 96
dominant/non-dominant hemisphere
    involvement 70
early life factors 24
endogenous 49
exotic syndromes 205–6
following bereavement 30
from cancer therapies 173
'functional' origin 48
in Alzheimer's disease 106–7
in childhood 219–22
    types 219–20
in Huntington's chorea 105–6
in immigrant communities 216–17
in mental handicap 218
in schizophrenia 97–8
in the elderly 222–5
incidence: cultural variation 204, 206–10
    historical 203–4
    racial 203
    sex variations 51–2, 209
interaction of factors 22
masked 59
nature 47
    controversies 230–4
physical manifestations 57
primary and secondary 48
psychoanalytic views 19–20
psychotic/neurotic distinction 50–1
'pure'/'depressive spectrum disease'
    distinction 46, 51
referral to psychiatrists 28–9
related to malignancy: common properties
    174–5
    course of cancer 171–2
    history 159–60
management 172–4
    onset of cancer 167–71
    preceding cancer 161–5
    psychological factors 165–7
    risk factors 162
    secondary to cancer 160–1
related to other cerebral disorders 112–17
risk factors 52
    managing 119
significant limbic system components 68–9
sociological causes 24, 41
somatic presentation 210–15
spontaneous remission 130–1
stigma in Asian countries 212–13
stress and vulnerability combined 44
typology, and response to amitriptyline 102
unipolar and bipolar 24
    clinical features 53

risk factors 52–3
variations in religious attitudes 215–16
with associated dementia 107–12
see also affective psychoses; distress
    management of depression;
    melancholia; senile depression;
    symptomatology; unhappiness;
    vulnerability factors
depressive equivalents 60
desipramine 86, 121, 127
    noradrenaline response 77
despair 56
developing countries
    attitudes to treatment 212
    impact of mental illness 207–9
    somatization of depression 211–12
    stigma of mental idsorders 212–3
devil, possession by 7–, 9
    see also witches
dexamethasone 87
    suppression test (DST) 88–9, 127–8
        dementia assessment 110–11
distress
    coping ability 27
    distinguished from depression 27
    nature and symptoms 26–7
    'simple' and 'morbid' 26–7
L-dopa, in Parkinson's disease therapy 103,
    104
dopamine 77, 78
dothiepin 120
doxepin 120
Dreyssig 11

elderly people, depression in 222–5
electroconvulsive therapy (ECT) 139–46
    and MAO inhibitors 132
    case histories 145–6
    clinical evaluation 130
    clinical practice 143–4
    complications 142–3
    contraindications 141–2
    depression in schizophrenia 99
    effects on memory 69
    efficacy 144–5
    for suicidal patients 198
    historical background 54, 140
    indications 141
    involutional melancholia 17
    mode of action 140–1
electroencephalography 74–6
emotions
    change, fictional accounts 236
    disorders in children 219
    manifestations related to arousal levels
        179–80
    neuroendocrine response 164
    lability 117

suppression, link with cancer 168–9
uncontrolled 113
endocrine disorders 115
energy loss 56
epilepsy 116
  lithium salts 135
Esquirol 12

fatiguability see energy loss
Ferriar, John 11
flupenthixol 129
Freud, Sigmund 19–20

Galen 3–4
general practice, treatment of distress
  and depression 28
genetic factors 246–7
  Burton's thesis 9
  in vulnerability 17, 41, 42
  monozygous and dizygous twins 44
  morbidity risk to relatives 43–4, 46
  multifactorial theory 45
  observed in the elderly 224
  sex-related incidence 44
  two-threshold transmission model 46
  X-linked dominant inheritance 44, 45
glaucoma 126
glucose-6-phospohate dehydrogenase
  (G6PD) deficiency, link with manic-
  depressive psychosis 45
Goes, Hugo van der 5
grief
  ambivalent syndrome 32
  chronic 32
  classification 31–2
  expression 34
  limitations of drug therapy 32
  link with depression 19–20
  mourning rituals 32
  repression 30
  therapies 34
  unexplained 32
  see also bereavement
Griesinger, Willhelm 13
growth hormone 90–1
  related to sleep cycle 92–3
Guillain-Barré syndrome 126
guilt feelings 56
  see also self-depreciation

hallucinations 20, 25, 56
  in bereavement 34
  in bipolar illness 50
  in depression with Cushing's syndrome
    115
  in schizo-affective psychoses 96
haloperidol 137, 199
Handel, George Frederic 244

Haydn, Franz Joseph 239
head injury 114
headache 57
heart
  effects of antidepressants 125
  lithium effects 137
heredity see genetic factors
Hill, George Nesse 12
Hippocrates 3
homicide 184
  female incidence 184
  relationship to suicide 186–7
  see also violence
hospital admissions 157
  for suicidal patients 198
5-HT see serotonin
Huntington's chorea 67, 95, 105–6, 247
  dementia 112
hydrocephalus, normal pressure (NPH) 113
hyperactivity, in children 221
hyperparathyroidism 115–16
hypersomnia see sleep disturbance
hypertension 38
hypochondriasis 10
  in the elderly depressive 223
  involutional melancholia 15, 18
  masking depression 59
hypochondrium, as source of melancholia 5
hypoglycaemia 90
hypopituitarism 115
hypothalamo-pituitary-adrenocortical (HPA)
  function 87
hypothalamus, effect on violence 178, 179
hypothyroidism 74

imipramine 86, 120, 121, 127
  anti-aggression properties 182
  binding sites 86
  clinical evaluation 130
  noradrenaline response 77
immune system
  effects of depression 82–3
  in malignancy 163–4
inherited factors see genetic factors
insomnia see sleep disturbance
intellectual function impairment 25
iproniazid 83, 132
irritability 114, 117, 185
isocarboxazid 120, 132
isoniazid 83, 100

James I, King 7
Johnson, Samuel 239–41

Kekulé, August von 232
koro 205
Korsakoff's syndrome 67

Laurentius, Andreas 5
Leigh, Vivien 228
libido
  grief and depression compared 20
  involutional melancholia/ 18
  oral fixation 20
life events
  categories 36, 39
  in old age 224
  related to depression 35–6
    in developing countries 210
  related to feelings of hopelessness 170
  related to organic disorders 37–8
light response 91, 92
limbic system
  common base for depression and
      aggression 183
  functional role 68–9
  in depressive vilence 178
  links with hypothalamus 89
  structure 67–8
lithium salts 120, 135
  adverse reactions 137–8
  antidepressant and antimanic action 84
  clinical practice 138–9
  effect on circadian rhythms 92
  effects on creativity 244–6
  introduction 54
  metabolism 135
  mode of action 135–7
  serotonin response 84
  treatment of aggression 183–4
liver dysfunction 125
Loewe, Otto 232
lofepramine 120, 121
lypemania 12

magnesium 82
malignancy 116
  hormone profiles 164
  personality factors: and prognosis 172
    compared with benign neoplasm patients
      170
  psychological factors 168–9
  related to depression 31, 159–60
    onset of cancer 167–71
  related to life events 37
  stress and tumour growth 164
  see also brain: tumours; cancer; depression;
      related to malignancy
management of depression
  factors 119
  physical treatment 120–50
  see also antidepressant drugs;
      electroconvulsive therapy (ECT);
      psychosurgery
mania 100–1
  associated with melancholia 7, 10, 12

diagnosis 101
drug side-effect 126
Esquirol's classification 12
lithium salts 135
primary/secondary divisions 100
symptoms 100
manic-depressive psychosis
  children with schizophrenia 47
  endogenous and exogenous 21, 22
  morbidity risk for relatives 43–4
  psychological testing 72
  resemblance to schizophrenia 95, 99
  sleep patterns 76
  unipolar/bipolar distinction 46, 50, 100
  Vivien Leigh 228
  with G6PD deficiency 45
maprotiline 129
Margaret of Corona, Saint 4–5
Maudsley, Henry 13
Mead, Richard 7
melancholia
  as 'English malady' 9
  associated with mania 7, 10, 12
  Burton's classification 8
  classification of symptoms 11
  concepts 1
  distinguished from hypochondriasis 11
  historical perspective 2
    early days and Middle Ages 2–7
    17th–18th centuries 8–11
    late 18th–20th centuries 11–14
  involutional: age relationship 14, 16
    criteria 15
    criticisms of concept 15–16
    cultural effects 19
    incidence 14
    symptoms and temperament distinguished
      5, 8
  true and false states 11
  see also depression
melatonin secretion 92
memory impairment 25, 66, 71
  ECT results 69, 142
  role of vasopressin 82
menstrual disturbance 58
mental disorders, classification 65
mental handicap 218
Mental Health Act (1983) 198, 200
Mercurialis, Hieronymus 5–6
Meynert, 13
mianserin 86, 120, 128–9
Michelangelo 238–9
monoamine oxidase inhibitors (MAOI) 59,
      132–5
  clinical evaluation 134–5
  metabolism 132–3
  mode of action 133
  side-effects and adverse reactions 133

monomania 12
mood changes 116-17
    children 219
    effect on memory 156
    effect on stressful events 35
    elderly people 223
    following bereavement 31
    language differences 214-15
    mania 100-1
    orchestral players 228
    related to symptoms 54-5
motility 247-8
mourning rituals 32
multiple sclerosis 112, 113

narcolepsy 85
nephropathy 137
neurobiological basis of depression 49
neurochemistry 76-86
neuro-endocrinology 87-91
    sleep disturbance 92
neurohistology 13
neuroleptics
    treatment of delusions 131
    treatment of schizophrenia with
        depression 99
neuroradiology 73-4
neurotic illness 22
nomifensine 129
noradrenaline (NA) 77-8, 84, 89
nortriptyline 86

obsessive-compulsive behaviour 56
out-patient treatment 158

palpitations 58
palsy, progressive supranuclear 67
Paracelsus 5
paresis 10
Parkinson's disease 67, 99, 102-5, 247
    antidepressant agent effects 124
    dementia 103-4, 111-12
    genetic factors 18
    prevalence in depression 102
periodic insanity 14
personality
    abnormal, with propensity to depression
        233-5
    changes 66
    defects 27
        in reactive psychosis 43
        tending to depression 52
        see also vulnerability factors
    impact of loss 166-7
    of cancer-prone individuals 160, 167-8, 172
    of homicidal patients 185
phases, in depression 53
phenelzine 120, 132

phenothiazines 54
physostigmine 89
piblokto 206
Poincaré, Henri 231-2
pregnancy 137
prolactin levels, during sleep 92
psychoanalysis, views of depression 19-20
psychological testing 71-2
psychopathy 46
psychosurgery 146-50
    indications and clinical practice 147-50
    lobotomies 146, 147
    stereotactic methods 147
psychotherapy 150
    Biblical references 2-3
    cognitive therapy 155-7
    combined with drugs 154-5
    developing treatment 152-4
    history-taking 151-2
    pathological grief 34
psychotic depression, genetic factors 22
puerperal psychosis 65
    see also childbirth

reactive depressive psychosis 38-9, 62-3, 65,
        100
    multiple stresses 40
    personality defects 43
    see also stress
reactivity 55-6
    in response to environmental changes 21-2
rehabilitation 157-8
remission
    natural 53-4
    therapy 54
reserpine 45, 83
risk factors 52
    see also vulnerability factors
Robinson, Nicholas 9
Rossine, Gloacchino Antonio 244
Rush, Benjamin 11

St Bartholomew's Hospital 4
schizo-affective psychoses 96, 99, 100
schizophrenia 95-100, 247
    creative ability 227
    genetic factors 17, 18
    homicide 184
    in children of manic-depressives 47
    mutability 99
    overlap with affective psychoses 95
    related to involutional melancholia 17
    risk of suicide 98, 190-1
    symptoms developed from depression 54
    with depressed first-degree relatives 97
school refusal 221
Schroeder van der Kolk, 13
Schumann, Robert 228, 243-4

scientists, incidence of mental illness 229
Scot, Reginald 7–8
seasonal variations 91–2
    suicide 189–90
self-depreciation 56
    see also guilt feelings
self-esteem, loss 20
self-harm, deliberate 192–6
    agents used 193–4
    among children 195
    assessment after act 200
    distinguished from attempted suicide 194
    predictive features 194–5
    reasons given 195
Sellers, Peter 234–5
senile dementia 223
    neuroradiology 73
senile depression 75
serotonin 78–81, 84
    effect of lithium 136
    metabolism 79
sexual dysfunction 58, 126
Sharif, Omar 235
skin reactions 125
sleep
    associated with creative thought 231–2
    related to retardation in depression 231
    stages 93
sleep disturbance 57, 75–6, 92–3
    antidepressant agent effects 126
    circadian rhythms 91
    effect on stages 93
    factors influencing 92
    following bereavement 31
    pattern of REM sleep 93
    serotonin activity 85, 86
Smart, Christopher 240
social factors in depression 24, 246, 248–9
    class, as risk factor 52
    disordered functioning 58, 59
    in prevention of depression 209
    relationships 42
    study of violence 177
sodium retention 82
somatic presentation 210
    cultural differences 211
    language pitfalls 213–15
    symptoms 211
somatostatin 81–2
speech impairment 117, 118
spleen, involvement inmelancholia 5
Stahl, G. E. 7
Stockhausen, Karlheinz 235
stress
    definition 39
    levels of interpretation 34–5
    long-term 37
    non-threatening types 36–7

orchestral players 228
    quantified effects 36
    related to depression 130
    related to tumour growth 164, 166
    response mediation 89
    sex variations 39
    see also reactive psychoses
strokes, associated depression 69–70
stupor 57
subarachnoid haemorrhage 118
success, striving for 41–2
suicide 25, 114, 187–201
    as form of aggression 180–1
    associated with cancer 161
    children 195
    double 187
    factors positively correlated 196
    gifted people 227
    in medical profession 191–2
    in secure institutions 190, 198
    incidence 188–9
        before and after puberty 221
    previous violence 190
    related to homicide 186–7
    risk assessment 56, 188, 196–7
        in bipolar/unipolar conditions 53
        in Huntington's chorea 105
        in schizophrenia 98
    seasonal variation 189–90
    sociological groupings 191
    transcultural elements 191
    see also self-harm, deliberate
symptomatology
    common to depression and mania 84
    normal and abnormal symptoms 25
    see also aggression; anxiety; circadian
        rhythms; delusions; memory
        impairment; mood changes; sleep
        disturbance

thyroid function 90
Tolstoy, Leo 236
tranylcypromine 120, 132
trimipramine 120
tryptophan
    dosage 80
    metabolism 79–80, 115
    L-tryptophan 129
Tuke, Samuel 12
tyramine, reaction to MAO inhibitors 133–4
typrosine, synthesis 77

unemployment
    factor in vulnerability 41
    related to suicide 188
    see also work
unhappiness, depression compared with 25–6
    see also anhedonia

vanadium 82
vasopressin 82
viloxazine 129
violence
  animal studies 178
  biological aspects 178–84
  management 197–201
  multifactorial origin 177–8
  sedation 199–200
  sociological factors 177
  see also aggression; homicide; suicide
vulnerability factors 40–41
  heredity 44–5
  in developing countries 210
  sex-related incidence 41, 42
  social relationships 42

Wallace, Alfred Russel 232

Webster, John 8
weeping 55
  see also grief
weight loss 57–8
Weyer, Johann 8
Willis, Thomas 6
Windigo 206
witches
  depressive states, 4, 7–8
  involutional melancholia 19
Woolf, Virginia 241–2
work
  protection against depression 20
  therapeutic value 157, 188
  to earn acclaim 237
  see also creative ability; unemployment
worthlessness *see* self-depreciation